Diagnosis and Management of Addiction and Other Mental Disorders (Dual Disorders)

Diagnosis and Management of Addiction and Other Mental Disorders (Dual Disorders)

Editors

Ana Adan
Marta Torrens

MDPI • Basel • Beijing • Wuhan • Barcelona • Belgrade • Manchester • Tokyo • Cluj • Tianjin

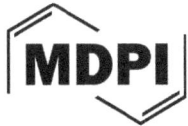

Editors

Ana Adan
1. Department of Clinical Psychology and Psychobiology;
2. Institute of Neurosciences
University of Barcelona
Barcelona
Spain

Marta Torrens
1. Addiction Program-Hospital del Mar, Department of Psychiatry;
2. Neuroscience Research Program-IMIM (Hospital del Mar Medical Research Institute)
Universitat Autònoma de Barcelona
Barcelona
Spain

Editorial Office
MDPI
St. Alban-Anlage 66
4052 Basel, Switzerland

This is a reprint of articles from the Special Issue published online in the open access journal *Journal of Clinical Medicine* (ISSN 2077-0383) (available at: www.mdpi.com/journal/jcm/special_issues/Addiction_Dual_Disorders).

For citation purposes, cite each article independently as indicated on the article page online and as indicated below:

LastName, A.A.; LastName, B.B.; LastName, C.C. Article Title. *Journal Name* **Year**, *Volume Number*, Page Range.

ISBN 978-3-0365-1283-9 (Hbk)
ISBN 978-3-0365-1282-2 (PDF)

© 2021 by the authors. Articles in this book are Open Access and distributed under the Creative Commons Attribution (CC BY) license, which allows users to download, copy and build upon published articles, as long as the author and publisher are properly credited, which ensures maximum dissemination and a wider impact of our publications.

The book as a whole is distributed by MDPI under the terms and conditions of the Creative Commons license CC BY-NC-ND.

Contents

About the Editors . . . . **vii**

Preface to "Diagnosis and Management of Addiction and Other Mental Disorders (Dual Disorders)" . . . . **ix**

Ana Adan and Marta Torrens
Special Issue: Diagnosis and Management of Addiction and Other Mental Disorders (Dual Disorders)
Reprinted from: *Journal of Clinical Medicine* 2021, *10*, 1307, doi:10.3390/jcm10061307 . . . . **1**

Jolanta Masiak, Jolanta Chmielowiec, Krzysztof Chmielowiec and Anna Grzywacz
DRD4, *DRD2*, *DAT1*, and *ANKK1* Genes Polymorphisms in Patients with Dual Diagnosis of Polysubstance Addictions
Reprinted from: *Journal of Clinical Medicine* 2020, *9*, 3593, doi:10.3390/jcm9113593 . . . . **5**

Deborah Hasin and Claire Walsh
Cannabis Use, Cannabis Use Disorder, and Comorbid Psychiatric Illness: A Narrative Review
Reprinted from: *Journal of Clinical Medicine* 2020, *10*, 15, doi:10.3390/jcm10010015 . . . . **21**

Julia E. Marquez-Arrico, José Francisco Navarro and Ana Adan
Health-Related Quality of Life in Male Patients under Treatment for Substance Use Disorders with and without Major Depressive Disorder: Influence in Clinical Course at One-Year Follow-Up
Reprinted from: *Journal of Clinical Medicine* 2020, *9*, 3110, doi:10.3390/jcm9103110 . . . . **41**

Adriana Farré, Judit Tirado, Nino Spataro, María Alías-Ferri, Marta Torrens and Francina Fonseca
Alcohol Induced Depression: Clinical, Biological and Genetic Features
Reprinted from: *Journal of Clinical Medicine* 2020, *9*, 2668, doi:10.3390/jcm9082668 . . . . **61**

Francina Fonseca, Joan-Ignasi Mestre-Pintó, Àlex Gómez-Gómez, Diana Martinez-Sanvisens, Rocío Rodríguez-Minguela, Esther Papaseit, Clara Pérez-Mañá, Klaus Langohr, Olga Valverde, Óscar J. Pozo, Magí Farré, Marta Torrens and on behalf of NEURODEP GROUP
The Tryptophan System in Cocaine-Induced Depression
Reprinted from: *Journal of Clinical Medicine* 2020, *9*, 4103, doi:10.3390/jcm9124103 . . . . **79**

Laura Río-Martínez, Julia E. Marquez-Arrico, Gemma Prat and Ana Adan
Temperament and Character Profile and Its Clinical Correlates in Male Patients with Dual Schizophrenia
Reprinted from: *Journal of Clinical Medicine* 2020, *9*, 1876, doi:10.3390/jcm9061876 . . . . **93**

Paul Brunault, Kevin Lebigre, Fatima Idbrik, Damien Maugé, Philippe Adam, Servane Barrault, Grégoire Baudin, Robert Courtois, Hussein El Ayoubi, Marie Grall-Bronnec, Coraline Hingray, Nicolas Ballon and Wissam El-Hage
Childhood Trauma Predicts Less Remission from PTSD among Patients with Co-Occurring Alcohol Use Disorder and PTSD
Reprinted from: *Journal of Clinical Medicine* 2020, *9*, 2054, doi:10.3390/jcm9072054 . . . . **109**

Laura Blanco, Albert Sió, Bridget Hogg, Ricard Esteve, Joaquim Radua, Aleix Solanes, Itxaso Gardoki-Souto, Rosa Sauras, Adriana Farré, Claudio Castillo, Alicia Valiente-Gómez, Víctor Pérez, Marta Torrens, Benedikt L. Amann and Ana Moreno-Alcázar
Traumatic Events in Dual Disorders: Prevalence and Clinical Characteristics
Reprinted from: *Journal of Clinical Medicine* **2020**, *9*, 2553, doi:10.3390/jcm9082553 . . . . **125**

Carlos Roncero, Llanyra García-Ullán, Alberto Bullón, Diego Remón-Gallo, Begoña Vicente-Hernández, Ana Álvarez, Amaya Caldero, Andrea Flores and Lourdes Aguilar
The Relevance of Dual Diagnoses among Drug-Dependent Patients with Sleep Disorders
Reprinted from: *Journal of Clinical Medicine* **2020**, *9*, 2862, doi:10.3390/jcm9092862 . . . . **139**

Gianina Luca and Lola Peris
Sleep Quality and Sleep Disturbance Perception in Dual Disorder Patients
Reprinted from: *Journal of Clinical Medicine* **2020**, *9*, 2015, doi:10.3390/jcm9062015 . . . . **153**

Matteo Pacini, Angelo G. I. Maremmani and Icro Maremmani
The Conceptual Framework of Dual Disorders and Its Flaws
Reprinted from: *Journal of Clinical Medicine* **2020**, *9*, 2098, doi:10.3390/jcm9072098 . . . . **167**

Syune Hakobyan, Sara Vazirian, Stephen Lee-Cheong, Michael Krausz, William G. Honer and Christian G. Schutz
Concurrent Disorder Management Guidelines. Systematic Review
Reprinted from: *Journal of Clinical Medicine* **2020**, *9*, 2406, doi:10.3390/jcm9082406 . . . . **179**

About the Editors

Ana Adan

Ana Adan is a full professor at the Department of Clinical Psychology and Psychobiology of the University of Barcelona (UB). She directs the Substance Use and Dual Disorders research line integrated in the Consolidated Group of Neuropsychology and the Institute of Neurosciences of the UB, and she has published more than two hundred scientific papers (index h of 34). Her research has been supported by 21 projects/networks, and she was recognized by three extraordinary awards for the PhD researches she supervised. She is a member of the editorial board of various specialized journals and has served on the scientific committee for clinical trials. She developed extensive teaching work in master's and doctoral courses and currently coordinates the compulsory subject of psychopharmacology for the degree of Psychology and that of addictions for the master's degree in general health psychology at UB. She is the director of the online degree Master in Drug Addiction of IL3-UB.

Marta Torrens

Marta Torrens, MD, PhD, and Specialist in Psychiatry, is a professor of the Department of Psychiatry and Legal Medicine at the Universidad Autònoma de Barcelona, the director of the Addiction Department at the Institute of Neuropsychiatry and Addictions of the Parc de Salut Mar in Barcelona, an elected member of the Scientific Committee of the European Monitoring Centre for Drugs and Drug Addiction and the Informal Scientific Network of UNODC and WHO, and a member of the executive of the Dual Pathology and Addiction Psychiatry section of the WPA. With respect to research, her main areas of interest are assessment and treatment of substance addictions diagnosis and its comorbidity, and the gender perspective in addictions. The results of her research have been published in main specialised journals with an h factor of 41. She has received several international and national awards, including "Honorary Member" of the Spanish Society of Dual Pathology (2013) and the EUFAS European Addiction Research Award 2020.

Preface to "Diagnosis and Management of Addiction and Other Mental Disorders (Dual Disorders)"

Addiction is a mental disorder that causes clinically and functionally significant impairment in affected individuals and for their families and constitutes a major global health problem. The link between addiction and other mental disorders, characterizing so-called "dual disorders", has been increasingly recognized. Patients with "dual disorders" show more clinical and social severity and poorer treatment outcomes compared with patients with only one disorder. Although interest in the study of addiction and dual disorders has increased in recent years, possible factors related to the etiology, adherence to treatment, course of pathology, and follow-up of relapses remain to be elucidated. There is also a need for more and better information on how to approach treatment of these patients, which must undoubtedly be based on the precision psychiatry model. The aim of this book is to highlight new advances regarding biological as well as psychological or social aspects in the diagnosis and treatment of addiction—mainly to substances (substance use disorders)—and dual disorders and to suggest lines for future research.

Ana Adan, Marta Torrens
Editors

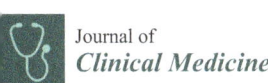

Editorial

Special Issue: Diagnosis and Management of Addiction and Other Mental Disorders (Dual Disorders)

Ana Adan [1,2,*] and Marta Torrens [3,4,5]

1. Department of Clinical Psychology and Psychobiology, School of Psychology, University of Barcelona, Passeig de la Vall d'Hebrón 171, 08035 Barcelona, Spain
2. Institute of Neurosciences, University of Barcelona, 08035 Barcelona, Spain
3. Addiction Research Group (GRAd), Neuroscience Research Program, Hospital del Mar Medical Research Institute (IMIM), 08003 Barcelona, Spain; MTorrens@parcdesalutmar.cat
4. Institut de Neuropsiquiatria i Addiccions, Hospital del Mar, 08003 Barcelona, Spain
5. Psychiatry Department, Universitat Autònoma de Barcelona (UAB), Cerdanyola del Vallès, 08093 Barcelona, Spain
* Correspondence: aadan@ub.edu; Tel.: +34-933-125-060

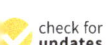

Citation: Adan, A.; Torrens, M. Special Issue: Diagnosis and Management of Addiction and Other Mental Disorders (Dual Disorders). *J. Clin. Med.* 2021, 10, 1307. https://doi.org/10.3390/jcm10061307

Received: 17 March 2021
Accepted: 20 March 2021
Published: 22 March 2021

Publisher's Note: MDPI stays neutral with regard to jurisdictional claims in published maps and institutional affiliations.

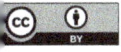

Copyright: © 2021 by the authors. Licensee MDPI, Basel, Switzerland. This article is an open access article distributed under the terms and conditions of the Creative Commons Attribution (CC BY) license (https://creativecommons.org/licenses/by/4.0/).

The term "dual disorder" (DD) refers to the coexistence or concurrence of at least one substance use disorder (SUD) and another mental disorder in the same person, as the World Health Organization established in its lexicon of alcohol and drug terms [1]. At the beginning of the last decade, the World Psychiatric Association (WPA) created a new section for this topic, deciding to use the term dual disorder/pathology.

DD has been associated with a worse prognosis in affected people. Compared with patients with a single disorder, SUD or another psychiatric disorder, patients with DD show greater psychopathological severity, greater attendance at emergency services, as well as a higher frequency of psychiatric admissions and a higher prevalence of suicide. In addition, DD patients present more risk behaviors, which are linked to infections like HIV and hepatitis B and C, as well as to unemployment, homelessness and illegal behaviors. Thus, taking into account the burden it places on the health and legal systems, psychiatric comorbidity among persons who use drugs carry high costs for society. Studies have shown that comorbid disorders are reciprocally interactive and cyclical, and a poor prognosis can be expected for both SUD and other mental disorders if treatment does not address DD in an integrated way [2–4].

DD is common, with different prevalence figures for different combinations of mental disorders and SUDs. The most frequent DDs are depression, anxiety (mainly panic disorder and generalized anxiety disorders), post-traumatic stress disorder, psychotic spectrum disorders, attention deficit disorder with or without hyperactivity, and personality disorders (mainly antisocial and borderline). These are combined with the different SUDs, both for the consumption of legal substances (i.e., tobacco, alcohol) and illegal substances (e.g., heroin, cocaine and methamphetamine).

The etiology and phenotypic expression of DDs adds difficulty to the already complex model of multiple risk and protective factors associated with any of the mental disorders. To date, the correct detection, diagnosis and therapeutic intervention in DD patients is a complicated task and a pending challenge among professionals in the field of mental health and addictions.

Providing effective treatments for DDs is a relevant concern not only because of the clinical and social severity of the patients but also because of the difficulties in accessing and coordinating the services where they receive treatment. Although specialized treatment units are advocated, these are scarce or non-existent, depending on the country. The usual thing is to manage patients either in mental-health care centers or in centers specializing in the treatment of SUDs. In both cases, there is a shortage of DD specialists. The differences

in the therapeutic approach are important, but it is not always possible to carry o
communication that allows multidisciplinary work between centers.

This special issue aims to contribute to the knowledge of patients with a DD, with n
advances that facilitate the development of possible preventive interventions and mo
individualized therapeutic strategies. For this, we have had the participation of vario
prestigious DD groups that have contributed to a variety of studies, from neurobiology
psychological and social aspects, which suggests lines for future research.

The most frequent pattern in both SUD and DD patients is polydrug use, whi
makes it difficult to determine the effect of the different substances and even determi
the main substance of dependence in a cross-sectional study. Starting from this reali
prioritizing the influence and differential aspects of comorbid psychiatric disorder, rega
less of consumption, seems the most practical approach. Thus, Masiak and colleagues
have explored the prevalence of certain polymorphisms in candidate genes associat
with dopaminergic receptors and transporters in polydrug users with various comorb
disorders. The most robust result was obtained for DRD4 Ex3 gene polymorphism, wi
the s/s genotype and the s alleles as more common for comorbid psychotic disorders a
generalized anxiety. In addition, the s alleles also appeared more common in comorb
depressive episode and dysthymia. Advances in this line can be expected to crystallize
pharmacogenetic findings for a better approach for patients with DD.

If one substance does deserve special attention for its high worldwide consumption a
controversy regarding the benefits and risks of its use, it is cannabis. The Hasin and Wal
review [6] confirms strong evidence for an increased risk of developing a comorbid psycho
disorder and, to a lesser extent, other comorbidities such as mood, anxiety and personal
disorders in cannabis users. More research is required in the immediate future on the etiolo
and course of DD with cannabis use since in therapeutic centers, the prevalence of cases
relevant, and both the approach and the prognosis present differential characteristics.

Comorbidity between SUD and major depression (MD) is the most common DD
the field of substance addiction. Three contributions from this special issue have focus
on the study of this comorbidity, which we will refer to as dual depression. The resear
by Marquez-Arrico et al. [7] found that various dimensions of a health-related quali
of life in patients with dual depression are worse than those with only SUD althoug
the presence of depressive symptoms and not DD explains the differences observed
physical functioning and health change. In addition, the quality of life shows the predicti
capacity of a relapse at a one-year follow-up differential according to the diagnosis. Wh
physical functioning is sensitive in SUD patients, general health is the indicator in t
case of asymptomatic dual depressive patients. The Farre et al. [8] study was aimed
investigating the clinical, biological and genetic source of alcohol-induced depressio
in respect of depression without an SUD. In patients with alcohol-induced depressio
they found differences among groups with a greater family history of alcoholism or oth
SUD, while patients with only depression showed a greater family history of depressio
Also, lifetime stressors like physical abuse, childhood abuse and intimate partner violen
difficulties in concentration and suicidal thoughts were more frequent in patients wi
alcohol-induced depression than in patients with only depression. However, non-gene
differences were found.

Continuing with the neurobiology of drug-induced depression, the study
Fonseca et al. [9] assessed the tryptophan–serotonin (Trp/5-HT) system by means of t
acute tryptophan depletion test (ATD), and the kynurenine pathway in subjects who ha
cocaine-induced depression, cocaine-primary depression, only depression, or were healt
controls. Interestingly, the results suggested that the neurobiological basis for cocair
induced depression does not seem to be primarily mediated by 5-HT dysfunction, but
probably more related to other neurotransmitters. Deepening this line of work may me
not only improving the understanding of the neurofunctional aspects of dual depressio
but also making progress towards a more effective psychopharmacological approach
these patients.

Two other empirical studies explored the existence of indicators of easy clinical evaluation in high prevalence comorbidities such as schizophrenia and post-traumatic stress. Río-Martinez et al. [10] have shown an endophenotype of personality traits characteristic of dual schizophrenia, which is related to more problematic clinical characteristics. The personality traits are modifiable and their consideration may be useful for designing specific intervention strategies. Brunault et al. [11] observed that the existence of childhood trauma is more related to the clinical remission of patients with a diagnosis of alcohol-use disorder and post-traumatic stress disorder than the severity of both diagnoses. Along the same line is the contribution of Blanco et al. [12], which points to childhood maltreatment as a predictor of both developing a DD and a more complex and severe clinical profile. In DD patients, the evaluation of traumatic events in childhood and integrating specific therapy into the treatment is an option for a better prognosis.

The research of Roncero et al. [13] and Luca and Peris [14] provided us with data on the presence of sleep disorders in DD patients, greater than 50%, an area that has very few previous studies. The evidence leaves no doubt about the role of altered sleep patterns (delayed sleep induction, sleep fragmentation, early awakening) in low sleep quality, which is more severe in outpatients and in those with comorbid depression. Incorporation in the diagnostic evaluation of sleep disturbances seems mandatory and both studies show us that it can be performed in a reliable and valid way with standardized self-applied or hetero-applied instruments that do not require a great deal of time or the involvement of specific units for sleep disorders. Detecting the type and magnitude of sleep impairment at the beginning of treatment should lead to the incorporation of chronobiological approach strategies (time habits), which can minimize the need to administer hypnotic or sedative drugs in patients diagnosed with both an SUD and a DD. Successfully addressing sleep disorders improves daytime arousal and mood. This can be positive for alleviating withdrawal symptoms and the symptoms of the comorbid disorder.

Finally, two contributions focus on the current state of the clinical evaluation and management of DD patients. Pacini and colleagues [15] developed a specific hierarchical algorithm to be followed for treating DD in heroin use disorder patients, a complex comorbidity that with different consumption patterns has shown an emerging state in recent years. The review on the quality of the clinical recommendation management guidelines, carried out by Hakobyan et al. [16], suggests the use of the NICE guideline to better meet the standards although it shows a clear need to improve the evidence-based recommendations for integrated treatment in DDs. In this sense, much remains to be done as the United Nations Commission on Narcotic Drugs–World Health Organization (WHO) has recently urged United Nations member states [4].

Author Contributions: Conceptualization, A.A. and M.T.; writing—original draft preparation, A.A. and M.T.; writing—review and editing, A.A. and M.T. All authors have read and agreed to the published version of the manuscript.

Funding: This research was funded by the Spanish Ministry of Economy, Industry and Competitiveness (PSI2015-65026-MINECO/FEDER/UE), the Generalitat de Catalunya (2017SGR-748 and 2017 SGR-530), the Spanish Ministry of Economy and Business (PSI2017-90806-REDT), and Instituto de Salud Carlos III–ISCIII Red de Trastornos Adictivos 2016 (RD16/0017/0010).

Conflicts of Interest: The authors declare no conflict of interest.

References

1. World Health Organization. *Lexicon of Alcohol and Drug Terms*; World Health Organization: Geneva, Switzerland, 1994.
2. Torrens, M.; Mestre-Pintó, J.I.; Montanari, L.; Vicente, J.; Domingo-Salvany, A. Patología dual: Una perspectiva europea. *Adicciones* **2017**, *29*, 3–5. [CrossRef] [PubMed]
3. Torrens, M.; Mestre-Pintó, J.J.; Domingo-Salvany, A. *Comorbidity of Substance Use and Mental Disorders in Europe, Insights*; European Monitoring Centre for Drug and Drug Addiction (EMCDDA); Publications Office of the European Union: Luxembourg, 2015.
4. Volkow, N.D.; Torrens, M.; Poznyak, V.; Sáenz, E.; Busse, A.; Kashino, W.; Krupchanka, D.; Kestel, D.; Campello, G.; Gerra, G. Managing dual disorders: A statement by the Informal Scientific Network, UN Commission on Narcotic Drugs. *World Psychiatry* **2020**, *19*, 396–397. [CrossRef] [PubMed]

5. Masiak, J.; Chmielowiec, J.; Chmielowiec, K.; Grzywacz, A. DRD4, DRD2, DAT1 and ANKK1 genes polymorphisms in patient with dual diagnosis of polysubstance addictions. *J. Clin. Med.* **2020**, *9*, 3593. [CrossRef] [PubMed]
6. Hasin, D.; Walsh, C. Cannabis use, cannabis use disorder, and comorbid psychiatric illness: A narrative review. *J. Clin. Med.* **202** *10*, 15. [CrossRef] [PubMed]
7. Marquez-Arrico, J.E.; Navarro, J.F.; Adan, A. Health-Related Quality of Life in male patients under treatment for substance us disorders with and without major depressive disorder: Influence in clinical course at one-year Follow-up. *J. Clin. Med.* **2020**, 3110. [CrossRef] [PubMed]
8. Farré, A.; Tirado, J.; Spataro, N.; Alías-Ferri, M.; Torrens, M.; Fonseca, F. Alcohol induced depression: Clinical, biological an genetic features. *J. Clin. Med.* **2020**, *9*, 2668. [CrossRef] [PubMed]
9. Fonseca, F.; Mestre-Pintó, J.I.; Gómez-Gómez, A.; Martinez-Sanvisens, D.; Rodríguez-Minguela, R.; Papaseit, E.; Pérez-Mañá, C Langohr, K.; Valverde, O.; Pozo, Ó.J.; et al. The tryptophan system in cocaine-induced depression. *J. Clin. Med.* **2020**, *9*, 410 [CrossRef] [PubMed]
10. Río-Martínez, L.; Marquez-Arrico, J.E.; Prat, G.; Adan, A. Temperament and character profile and its clinical correlates in mal patients with dual schizophrenia. *J. Clin. Med.* **2020**, *9*, 1876. [CrossRef] [PubMed]
11. Brunault, P.; Lebigre, K.; Idbrik, F.; Baugé, D.; Adam, P.; Barrault, S.; Baudin, G.; Courtois, R.; El Ayoubi, H.; Grall-Bronnec, M et al. Childhood trauma predicts less remission from PTSD among patients with co-occurring alcohol use disorder and PTSD. *Clin. Med.* **2020**, *9*, 2054. [CrossRef] [PubMed]
12. Blanco, L.; Sió, A.; Hogg, B.; Esteve, R.; Radua, J.; Solanes, A.; Gardoki-Souto, I.; Sauras, R.; Farré, A.; Castillo, C.; et al. Traumati events in dual disorders: Prevalence and clinical characteristics. *J. Clin. Med.* **2020**, *9*, 2553. [CrossRef] [PubMed]
13. Roncero, C.; García-Ullán, L.; Bullón, A.; Remón-Gallo, D.; Vicente-Hernández, B.; Álvarez, A.; Caldero, A.; Flores, A.; Aguilar, The relevance of dual diagnoses among drug-dependent patients with sleep disorders. *J. Clin. Med.* **2020**, *9*, 2862. [CrossRe [PubMed]
14. Luca, G.; Peris, L. Sleep quality and sleep disturbance perception in dual disorder patients. *J. Clin. Med.* **2020**, *9*, 2015. [CrossRe [PubMed]
15. Pacini, M.; Maremmani, A.G.I.; Maremmani, I. The conceptual framework of dual disorders and its flaws. *J. Clin. Med.* **2020**, 2098. [CrossRef] [PubMed]
16. Hakobyan, S.; Vazirian, S.; Lee-Cheong, S.; Krausz, M.; Honer, W.G.; Schutz, C.G. Concurrent disorder management guideline *Syst. Rev. J. Clin. Med.* **2020**, *9*, 2406.

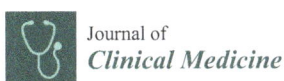

Article

DRD4, *DRD2*, *DAT1*, and *ANKK1* Genes Polymorphisms in Patients with Dual Diagnosis of Polysubstance Addictions

Jolanta Masiak [1], Jolanta Chmielowiec [2], Krzysztof Chmielowiec [2] and Anna Grzywacz [3],*

[1] Neurophysiological Independent Unit, Department of Psychiatry, Medical University of Lublin, 20-093 Lublin, Poland; jolantamasiak@wp.pl
[2] Department of Hygiene and Epidemiology, Collegium Medicum, University of Zielona Góra, 65-046 Zielona Góra, Poland; chmiele1@o2.pl (J.C.); chmiele@vp.pl (K.C.)
[3] Independent Laboratory of Health Promotion, Pomeranian Medical University in Szczecin, 70-204 Szczecin, Poland
* Correspondence: grzywacz.anna.m@gmail.com; Tel.: +48-91441-47-46

Received: 24 September 2020; Accepted: 5 November 2020; Published: 8 November 2020

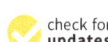

Abstract: Background: Approximately 25–50% of people diagnosed with substance use disorder experience psychiatric disorders, and this percentage is even higher if subclinical psychopathological symptomatology is taken into consideration. "Dual diagnosis" implies the comorbidity of two disorders (mental disorder and addiction), but in a clinical setting, numerous dual diagnoses involve multiple addictions (polysubstance use means the concurrent use of more than one psychoactive substance). Clinical observations and epidemiological studies showed that the use of stimulants in combination with other substances results in additional risks. Apart from the clinical significance of the specificity of stimulants used in combination with other substances, only non-exhaustive research on the specificity of this comorbidity has been performed to date. The aim of the study was to analyze polymorphisms of the genes (DRD4 VNTR in exon III Ex3, DRD2 rs1076560, rs1800498, rs1079597, rs6276, as well as in the PROM promoter region (rs1799732, ANKK1 Tag1A rs1800497, DAT) in a group of patients diagnosed with polysubstance use disorder, including addiction to stimulants, and the co-occurrence of specific mental disorders in a group of patients diagnosed with polysubstance use disorder, including addiction to stimulants, compared to the group of patients diagnosed with polysubstance use disorder. **Methods:** The study group consisted of 601 male volunteers with psychoactive substance dependence (*n* = 300) and non-dependent controls (*n* = 301). The genomic DNA was extracted from venous blood using standard procedures. Genotyping was conducted with the real-time PCR method. All computations were performed using STATISTICA 13. **Results:** Psychotic disorders were significantly more common in the group of males with polysubstance addiction, including addiction to stimulants, compared to the group of males with polysubstance addiction without addiction to stimulants. In our own research, different statistical significances were found in the frequency of the DRD4 Ex3 gene polymorphism: s/s was more common in the study group. Psychotic disorders were more common in people addicted to stimulants compared to people addicted to other substances. **Conclusions:** In our study, psychotic disorders occurred more frequently in the study group of patients with polysubstance addiction, including addiction to stimulants, compared to the control group of patients with polysubstance addiction, but with no addiction to stimulants. Different statistical significances were found in the frequency of the DRD4 Ex3 gene polymorphism: s/s was more common in the study group, while the l/l genotype was less frequent in the study group. In DRD2 PROM rs 1799732, the del allele occurred more often than the ins allele in the study group. In the DRD4 Ex3 gene polymorphism, the s allele was more common in the study group, and the l allele was less frequent. In the DRD4 Ex3 gene polymorphism for the s/s genotype, psychotic disorders and generalized anxiety were more common, while for the s/l and l/l genotype, they were less frequent. The DRD4 Ex3 polymorphism s alleles were more common for depressive episode, dysthymia, and psychotic disorders as well as generalized anxiety disorder. We see a clear genetic aspect here. However, we want to be careful and draw no definite conclusions.

Keywords: dual diagnosis; polysubstance addictions; gene polymorphisms

1. Introduction

In 2018, the dual diagnosis, i.e., co-occurrence of mental disorder and substance use disorders was found in approximately 9.2 million US adults aged 18 or older (3.7 percent of adults). In 2018, 3.2 million adults in the US experienced a comorbidity of substance use disorder as well as a serious mental illness, while in 2018, 11.4 million adults in the US were diagnosed with a serious mental illness [1]. Approximately 25–50% of people diagnosed with substance use disorder experience a mental disorder at the same time [2], and this percentage is even higher if subclinical psychopathological symptomatology is taken into consideration [3]. The results of The Epidemiologic Catchment Area Survey (ECA) reported that nearly 30% of patients with a psychiatric diagnosis suffered from substance use disorder. In addition, 48% of people diagnosed with schizophrenia, 55% of patients diagnosed with bipolar disorder, 90% of patients diagnosed with personality disorder, and more than 50% of patients with substance use disorder also developed a mental disorder during their lifetime [4]. Pre-existing mental disorders are significantly associated with an increased risk of developing substance use disorder related to alcohol, cannabis, as well as stimulants [5]. "Dual diagnosis" implies the comorbidity of two disorders (mental disorder and addiction), but in a clinical setting, numerous dual diagnoses involve multiple addictions (polysubstance use means the concurrent use of more than one psychoactive substance, or [6]) with one or more mental disorders consecutively [7]. As a result of the complexity of that multiple co-occurrence of psychiatric and substance use disorders, the concept of multimorbidity was formulated. Multimorbidity involves multiple mental disorders, substance use disorders, and general medical conditions [8]. These "complex" dual diagnoses present significant treatment challenges, with more severe illnesses and insufficiently integrated care for patients as well as a faster progression from regular use to substance use disorder [9,10]. Clinical observations and epidemiological studies showed that use of stimulants in combination with other substances results in additional risks. SAMHSA (Substance Abuse and Mental Health Services Administration) reports on increasing emergency department visits related to the use of stimulants, and 62% of the patients used stimulants with at least one more additional substance [11]. Apart from the clinical significance of the specificity of stimulants used in combination with other substances, inexhaustive research on the specificity of this comorbidity has been performed to date. One study showed that individuals with stimulant polysubstance use have a lower emotional empathy and a smaller social network compared to healthy controls [12]. The aim of the study was to analyze the polymorphisms of the genes (DRD4 Ex3, DRD2 (rs1076560, rs1800498, rs1079597, rs6276, rs1799732), ANKK1 Tag1A rs1800497, DAT1) and co-occurrence of specific mental disorders in the group of patients diagnosed with polysubstance use disorder, including stimulants, compared to the group of patients diagnosed with polysubstance use disorder. From the scientific point of view, it was also very interesting for us to learn about the specificity of co-occurring mental disorders in people who used stimulants in combination with other substances.

To advance the treatment of these complex conditions, more research is needed to reveal biological mechanisms of mental disorders and polysubstance addiction vulnerability [13,14]. Of course, we must bear in mind the importance of GWAS studies in the context of deliberations on addiction genetics and research methodology. The current studies on the brain-based linkages between these comorbidities are not intensive. Substance use disorder has a multifactorial etiopathology in which various factors are taken into consideration, including the individual genetic account for 40–60% of the susceptibility as well as environmental factors [15–18].

Attempts to understand these complex interactions are currently being made by means of analyzing, among other things, possible genetic factors that constitute the common background for this comorbidity. In the search for possible genetic risk factors related to substance use disorders, new molecular techniques are used to identify candidate genes involved in the regulation of neurotransmission and different processes modulated by dopamine [19]. It is well recognized that it is not only dopamine neurotransmission that is involved in substance use disorder. However, the role of dopamine transmission is unquestionable [20]. One of the candidate genes is the gene coding dopamine receptor 4 (DRD4). The DRD4 gene is located in chromosome 11p near the telomere, and it encodes the seven transmembrane G-protein coupled receptor, which responds to endogenous dopamine [21,22]. The variable number tandem repeat (VNTR) polymorphism occurs in exon III of the DRD4 gene. There is a 48 base pair sequence with a range of 2–11 repeats which manifests itself as either a "short" variant (five or fewer repeats—DRD4S) or a "long" variant (six or more repeats—DRD4L). The two, four, and seven repeats are considered as the most common genotypes [23]; the length of the variant has functional effects on the dopamine receptor. Repeats seven and more were correlated with blunted intracellular sensitivity and responsiveness to dopamine, which may contribute to the differences in motivation, sensation-seeking, and impulsivity often observed among carriers of DRD4S and DRD4L [24]. DRD4 exon III (VNTR) polymorphism was reported as a candidate genetic variant associated with substance use disorder (SUD) susceptibility in different populations [25] as well as a number of approach-oriented behavioral phenotypes and psychiatric disorders. Another candidate gene is the gene coding dopamine receptor 2 (DRD2). There is a continuing controversy concerning the role of the dopamine D2 receptor gene (DRD2) in association with alcohol use disorder (AUD) and other psychopathologies [26]. The research confirmed the role of dopaminergic transmission through the D2 receptor in addiction: it determines the expression of reward, diminishes alcohol consumption in animal studies, and has associations with vulnerability to addiction [27,28]. The gene of the dopamine receptor D2 (DRD2) is located in the chromosome 11q23 and spans 65,56 kilobase. The DRD2 gene includes eight exons that undergo transcription to messenger RNA of 2713 kb that is translated to 443 amino acid proteins. Skipping the sixth exon results in the formation of a short form of a receptor when the long variant of the receptor protein is constituted of 29 amino acids. The two isoforms of the D2 receptors have a different affinity with inhibitory G-proteins [29]. Polymorphic versions of the DRD2 gene rs1076560 located in its 6th intron are considered important factors in the genetics of mental disorders and behavior. The presence of the A allele of rs1076560 is associated with a lower expression of the short isoform relative to the long isoform in the prefrontal cortex and caudate putamen. A low activity of D2 receptors was observed in patients with alcohol dependence and cocaine and opiates abuse [30–32].

The aim of the study was to analyze polymorphisms of the genes (DRD4 Ex3, DRD2 (rs1076560, rs1800498, rs1079597, rs6276, rs1799732), ANKK1 Tag1A rs1800497, DAT1) and co-occurrence of specific mental disorders in the group of patients diagnosed with polysubstance use disorder including stimulants, compared to the group of patients diagnosed with polysubstance use disorder.

2. Experimental Section

2.1. Subjects

The study group consisted of 601 male volunteers with psychoactive substance dependence ($n = 300$; mean age = 28.18, SD = 6.45) and non-dependent controls ($n = 301$; mean age = 22; SD = 4.57). From the group of patients with psychoactive substance dependence, those dependent on stimulants (F15.2 $n = 247$; mean age = 27.6, SD = 5.75) and other psychoactive substances ($n = 53$; mean age = 31, SD = 8.52) were distinguished. Only men were included in the study, as it was a section of a larger study in which fluctuations in women's sex hormone cycles may have affected the examined properties. For further analysis, a group of men dependent on many substances, including stimulants, were selected in order to achieve the aim of the study.

The psychiatric examination was also performed on the control group. The occurrence of mental disorders in that group was evaluated. The occurrence of any mental disorder in a candidate for the control group was a disqualifying criterion.

The percentage distribution of a particular type of addiction in the patients under study is shown in Table 1. After obtaining the approval of the Bioethics Committee of the Pomeranian Medical University in Szczecin (KB-0012/106/16) and an informed, written consent of the participants, the study was conducted in the Independent Laboratory of Health Promotion. Patients with psychoactive substance dependence were recruited after at least 3 months of abstinence in addiction treatment facilities. We did not differentiate the simultaneous co-ingestion of different substances from concurrent (different substances used on the same or separate occasions within the same period) polysubstance use.

Table 1. Type of use of psychoactive substances in addicts.

Type of Substance/Addiction Used	All Addicted ($n = 300$)		Addicted to Stimulants ($n = 247$)		Addicted to Other Psychoactive Substances ($n = 53$)	
	n	%	n	%	n	%
Behavioral addiction	128	43	107	43	21	40
Designer drugs	73	24	56	23	17	32
F10.2-alcohol	166	55	134	54	32	60
F11.2-opiates	61	20	44	18	17	32
F12.2-cannabinols	214	71	181	73	33	62
F13.2-sedatives and hypnotics	38	13	22	9	16	30
F14.2-cocaine	31	10	29	12	2	4
F15.2-stimulants	247	82	247	100	-	-
F16.2-hallucinogenic	31	10	31	13	0	0
F19.2-mixed addictions	172	57	156	63	16	30

The total is not 100%. It was found that the addicts used various psychoactive substances.

The dependent patients and controls were clinically tested by psychiatrists for the following disorders: depressive episode, dysthymia, suicide attempt, hypo or manic episode, panic-related disorders, agoraphobia, social phobia, obsessive-compulsive disorder (OCD), post-traumatic stress disorder (PTSD), psychotic disorder, and generalized anxiety.

The history of dependence was collected using the Polish version of ICD-10, authors' survey, and the medical history. DNA was provided from the venous blood.

2.2. Genotyping

The genomic DNA was extracted from venous blood using standard procedures. Genotyping was conducted with the real-time PCR method.

The LightCycler® 480 II System (Roche Diagnostic, Basel, Switzerland) was applied to perform the fluorescence resonance energy into the genotypic data. The data related to the DRD2 gene polymorphism were obtained under the following conditions: PCR was performed with 50 ng DNA of each sample in a final volume of 20 µl containing 2 µl reaction mix, 0.5 mM of each primer, 0.2 mM of each hybridization probe, and 2 mM of MgCl2 according to the manufacturer's instructions with initial denaturation (95 °C for 10 min) and then 35 cycles of denaturation (95 °C for 10 s), annealing (60 °C for 10 s), and extension (72 °C for 15 s). After amplification, a melting curve was generated by holding the reaction at 40 °C for 20 s and then heating slowly to a level of 95 °C. The fluorescence signal was plotted against temperature to provide melting curves for each sample.

The peaks for rs1800497 were obtained at 58.95 °C for the T allele and 67.17 °C for the C allele. For rs6276, they were at 59.14 °C for the G allele and at 67.66 °C for the A allele. For rs1076560, the peaks were obtained at 57.13 °C for the A allele and 64.40 °C for the C allele. For rs1800498, the peaks were obtained at 57.87 °C for the T allele and 66.34 °C for the C allele. For rs1079597, the peaks were obtained at 57.41 °C for the G allele and 62.25 °C for the A allele. For ANKK1 rs1800497, they were obtained at 58.95 °C for the T (A1) allele and at 67.17 °C for the °C (A2) allele.

The DAT1 genotypes were grouped according to the presence of nine or 10 repeat variants. Genotyping was performed using the PCR-VNTR method, with primers: F: 50-TGT GGT GTA GGG AAC GGC CTG Ag 30, R: 50-CTT CCT GGA GGT CAC GGC TCA AGG 30; in the final volume of 25 L PCR mix per reaction, with l00 ng genomic DNA, 10 pmol of primers, 50 mM KCl, 10 mM TrisHCl, 1.5 mM MgCl2, 200 M dATP, dCTP, dTTP, dGTP, and 0.8 U of the Tag polymerase. The conditions for the reaction were as follows: 5 min of initial denaturation in 94 °C, 55 s of denaturation in 94 °C, 50 s of primer hybridization in 55 °C, and 1 min of elongation in 72 °C, repeated in 30 cycles, with 10 min of final elongation in 72 °C. The amplified products were visualized using ethidium bromide stained gel electrophoresis (3% agarose) and UV photography. The products were 450 bp in length for 10 repeat alleles and 410 bp for nine repeat alleles.

The DRD4 genotypes were grouped based on the presence of the short (2–5 repeat) and long (6–11 repeat) variants. Genotyping was performed using the PCR-VNTR method with the following primers: F: 50-GCG ACT ACG TGG TCT ACT CG 3 0, R: 50-AGG ACC CTC ATG GCC TTG 3 0; in the final volume of 25 μL PCR mix per reaction, with l00 ng genomic DNA, 10 pmol of primers, 50 mM KCl, 10 mM TrisHCl, 1.5 mM MgCl2, 200 μM dATP, dCTP, dTTP, dGTP and 0.8 U of the Tag polymerase. The conditions for the reaction: 3 min of initial denaturation in 95 °C, cycling 30 s of denaturation in 95 °C, 1 min of primers hybridization in 63 °C and 30 s of elongation in 72 °C, repeated in 35 cycles, 5 min of final elongation in 72 °C. The amplified products were visualized using ethidium bromide stained gel electrophoresis (3% agarose) and UV photography. The products ranged from 379 bp (2 repeats) to 811 (11 repeats). The products were divided into two groups: short alleles (S, 2–5 repeats) and long alleles (L, 6–11 repeats).

2.3. Statistical Analysis

The relations between DRD4 Ex3, DRD2 rs1076560, DRD2 Tag1D rs1800498, DRD2Tag1B rs1079597, DRD2 Ex8 rs6276, DRD2 PROM. rs1799732, ANKK1 Tag1A rs1800497, DAT1 variants, in control subjects with dependence on stimulants and the occurrence of mental disorders were tested with the chi square test. No statistically significant associations were found between the polymorphism of the DRD2 rs1076560, DRD2 Tag1D rs1800498, DRD2Tag1B rs1079597, DRD2 Ex8 rs6276, DRD2 PROM.rs1799732, ANKK1 Tag1A rs1800497, DAT genes, and psychiatric disorders in patients addicted to stimulants and in the control group. In the study group, further analysis of the relationship between mental disorders was performed only for the DRD4 Ex3 gene polymorphism. In that case, the chi square test was also used. For these variables, the Bonferroni multiple comparisons correction was applied, and the accepted level of significance was 0.0045 (0.05/11). All computations were performed using STATISTICA 13 (Tibco Software Inc, Palo Alto, CA, USA) for Windows (Microsoft Corporation, Redmond, WA, USA).

3. Results

Significant differences were found in the DRD4 Ex3 polymorphism for addiction-stimulating substances and the control group genotypes (s/l 0.31 vs s/l 0.33, s/s 0.65 vs. s/s 0.59, l/l 0.04 vs. l/l 0.09, $\chi^2 = 6.27$, $p = 0.043$) and the frequency of DRD4 Ex3 alleles (s 0.81 vs. s 0.75, l 0.19 vs. l 0.25, $\chi^2 = 5.05$, $p = 0.025$). Statistically significant differences were also found only in the frequency of the DRD2 PROM allele rs1799732 between addiction-stimulating substances and control groups (del 0.15 vs. del 0.11, ins 0.85 vs. ins 0.89, $\chi^2 = 5.07$, $p = 0.024$). For other gene polymorphisms (DRD2 rs1076560, DRD2 Tag1D rs1800498, DRD2Tag1B rs1079597, DRD2 Ex8 rs6276, ANKK1 Tag1A rs1800497, DAT1) and their allele distribution, no significant statistical differences were found (Table 2).

Table 2. Genetic polymorphism dopamine receptor (DRD4 Ex3), dopamine receptor 2 (DRD2) in addicts, and coexisting F15.2-stimulants.

	Genotype			Allele	
	DRD2 rs1076560				
	C/C n (%)	A/C n (%)	A/A n (%)	C n (%)	A n (%)
Addiction-stimulating substances n = 247	160 (64.78%)	77 (31.17%)	10 (4.05%)	397 (80.36%)	97 (19.64%)
Control n = 301	208 (69.10%)	82 (27.24%)	11 (3.65%)	498 (82.72%)	104 (17.28%)
Pearson's χ^2 (p value)		1.155 (0.561)			1.010 (0.315)
	DRD2 Tag1D rs1800498				
	T/T n (%)	C/T n (%)	C/C n (%)	T n (%)	C n (%)
Addiction-stimulating substances n = 247	77 (31.17%)	118 (47.77%)	52 (21.05%)	272 (55.06%)	222 (44.94%)
Control n = 301	108 (35.88%)	142 (47.18%)	51 (16.94%)	358 (59.47%)	244 (40.53%)
Pearson's χ^2 p value		2.119 (0.347)			2.160 (0.142)
	DRD2Tag1B rs1079597				
	G/G n (%)	A/G n (%)	A/A n (%)	G n (%)	A n (%)
Addiction-stimulating substances n = 247	165 (66.80%)	74 (29.96%)	8 (3.24%)	404 (81.78%)	90 (18.22%)
Control n = 301	207 (68.77%)	83 (27.57%)	11 (3.65%)	497 (82.56%)	105 (17.44%)
Pearson's χ^2 p value		0.414 (0.813)			0.110 (0.738)
	DRD2 Ex8 rs6276				
	A/G n (%)	A/A n (%)	G/G n (%)	A n (%)	G n (%)
Addiction-stimulating substances n = 247	118 (47.77%)	100 (40.49%)	29 (11.74%)	336 (68.02%)	158 (31.98)
Control n = 301	129 (42.86%)	127 (42.19%)	45 (14.95%)	385 (63.95%)	217 (36.05%)
Pearson's χ^2 p value		1.857 (0.395)			1.990 (0.158)
	DRD2 PROM. rs1799732				
	del/del n (%)	ins/ins n (%)	ins/del n (%)	del n (%)	ins n (%)
Addiction-stimulating substances n = 247	9 (3.64%)	181 (73.28%)	57 (23.08%)	75 (15.18%)	419 (84.82%)
Control n = 301	4 (1.33%)	241 (80.07%)	56 (18.60%)	64 (10.63%)	538 (89.37%)
Pearson's χ^2 p value		5.192 (0.074)			5.07* (0.024)

Table 2. *Cont.*

	Genotype			Allele	
	\multicolumn{5}{c}{ANKK1 Tag1A rs1800497}
	C/C n (%)	C/T n (%)	T/T n (%)	C n (%)	T n (%)
Addiction-stimulating substances n = 247	154 (62.35%)	82 (33.20%)	11 (4.45%)	390 (78.95%)	104 (21.05%)
Control n = 301	199 (66.33%)	95 (31.33%)	7 (2.33%)	493 (81.89%)	109 (18.11%)
Pearson's χ^2 p value	2.330 (0.312)			1.500 (0.220)	
	\multicolumn{5}{c}{DAT1}
	9/10 n (%)	9/9 n (%)	10/10 n (%)	9 n (%)	10 n (%)
Addiction-stimulating substances n = 247	101 (40.89%)	7 (2.83%)	139 (56.28%)	115 (23.28%)	379 (76.72%)
Control n = 301	114 (37.87%)	19 (6.31%)	168 (55.81%)	152 (25.25%)	450 (74.75%)
Pearson's χ^2 p value	3.779 (0.151)			0.570 (0.450)	
	\multicolumn{5}{c}{DRD4 Ex3}
	s/l n (%)	s/s n (%)	l/l n (%)	s n (%)	l n (%)
Addiction-stimulating substances n = 247	77 (31.17%)	161 (65.18%)	9 (3.64%)	399 (80.77%)	95 (19.23%)
Control n = 301	98 (32.56%)	177 (58.80%)	26 (8.64%)	452 (75.08%)	150 (24.92%)
Pearson's χ^2 p value	6.274 * (0.043)			5.050 * (0.025)	

* Significant statistical differences.

By comparing the frequency of occurrence of particular mental disorders between people addicted to stimulants and people dependent on other psychoactive substances, statistically significant differences were shown only in the frequency of psychotic disorders. Psychotic disorders occurred more frequently in people addicted to stimulants (0.49 vs. 0.22, $\chi^2 = 13.24$, $p = 0.0003$, Table 3).

A relationship was found between the presence or absence of psychotic disorders (the study group and the control group in total $n = 601$) and the polymorphism of the DRD4 Ex3 genotype (s/l 0.25 vs. s/l 0.34, s/s 0.72 vs. s/s 0.59, l/l 0.03 vs. l/l 0.07, $\chi^2 = 7.19$, $p = 0.027$) and the frequency of DRD4 Ex3 alleles (s 0.84 vs. s 0.76, l 0.16 vs. l 0.24, $\chi^2 = 7.72$, $p = 0.006$). A relationship was also found between the presence of generalized anxiety or its absence and polymorphism of the DRD4 Ex3 genotype (s/l 0.22 vs. s/l 0.33, s/s 0.78 vs. s/s 0.59, l/l 0.00 vs. l/l 0.07, $\chi^2 = 10.57$, $p = 0.005$) and the frequency of DRD4 Ex3 alleles (s 0.89 vs. s 0.76, l 0.11 vs. l 0.24, $\chi^2 = 11.40$, $p = 0.0007$). However, only significant differences were found for the frequency of the DRD4 Ex3 allele in people with a diagnosed depressive episode (s 0.84 vs. s 0.77, l 0.16 vs. l 0.23, $\chi^2 = 4.02$, $p = 0.045$) and dysthymia (s 0.86 vs. s 0.77, l 0.14 vs. l 0.23, $\chi^2 = 4.71$, $p = 0.03$) compared to people without those mental disorders. After the Bonferroni correction was applied, a relationship was also found between the presence of generalized anxiety or its absence and the polymorphism of the DRD4 Ex3 alleles (Table 4).

Table 3. Mental disorders in addicts and coexisting addiction F15.2-stimulants.

Mental Disorders	Addiction	Not n (%)	Yes n (%)	Pearson's χ^2 p Value
Depressive episode	other addictions n = 54	37 (68.52%)	17 (31.48%)	0.0002 (0.989)
	addiction-stimulating substances n = 247	169 (68.42%)	78 (31.58%)	
Dysthymia	other addictions n = 54	47 (87.04%)	7 (12.96%)	1.242 (0.265)
	addiction-stimulating substances n = 247	199 (80.57%)	48 (19.43%)	
Suicide attempts	other addictions n = 54	51 (94.44%)	3 (5.56%)	0.001 (0.974)
	addiction-stimulating substances n = 247	233 (94.33%)	14 (5.67%)	
Hypomanic or manic episode	other addictions n = 54	38 (70.37%)	16 (29.63%)	0.0001 (0.991)
	addiction-stimulating substances n = 247	174 (70.45%)	73 (29.55%)	
Panic-related disorder	other addictions n = 54	49 (90.74%)	5 (9.26%)	0.196 (0.658)
	addiction-stimulating substances n = 247	219 (88.66%)	28 (11.34%)	
Agoraphobia	other addictions n = 54	49 (90.74%)	5 (9.26%)	0.078 (0.779)
	addiction-stimulating substances n = 247	227 (91.90%)	20 8.10% ()	
Social phobia	other addictions n = 54	48 (88.89%)	6 (11.11%)	1.749 (0.186)
	addiction-stimulating substances n = 247	201 (81.38%)	46 (18.62%)	
OCD	other addictions n = 54	47 (87.04%)	7 (12.96%)	0.856 (0.355)
	addiction-stimulating substances n = 247	202 (81.78%)	45 (18.22%)	
PTSD	other addictions n = 54	50 (92.59%)	4 (7.41%)	0.029 (0.865)
	addiction-stimulating substances n = 247	227 (91.90%)	20 (8.10%)	
Psychotic disorders	other addictions n = 54	42 (77.78%)	12 (22.22%)	13.244*# (0.0003)
	addiction-stimulating substances n = 247	125 (50.61%)	122 (49.39%)	
Generalized anxiety	other addictions n = 54	44 (81.48%)	10 (18.52%)	1.440 (0.230)
	addiction-stimulating substances n = 247	182 (73.68%)	65 (26.32%)	

* Significant statistical differences. # Bonferroni correction was used, and the p value was reduced to 0.0045 (p = 0.05/11 (number of statistical tests conducted)).

Table 4. Polymorphism of the DRD4 Ex3 gene in the study group (people addicted to stimulants and the control group), including mental disorders.

	Genotype			Allele	
	DRD4 Ex3				
	s/l n (%)	s/s n (%)	l/l n (%)	s n (%)	l n (%)
Depressive episode - not n = 468	153 (32.69%)	282 (60.26%)	33 (7.05%)	717 (76.60)	219 (23.40%)
Depressive episode - yes n = 80	22 (27.50%)	56 (70.00%)	2 (2.50%)	134 (83.75)	26 (16.25)
Pearson's χ^2 p value		3.844 (0.146)			4.020* (0.045)
Dysthymia - not n = 500	164 (32.80%)	302 (60.40%)	34 (6.80%)	768 (76.80%)	232 (23.20%)
Dysthymia - yes n = 48	11 (22.92%)	36 (75.00%)	1 (2.08%)	83 (86.46%)	13 (13.54%)
Pearson's χ^2 p value		4.379 (0.112)			4.710* (0.030)
Suicide attempts - not n = 535	171 (31.96%)	329 (61.50%)	35 (6.54%)	829 (77.48%)	241 (22.52%)
Suicide attempts - yes n = 13	4 (30.77%)	9 (69.23%)	0 (0.00%)	22 (84.62%)	4 (15.38%)
Pearson's χ^2 p value		0.979 (0.612)			0.750 (0.388)
Hypo or manic episode - not n = 477	154 (32.29%)	290 (60.80%)	33 (6.92%)	734 (76.94%)	220 (23.06%)
Hypo or manic episode - yes n = 71	21 (29.58%)	48 (67.61%)	2 (2.82%)	117 (82.39%)	25 (17.61%)
Pearson's χ^2 p value		2.234 (0.327)			2.120 (0.145)
Hypo or manic episode - not n = 520	167 (32.12%)	318 (61.15%)	35 (6.73%)	802 (77.21%)	237 (22.79%)
Hypo or manic episode - yes n = 28	8 (28.57%)	20 (71.43%)	0 (0.00%)	48 (85.71%)	8 (14.29%)
Pearson's χ^2 p value		2.444 (0.295)			2.220 (0.136)
Agoraphobia - not n = 527	168 (31.88%)	324 (61.48%)	35 (6.64%)	816 (77.42%)	238 (22.58)
Agoraphobia - yes n = 21	7 (33.33%)	14 (66.67%)	0 (0.00%)	35 (83.33%)	7 (16.67%)
Pearson's χ^2 p value		1.496 (0.473)			0.810 (0.367)
Social phobia - not n = 502	158 (31.47%)	309 (61.55%)	35 (6.97%)	776 (77.29%)	228 (22.71%)
Social phobia - yes n = 46	17 (36.96%)	29 (63.04%)	0 (0.00%)	75 (81.52%)	17 (18.48%)
Pearson's χ^2 p value		3.618 (0.163)			0.870 (0.351)

Table 4. Cont.

	Genotype			Allele	
OCD -not n = 503 OCD - yes n = 45	164 (32.60%) 11 (24.44%)	305 (60.64%) 33 (73.33%)	34 (6.76%) 1 (2.22%)	774 (76.94%) 77 (85.56%)	232 (23.06%) 13 (14.44%)
Pearson's χ^2 p value		3.272 (0.195)			3.530 (0.060)
PTSD -not n = 528 PTSD - yes n = 20	169 (32.01%) 6 (30.00%)	325 (61.55%) 13 (65.00%)	34 (6.44%) 1 (5.00%)	819 (77.56%) 32 (80.00%)	237 (22.44%) 8 (20.00%)
Pearson's χ^2 p value		0.123 (0.939)			0.130 (0.716)
Psychotic disorder - not n = 425 Psychotic disorder - yes n = 123	144 (33.88%) 31 (25.20%)	250 (58.82%) 88 (71.54%)	31 (7.29%) 4 (3.25%)	644 (75.76%) 207 (84.15%)	206 (24.23%) 39 (15.85%)
Pearson's χ^2 p value		7.193* (0.027)			7.720* (0.006)
Generalized anxiety - not n = 483 Generalized anxiety - yes n = 65	161 (33.33%) 14 (21.54%)	287 (59.42%) 51 (78.46%)	35 (7.25%) 0 (0.00%)	735 (76.09%) 116 (89.23%)	231 (23.91%) 14 (10.77%)
Pearson's χ^2 p value		10.573* (0.005)			11.400*# (0.0007)

* Significant statistical differences. # Bonferroni correction was used, and the p value was reduced to 0.0045 (p = 0.05/11 (number of statistical tests conducted)).

4. Discussion

The initial consideration in our research was an assessment of the prevalence of certain polymorphisms in candidate genes in people addicted to multiple substances, including stimulants. We also investigated the presence of psychiatric disorders in people addicted to multiple substances, including stimulants, versus people addicted to multiple psychoactive substances.

An additional factor conditioning the clinical picture is the type of substance used by the patient. In our opinion, the most interesting result of the analyses is that psychotic disorders occurred more frequently in the study group of patients with polysubstance addiction, including addiction to stimulants, compared to the control group of patients with polysubstance addiction, but without addiction to stimulants (Table 3). Stimulants cause hallucinations and a delusional interpretation of reality, even in mentally healthy people. Stimulants are among the most popular psychoactive drugs used by people diagnosed with psychosis. Stimulants may cause psychotic states similar to schizophrenia in mentally healthy people or exacerbate symptoms of pre-existing psychoses. The symptoms include paranoid states and may recur in the form of flashbacks after long periods of abstinence [33,34].

Following the literature and the statement of "common susceptibility", for our analyses, we chose polymorphisms of genes associated with dopaminergic receptors and transporters. A significantly increased prevalence of substance use disorders in people diagnosed with psychotic disorders compared to general population is well confirmed by research. Theories explaining the comorbidity of addiction and schizophrenia include the primary addiction or "shared vulnerability" hypothesis of shared genetic and environmental risk factors and neurobiological dysfunctions within the meso-cortico-limbic dopamine system, which predisposes to schizophrenia but also to substance use disorder [35].

This hypothesis proposes that the genetic determinants of risk for the occurrence of schizophrenia predispose to substance use disorder which, in turn, serves as a risk factor for the development of schizophrenia symptomatology [36].

Genetic factors were studied in regard to susceptibility to the development of schizophrenia and co-occurring substance use disorder. It was also confirmed that polygenic risk scores for schizophrenia are associated with cannabis use, cocaine use, nicotine use, and severe alcohol use [37]. Since such a strong genetic correlation was found, our first analysis was justified.

In our own research, different statistical significances were found in the frequency of the DRD4 Ex3 gene polymorphism: s/s is more common in the study group, while the l/l genotype is less frequent in the study group (Table 2). On the other hand, in DRD2 PROM rs 1799732, the del allele occurs more often than the ins allele in the study group (Table 2). In the DRD4 Ex3 gene polymorphism, the s allele is more common in the study group, and the l allele is less frequent (Table 2). Such analysis shows us the genotypic and allelic characteristics in the study group. We found that in our group, some variants were statistically significantly more frequent, which confirmed the theory related to the aspect of a genetic component in addiction and pointed to which area of research should be explored. However, in our study, we wanted to get a broader picture of the group, not only in terms of genetic conditions, but mainly in terms of all differences related to clinical aspects of dual diagnosis. Table 3 shows an interesting aspect, where the difference at a level of statistical significance is shown. Specifically, psychotic disorders were more common in people addicted to stimulants compared to people addicted to other substances (Table 3). Interestingly, the literature includes reports on the widely described bipolar spectrum resulting from the use of stimulants. The bipolar spectrum was in fact the only profile that differentiated heroin users or people with alcohol dependence from healthy people [38,39].

In addition to research focused on addiction, other authors point to the use of stimulants (substances from the group of stimulants), possibly in combination with alcohol and cannabinoids, as characteristic of the bipolar spectrum. The concept of bipolarity resulting from the use of stimulants was proposed. The study shows that patients who had a significantly elevated mood in the bipolar spectrum had used stimulants for years before they developed more severe mood disorders, and the use of these stimulants resulted in a controlled and sustained subclinical rewarding mood condition. This was important both for the emergence of bipolar and dependence traits [40]. In our study group, no relationship of this kind was observed.

A similar study was carried out on a group of politoxicomaniac patients—where groups of patients with alcohol and heroin dependence, alcohol and cocaine dependence, and heroin and cocaine dependence were compared, respectively. The pattern of repeated use of alcohol is typical of people with bipolar disorder with a low intensity of mood swings [41–45]. Depressive disorders were not associated with any of the combinations. However, people addicted both to heroin and alcohol developed their addiction by skipping drug doses, ending treatment too early, or receiving insufficient pharmacological treatment, which appears to be a substitute for opioid use [46,47].

In our study, in the DRD4 Ex3 gene polymorphism for the s/s genotype, psychotic disorders and generalized anxiety were more common, while for the s/l and l/l genotype, they were less frequent (Table 4). We see a clear genetic aspect here. However, we want to be careful and draw no definite conclusions. The DRD4 Ex3 polymorphism s alleles were more common for depressive episode, dysthymia, psychotic disorders, and generalized anxiety disorder (Table 4).

Table 4 shows the results with Bonferroni's correction; differences in the distribution of alleles in the study group were found to be significantly more frequent in patients with generalized anxiety in the study group (using many psychoactive substances, including stimulants) and healthy individuals from the control group. Analogically, allele l was less frequent in people with generalized anxiety in this group. These results may indicate that generalized anxiety is related to the polymorphisms of the DRD4 gene, but it was found that significant differences in individuals dependent on multiple substances, including stimulants, are not only found in the DRD4 gene but also in the DRD2 gene in the RS 1799732 promoter. The short variant of the DRD4 VNTR exon III was associated with increased neurotic symptoms in healthy individuals [48].

In the promoter region of DRD2 rs1799732 in the group of patients diagnosed with polysubstance use disorder, including addiction to stimulants, allel del ins occurred significantly more often compared to the group of healthy controls, and allel ins occurred less often. It may be assumed that the more frequent occurrence of the s allele is connected with the more frequent occurrence of generalized anxiety and similarly, the s allele is more frequent in people dependent on many substances, including stimulants. Therefore, it is worth considering whether the presence of the s allele is not associated with greater susceptibility to mental disorders, such as generalized anxiety disorder and dependence on many substances, including stimulants.

Substance use disorders are also heterogeneous, since not all clinical images correspond to a chronic, recurrent loss of control over use (dependence). In addition, not all cases of multiple use have the same dynamics for primary dependence and comorbid psychiatric disorders; therefore, the biological aspect should also be considered. The biology of addictions is still unknown and based on the research we have carried out, we are aware of the need for further analyses. In the case of multigeneity and multifactoriality in addiction, the GWAS seems to be the most accurate analysis.

Large-scale GWAS are well powered to detect genetic effects in or near candidate genes, and their failure to implicate candidate genes—while implicating many other loci—is informative. Most promisingly, what has emerged (and is still emerging) from GWAS is a set of novel variants that provide clues to the etiology of psychiatric diseases [14]. GWAS will be the next stage of our research when gathering the appropriate group size. The deviation from the classical criteria of intoxication and particular substance withdrawal syndrome inspires performing a dual diagnosis.

5. Conclusions

In studies on addiction, we should be particularly sensitive to the criterion of dual diagnosis. The combination of different substances used simultaneously has a diagnostic and therapeutic significance as well. Moreover, the factors related to differentiating patients may lie in the biological aspect, e.g., in the differentiation of individual polymorphic variants of candidate genes. In our study, psychotic disorders occurred more frequently in the study group of patients with polysubstance addiction, including addiction to stimulants, compared to the control group of patients with polysubstance addiction, but without addiction to stimulants. Different statistical significances were found in the frequency of the DRD4 Ex3 gene polymorphism: s/s was more common in the study group of patients addicted to stimulants and other psychoactive substances, while the l/l genotype was less frequent in the study group. In DRD2 PROM rs 1799732, the del allele occured more often than the ins allele in the study group. In the DRD4 Ex3 gene polymorphism, the s allele was more common in the study group, and the l allele was less frequent. In the DRD4 Ex3 gene polymorphism for the s/s genotype, psychotic disorders and generalized anxiety were more common, while for the s/l and l/l genotype, they were less frequent. The DRD4 Ex3 polymorphism s alleles were more common for depressive episode, dysthymia, psychotic disorders, and generalized anxiety disorder. We see a clear genetic aspect here. However, we want to be careful and draw no definite conclusions.

Author Contributions: Conceptualization, A.G., K.C.; methodology, J.M., J.C.; formal analysis, A.G., K.C.; investigation, A.G., K.C., J.C., J.M.; resources, J.C.; data curation, J.C.; writing—original draft preparation, A.G., K.C., J.M., J.C.; writing—review and editing, A.G., K.Ch., J.M., J.C.; supervision, A.G.; project administration, A.G.; funding acquisition, A.G., J.M. All authors have read and agreed to the published version of the manuscript.

Funding: This research was funded by the National Science Center, Poland, grant number UMO-2015/19/B/NZ7/03691.

Conflicts of Interest: The authors declare no conflict of interest.

References

1. Substance Abuse and Mental Health Services Administration. *Results from the 2018 National Survey on Drug Use and Health: Detailed tables*; Center for Behavioral Health Statistics and Quality, Substance Abuse and Mental Health Services Administration: Rockville, MD, USA, 2019. Available online: https://www.samhsa.gov/data/ (accessed on 5 November 2020).
2. Teesson, M.; Slade, T.; Swift, W.; Mills, K.; Memedovic, S.; Mewton, L.; Grove, R.; Newton, N.; Hall, W. Prevalence, correlates and comorbidity of DSM-IV cannabis use and cannabis use disorders in Australia. *Aust. N. Z. J. Psychiatry* **2012**, *6*, 1182–1192. [CrossRef] [PubMed]
3. Guest, C.; Holland, M. Co-existing mental health and substance use and alcohol difficulties–why do we persist with the term "dual diagnosis" within mental health services? *Adv. Dual Diagn.* **2011**, *4*, 162–172. [CrossRef]
4. Regier, D.A.; Farmer, M.E.; Rae, D.S.; Locke, B.Z.; Keith, S.J.; Judd, L.L.; Goodwin, F.K. Comorbidity of mental disorders with alcohol and other drug abuse. Results from the Epidemiologic Catchment Area (ECA) Study. *JAMA* **1990**, *264*, 2511–2518. [CrossRef] [PubMed]
5. Marel, C.; Sunderland, M.; Mills, K.L.; Slade, T.; Teesson, M.; Chapman, C. Conditional probabilities of substance use disorders and associated risk factors: Progression from first use to use disorder on alcohol, cannabis, stimulants, sedatives and opioids. *Drug Alcohol Depend.* **2019**, *194*, 136–142. [CrossRef]
6. European Monitoring Centre for Drugs, & Drug Addiction. *Two Thousand and Two Annual Report on the State of the Drugs Problem in the European Union and Norway*; Office for Official Publications of the European Communities: Luxembourg, 2002.
7. Delgadillo, J.; Kay-Lambkin, F. Closing the science-practice gap: Introduction to the special issue on psychological interventions for comorbid addictions and mental health problems. *Adv. Dual Diagn.* **2016**, *9*. [CrossRef]
8. Bhalla, I.P.; Rosenheck, R.A. A change in perspective: From dual diagnosis to multimorbidity. *Psychiatr. Serv.* **2018**, *69*, 112–116. [CrossRef] [PubMed]
9. Torrens, M.; Mestre-Pintó, J.I.; Domingo-Salvany, A. *Comorbidity of Substance Use and Mental Disorders in Europe*; Publication Office of the European Union: Luxembourg, 2015.
10. Petrakis, M.; Robinson, R.; Myers, K.; Kroes, S.; O'Connor, S. Dual diagnosis competencies: A systematic review of staff training literature. *Addict. Behav. Rep.* **2018**, *7*, 53–57. [CrossRef]
11. Substance Abuse and Mental Health Services Administration. *The DAWN Report: Emergency Department Visits Involving Methamphet- Amine: 2007 to 2011*; Center for Behavioral Health Statistics and Quality: Rockville, MD, USA, 2014.
12. Kroll, S.L.; Wunderli, M.D.; Vonmoos, M.; Hulka, L.M.; Preller, K.H.; Bosch, O.G.; Quednow, B.B. Socio-cognitive functioning in stimulant polysubstance users. *Drug Alcohol Depend.* **2018**, *190*, 94–103. [CrossRef] [PubMed]
13. Sartor, C.E.; Kranzler, H.R.; Gelernter, J. Rate of progression from first use to dependence on cocaine or opioids: A cross-substance examination of associated demographic, psychiatric, and childhood risk factors. *Addict. Behav.* **2014**, *39*, 473–479. [CrossRef] [PubMed]
14. Duncan, L.E.; Ostacher, M.; Ballon, J. How genome-wide association studies (GWAS) made traditional candidate gene studies obsolete. *Neuropsychopharmacology* **2019**, *44*, 1518–1523. [CrossRef]
15. Uhl, G.R. Molecular genetic underpinnings of human substance abuse vulnerability: Likely contributions to understanding addiction as a mnemonic process. *Neuropharmacology* **2004**, *47*, 140–147. [CrossRef] [PubMed]
16. Suchanecka, A.; Chmielowiec, J.; Chmielowiec, K.; Masiak, J.; Sipak-Szmigiel, O.; Sznabowicz, M.; Czarny, W.; Michałowska-Sawczyn, M.; Trybek, G.; Grzywacz, A. Dopamine Receptor DRD2 Gene rs1076560, Personality Traits and Anxiety in the Polysubstance Use Disorder. *Brain Sci.* **2020**, *10*, 262. [CrossRef]
17. Suchanecka, A.; Chmielowiec, K.; Chmielowiec, J.; Trybek, G.; Masiak, J.; Michałowska-Sawczyn, M.; Nowicka, R.; Grocholewicz, K.; Grzywacz, A. Vitamin D Receptor Gene Polymorphisms and Cigarette Smoking Impact on Oral Health: A Case-Control Study. *Int. J. Environ. Res. Public Health* **2020**, *17*, 3192. [CrossRef] [PubMed]

18. Lachowicz, M.; Chmielowiec, J.; Chmielowiec, K.; Suchanecka, A.; Masiak, J.; Michałowska-Sawczyn, M.; Mroczek, B.; Mierzecki, A.; Ciechanowicz, I.; Grzywacz, A. Significant association of DRD2 and ANKK1 genes with rural heroin dependence and relapse in men. *Ann. Agric. Environ. Med.* **2020**, *27*, 269–273. [CrossRef] [PubMed]
19. Li, C.Y.; Mao, X.; Wei, L. Genes and (common) pathways underlying drug addiction. *PLoS Comput. Biol.* **2008**, *4*, e2. [CrossRef] [PubMed]
20. Volkow, N.D.; Koob, G.F.; McLellan, A.T. Neurobiologic advances from the brain disease model of addiction. *N. Engl. J. Med.* **2016**, *374*, 363–371. [CrossRef] [PubMed]
21. Van Tol, H.H.; Wu, C.M.; Guan, H.C.; Ohara, K.; Bunzow, J.R.; Civelli, O.; Kennedy, J.; Seeman, P.; Niznik, H.B.; Jovanovic, V. Multiple dopamine D4 receptor variants in the human population. *Nature* **1992**, *358*, 149–152.
22. Asghari, V.; Sanyal, S.; Buchwaldt, S.; Paterson, A.; Jovanovic, V.; Van Tol, H.H. Modulation of intracellular cyclic AMP levels by different human dopamine D4 receptor variants. *J. Neurochem.* **1995**, *65*, 1157–1165. [CrossRef]
23. Chmielowiec, J.; Chmielowiec, K.; Suchanecka, I.; Mroczek, B.; Trybek, G.; Małecka, I.; Grzywacz, A. Associations between the Dopamine D4 Receptor and DAT1 Dopamine Transporter Genes Polymorphisms and Personality Traits in Addicted Patients. *Int. J. Environ. Res. Public Health* **2018**, *15*, 2076. [CrossRef]
24. Ray, L.A.; Bryan, A.; MacKillop, J.; McGeary, J.; Hesterberg, K.; Hutchison, K.E. The dopamine D4 receptor (DRD4) gene exon III polymorphism, problematic alcohol use, and novelty seeking: Direct and mediated genetic effects. *Addict. Biol.* **2008**, *14*. [CrossRef]
25. Al-Eitan, L.N.; Alshudaifat, K.M.; Anani, J.Y. Association of the DRD4 exon III and 5-HTTLPR VNTR polymorphisms with substance abuse in Jordanian Arab population. *Gene* **2020**, *733*, 144267. [CrossRef]
26. Samochowiec, J.; Grzywacz, A. Case-control analysis of DRD2 gene polymorphisms in drug addicted patients. *Psychiatr. Pol.* **2018**, *6*, 1013–1022.
27. Blum, K.; Braverman, E.R.; Holder, J.M.; Lubar, J.F.; Monastra, V.J.; Miller, D.; Lubar, J.O.; Chen, T.J.; Comings, D.E. Reward deficiency syndrome: A biogenetic model for the diagnosis and treatment of impulsive, addictive, and compulsive behaviors. *J. Psychoact. Drugs* **2000**, *32* (Suppl. i–iv), 1–112. [CrossRef]
28. Jung, Y.; Montel, R.A.; Shen, P.H.; Mash, D.C.; Goldman, D. Assessment of the association of D2 dopamine receptor gene and reported allele frequencies with alcohol use disorders: A systematic review and meta-analysis. *JAMA Netw. Open* **2019**, *2*, e1914940. [CrossRef]
29. Khan, Z.U.; Mrzljak, L.; Gutierrez, A.; De La Calle, A.; Goldman-Rakic, P.S. Prominence of the dopamine D2 short isoform in dopaminergic pathways. *Proc. Natl. Acad. Sci. USA* **1998**, *95*, 7731–7736. [CrossRef]
30. Sasabe, T.; Furukawa, A.; Matsusita, S.; Higuchi, S.; Ishiura, S. Association analysis of the dopamine receptor D2 (DRD2) SNP rs1076560 in alcoholic patients. *Neurosci. Lett.* **2007**, *412*, 139–142. [CrossRef]
31. Moyer, R.A.; Wang, D.; Papp, A.C.; Smith, R.M.; Duque, L.; Mash, D.C.; Sadee, W. Intronic Polymorphisms Affecting Alternative Splicing of Human Dopamine D2 Receptor Are Associated with Cocaine Abuse. *Neuropsychopharmacology* **2010**, *36*, 753–762. [CrossRef]
32. Clarke, T.-K.; Weiss, A.R.D.; Ferarro, T.N.; Kampman, K.M.; Dackis, C.A.; Pettinati, H.M.; O'Brien, C.P.; Oslin, D.W.; Lohoff, F.W.; Berrettini, W.H. The dopamine receptor D2 (DRD2) SNP rs1076560 is associated with opioid addiction. *Ann. Hum. Genet.* **2013**, *78*, 33–39. [CrossRef] [PubMed]
33. Gordon, A. *Comorbidity of Mental Disorders and Substance Use: A Brief Guide for the Primary Care Clinician*; Drug and Alcohol Services South Australia (DASSA) Clinical Services and Research: Adelaide, Australia, 2010.
34. Simonienko, K.; Wygnał, N.; Cwalina, U.; Kwiatkowski, M.; Szulc, A.; Waszkiewicz, N. The reasons for use of cannabinoids and stimulants in patients with schizophrenia. *Psychiatr. Pol.* **2018**, *52*, 261–273. [CrossRef] [PubMed]
35. Alexander, P.D.; Gicas, K.M.; Cheng, A.; Lang, D.J.; Procyshyn, R.M.; Vertinsky, A.T.; Chan, T. A comparison of regional brain volumes and white matter connectivity in subjects with stimulant induced psychosis versus schizophrenia. *Psychopharmacology* **2019**, *236*, 3385–3399. [CrossRef]
36. Chambers, R.A.; Krystal, J.H.; Self, D.W. A neurobiological basis for substance abuse comorbidity in schizophrenia. *Biol. Psychiatry* **2001**, *50*, 71–83. [CrossRef]
37. Khokhar, J.Y.; Dwiel, L.L.; Henricks, A.M.; Doucette, W.T.; Green, A.I. The link between schizophrenia and substance use disorder: A unifying hypothesis. *Schizophr. Res.* **2018**, *194*, 78–85. [CrossRef]
38. Pacini, M.; Maremmani, I.; Vitali, M.; Santini, P.; Romeo, M.; Ceccanti, M. Affective temperaments in alcoholic patients. *Alcohol* **2009**, *43*, 397–404. [CrossRef] [PubMed]

39. Maremmani, I.; Pacini, M.; Popovic, D.; Romano, A.; Maremmani, A.G.; Perugi, G.; Deltito, J.; Akiskal, K.; Akiskal, H. Affective temperaments in heroin addiction. *J. Affect. Disord.* **2009**, *117*, 186–192. [CrossRef]
40. Camacho, A.; Akiskal, H.S. Proposal for a bipolar-stimulant spectrum: Temperament, diagnostic validation and therapeutic outcomes with mood stabilizers. *J. Affect. Disord.* **2005**, *85*, 217–230. [CrossRef]
41. Maremmani, I.; Pacini, M.; Perugi, G.; Deltito, J.; Akiskal, H. Cocaine abuse and the bipolar spectrum in 1090 heroin addicts: Clinical observations and a proposed pathophysiologic model. *J. Affect. Disord.* **2008**, *106*, 55–61. [CrossRef]
42. Pacini, M.; Maremmani, I.; Vitali, M.; Romeo, M.; Santini, P.; Vermeil, V.; Ceccanti, M. Cocaine Abuse in 448 Alcoholics: Evidence for a Bipolar Connection. *Addict Disord Their Treat.* **2010**, *9*, 164–335. [CrossRef]
43. Vitali, M.; Pacini, M.; Maremmani, I.; Romeo, M.; Ceccanti, M. Pattern of cocaine consumption in a sample of italian alcoholics. *Int. Clin. Psychopharmacol.* **2011**, *26*, e98. [CrossRef]
44. Maremmani, A.G.I.; Pacini, M.; Bacciardi, S.; Ceccanti, M.; Maremmani, I. Current use of cannabis and past use of heroin as predictors of alcohol and concomitant cocaine use disorder. *Alcologia* **2015**, *22*, 36–40.
45. Maremmani, A.G.I.; Pacini, M.; Pani, P.P.; Ceccanti, M.; Bacciardi, S.; Akiskal, H.S.; Maremmani, I. Possible trajectories of addictions: The role of bipolar spectrum. *Heroin Addict. Relat. Clin. Probl.* **2016**, *18*, 23–32.
46. Maremmani, I.; Shinderman, M.S. Alcohol, benzodiazepines and other drugs use in heroin addicts treated with methadone. Polyabuse or undermedication? *Heroin Addict. Relat. Clin. Probl.* **1999**, *1*, 7–13.
47. Pacini, M.; Maremmani, A.G.I.; Ceccanti, M.; Maremmani, I. Former heroin-dependent alcohol use disorder patients. Prevalence, addiction history and clinical features. *Alcohol Alcohol.* **2015**, *50*, 451–457. [CrossRef]
48. Tochigi, M.; Hibino, H.; Otowa, T.; Kato, C.; Marui, T.; Ohtani, T.; Umekage, T.; Kato, N.; Sasaki, T. Association between dopamine D4 receptor (DRD4) exon III polymorphism and neuroticism in the Japanese population. *Neurosci. Lett.* **2006**, *398*, 333–336. [CrossRef]

Publisher's Note: MDPI stays neutral with regard to jurisdictional claims in published maps and institutional affiliations.

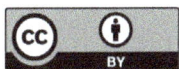

© 2020 by the authors. Licensee MDPI, Basel, Switzerland. This article is an open access article distributed under the terms and conditions of the Creative Commons Attribution (CC BY) license (http://creativecommons.org/licenses/by/4.0/).

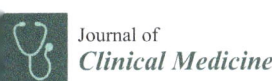

Review

Cannabis Use, Cannabis Use Disorder, and Comorbid Psychiatric Illness: A Narrative Review

Deborah Hasin [1,2,*] and Claire Walsh [1]

1. New York State Psychiatric Institute, New York, NY 10032, USA; claire.walsh@nyspi.columbia.edu
2. Department of Epidemiology, Mailman School of Public Health, Columbia University Medical Center, New York, NY 10032, USA
* Correspondence: dsh2@cumc.columbia.edu; Tel.: +1-646-774-7909

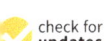

Citation: Hasin, D.; Walsh, C. Cannabis Use, Cannabis Use Disorder, and Co-morbid Psychiatric Illness: A Narrative Review. *J. Clin. Med.* **2021**, *10*, 5. https://dx.doi.org/10.3390/jcm10010015

Received: 26 October 2020
Accepted: 19 December 2020
Published: 23 December 2020

Publisher's Note: MDPI stays neutral with regard to jurisdictional claims in published maps and institutional affiliations.

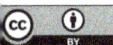

Copyright: © 2020 by the authors. Licensee MDPI, Basel, Switzerland. This article is an open access article distributed under the terms and conditions of the Creative Commons Attribution (CC BY) license (https://creativecommons.org/licenses/by/4.0/).

Abstract: Background: The landscape of attitudes, legal status and patterns of use of cannabis is rapidly changing in the United States and elsewhere. Therefore, the primary aim of this narrative review is to provide a concise overview of the literature on the comorbidity of cannabis use and cannabis use disorder (CUD) with other substance use and psychiatric disorders, and to use this information to accurately guide future directions for the field. Methods: A literature review of PubMed was conducted for studies relating to cannabis use, CUD, and a co-occurring psychiatric disorder. To provide an overview of representative data, the literature review focused on national-level, population-based work from the National Epidemiologic Survey on Alcohol and Related Conditions (NESARC) and National Survey on Drug Use and Health (NSDUH) surveys. Considering rapidly changing cannabis laws, recent (past five-year) studies were addressed. Results: A strong body of literature shows associations between cannabis use and CUD with other drug use, psychosis, mood disorders, anxiety disorders, and personality disorders. The strongest evidence of a potential causal relationship exists between cannabis use and psychotic disorders. While some evidence shows potential directionality between cannabis use and mood and anxiety disorders, results are inconsistent. Studies have established higher rates of CUD among those with personality disorders, but little about the specifics of this relationship is understood. Conclusions: Although the general population in the United States increasingly perceives cannabis to be a harmless substance, empirical evidence shows that cannabis use is associated both with CUD and comorbid psychiatric illness. However, there is mixed evidence regarding the role of cannabis in the etiology, course, and prognosis of a co-occurring disorder across all categories of psychiatric disorders. Future research should expand on the existing body of literature with representative, longitudinal data, in order to better understand the acute and long-term effects of cannabis on comorbid psychiatric illness.

Keywords: cannabis; comorbidity; cannabis use disorder; co-occurring disorder

1. Introduction

Cannabis is one of the most widely used psychoactive substances in the United States (U.S.), with around 43.5 million people over the age of 12 reporting past-year use and around 124 million people reporting lifetime use in 2018 [1,2]. The legal status of cannabis in the U.S. is rapidly changing, with a total of 33 U.S. states permitting adult use of medical cannabis and 11 states additionally permitting adult recreational use in 2020 [3]. Globally, an estimated 188 million people used cannabis within the past year in 2017, with trend rates in use rising substantially in the Americas and Asia [4]. Although trends in cannabis use have not increased at the same rate in Europe, cannabis remains the most commonly used illicit drug there [4]. For example, cannabis accounted for 71% of all illegal drug seizures in England and Wales in the fiscal year 2018–2019 [5]. Furthermore, the changing legalities in the United States has stimulated debate in Europe regarding the advantages and disadvantages of medical and recreational cannabis [6]. No country in the European

Union currently permits cannabis for medical or recreational use. However, cannabis use is decriminalized in countries such as Portugal and the Netherlands [7]. Data show that youth across Europe perceive cannabis use as risky, but this perception may be moderated by peer use [8]. Despite an increasing perception among the U.S. public of cannabis as a safe substance [9], both adverse mental and physiological effects of cannabis use can occur [10–13]. In the U.S. general population, the prevalence of medical and recreational cannabis use, as well as cannabis use disorder (CUD), is increasing [14]. Levels of delta-tetrahydrocannabinol (THC) concentration in cannabis products are also increasing in the U.S. [15], and in Europe [16–18]. Furthermore, while a commonly-held assumption is that few cannabis users will develop cannabis use disorder [19], CUD now occurs in 20–30% users [20–22].

Studies dating back to the 1980s show a high degree of comorbidity of substance and psychiatric problems among treated patients [23]. These findings were originally assumed to be due to Berkson's bias, i.e., that those with multiple conditions more likely to enter treatment than those with only a single condition of primary interest [24]. However, the first large-scale general population study of specific substance and psychiatric disorders in the U.S., the Epidemiologic Catchment Area (ECA) 5-site study [25], indicated that psychiatric and substance use disorders (SUDs) were also highly comorbid in adults in the general population [24,25]. Additional findings in several more recent nationally representative surveys have confirmed the association of psychiatric and substance use disorders, and expanded on the specificity of the associations [26–35]. In these general population studies, comorbidity was defined as evidencing both types of disorder within the past year, or on a lifetime basis. Understanding the comorbidity of substance and psychiatric disorders is important to guide clinicians, inform the delivery of treatment services and suggest etiological factors. With the changing legal landscape and increasing prevalence of cannabis use, examining the comorbidity of psychiatric disorders with cannabis use has become especially important.

Psychiatric and substance use disorders are each associated with disability and impaired functioning [27,30,31,36–38]. For example, those with depression and those with an SUD have been shown to score significantly below the population-based mean on the 12-Item Short-Form Health Survey version 2 (SF-12v2) [30,31], a reliable measure of social and emotional functioning, as well as disability. Thus, individuals with comorbid substance and psychiatric disorders may be at risk of greater disability and more greatly impaired functioning than those with single disorders [36,39]. Because of this, a closer examination of the current evidence regarding the association of CUD with other psychiatric illnesses warranted.

Although strong evidence has suggested that cannabis use and CUD are associated with psychiatric comorbidities [28], the complexities of this association are not fully understood, and even inconsistent at times. Specifically, national data have consistently shown that those with past-year and lifetime CUD are at an elevated risk of other illicit substance use, psychosis, mood disorders, anxiety disorders, and personality disorders in comparison to individuals with no CUD [28,40–44]. However, the nature of the relationship between cannabis use, CUD and other psychiatric disorders remains unclear, with empirical findings on the etiology and course of CUD with a co-occurring disorder producing mixed findings. Therefore, this narrative review provides an examination of the current literature on cannabis use, CUD, and dual diagnoses, in order to summarize what known from large scale, population-based studies, and establish future directions to guide research, practice and policy. The objectives of the review are to (1) provide an overview of information on the association of cannabis use and CUD with other psychiatric disorders and (2) concisely identify particular risk factors related to the course of the disorders when comorbid, and (3) summarize the related unclear or inconsistent results. This material organized by the category of psychiatric diagnosis.

2. Methods

A search of PubMed was conducted for studies pertaining to cannabis use, CUD, and co-occurring disorder using defined terms. PubMed was selected as the primary article database, since it is currently one of the largest collections of peer-reviewed, biomedical research, containing over 30 million sources as of writing [45]. A similar initial search was also conducted in the Google Scholar database. Upon screening of the first 100 search results, this database produced similar articles. Searches included the phrases "cannabis use", "cannabis use disorder", in combination with "comorbidity", "dual diagnosis", "psychiatric", and comorbid diagnoses of interest: "depression", "anxiety", "bipolar", "personality", "psychosis", "substance". Studies with samples smaller than 100 participants were excluded, as were studies of highly specific samples or subgroups (i.e., studies with a sample only consisting of individuals with a physical condition such as heart failure, or specific study settings such as group homes). While addressing cannabis use and comorbid psychopathologies within these specific groups is important, the primary aim of the review is to provide an overview of large, nationally representative data to remain generalizable. Additional exclusion criteria included non-English studies, commentaries, clinical trial protocol lists, case reports, and opinion pieces. These exclusion criteria and search terms were applied through the "My NCBI Filters" feature on PubMed. Selected search terms were required to be in the title, abstract, and/or key words of the articles. The non-empirical article types described above were automatically left out of the search through the computerized filter function. Although no formal range of dates was applied, studies published within the past five years were the focal point of the review, in light of rapidly changing cannabis policies. Older studies were incorporated as necessary to provide additional information or context. The exact search text used in PubMed is detailed in Figure 1.

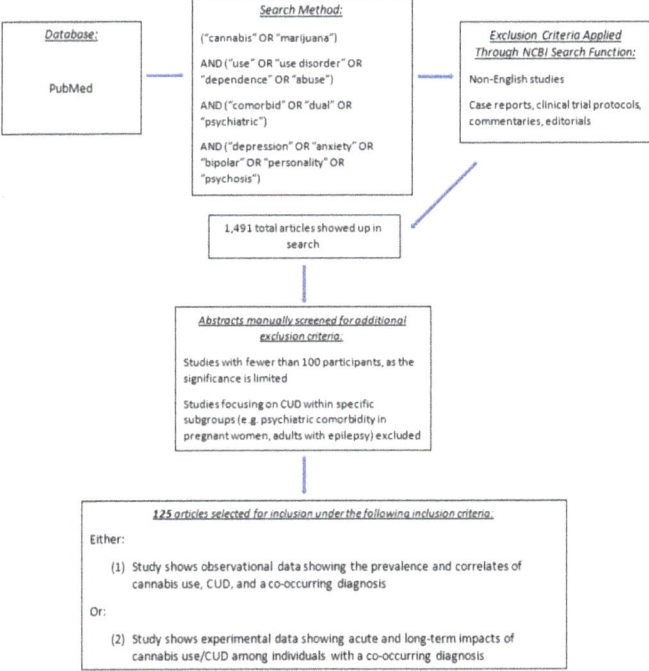

Figure 1. PubMed search strategy to identify studies or meta-analyses with data on cannabis use, cannabis use disorder (CUD), and a co-occurring disorder.

The search was conducted on 11 August 2020 and drew 1491 total results. Articles were sorted by recency of publication to prioritize the most relevant literature. Of the 1491 articles, the screening of article titles and abstracts was conducted by CW to determine eligibility for inclusion, e.g., studies that included fewer than 100 participants were excluded. Furthermore, in order to summarize relevant, nationally representative findings for the purpose of generalizability, articles that focused on cannabis use and a co-occurring disorder within specific subgroups (e.g., CUD and psychiatric comorbidity in pregnant women, adults with epilepsy, or those with chronic inflammation) were excluded. To organize the findings, relevant articles on cannabis use and comorbidity were added to a list on an Excel spreadsheet, and sorted by related dual diagnoses. After excluding articles on the basis described above, 125 articles were selected for inclusion.

After the PubMed search was conducted and relevant articles were incorporated, additional papers were retrieved to provide more specific information pertaining to specific points regarding cannabis policy, comorbid illnesses, and etiology of those illnesses.

Since many of the included studies used data from two major nationally representative US survey series, the surveys are described briefly here. One series consisted of the National Epidemiologic Survey on Alcohol and Related Conditions (NESARC) surveys [28,40]. These surveys included large, nationally representative samples of household residents who were assessed for patterns of lifetime and current alcohol use, illicit drug use, alcohol use disorders, drug use disorders, and many psychiatric disorders [46,47]. The surveys provide detailed data on substance use and psychiatric disorders. The 2001–2002 NESARC included 43,093 adults. Approximately a decade later, a survey was conducted with a similar sample design and measures, the NESARC-III, which included 36,309 adults.

Another important source of information on substance use and comorbidities is the series of National Survey on Drug Use and Health (NSDUH). These yearly surveys sponsored by the Substance Abuse and Mental Health Services Administration (SAMHSA) have provided national prevalences of substance use and related psychiatric and health issues since 1971 [48], and are therefore an important source for identifying comorbidity trends at the national level. The NSDUH surveys include considerable detail on drug use patterns, drug use disorders, and some information on alcohol use and alcohol use disorders. Some psychiatric conditions are also covered in NSDUH, although fewer and in less detail than the NESARC surveys. NSDUH surveys are often used to examine trends over time, in particular patterns of drug use and potentially related variables. Moreover, nationally representative trends data allows for identifying groups at an elevated risk of experiencing a comorbid psychiatric illness, for example youth [49,50], people in poverty [51], and non-medical opioid users [52].

3. Results

3.1. The Association of CUD with Other SUDs

CUD is highly comorbid with other SUDs. NESARC results (Table 1) show that around half of those with past-year CUD also met diagnostic criteria for an alcohol use disorder (OR 7.8) or nicotine dependence (OR 5.1) [40]. NESARC-III findings (Table 1) also show strong associations between past-year CUD and other SUD (OR 6.0–9.3) [28].

Later NESARC-III analyses have illustrated extensive polysubstance involvement, showing that DSM-5 CUD is associated with higher prevalences of other substance use disorders across all drug classes [42]. Notably, past-year CUD was associated with an elevated risk of a co-occurring cocaine (aOR 9.3), sedative (aOR 5.1), stimulant (aOR 4.3), club drug (aOR 16.1), and opioid (aOR 4.6) use disorders [42]. However, CUD and a concurrent heroin or other drug use disorder were not significantly associated [42]. In addition, age at onset of cannabis use was two years earlier, on average, among those with CUD compared to those without CUD (15.7 years old and 17.7 years old, respectively) [42]. Finally, cannabis was used prior to any other substance class regardless of CUD status [42].

Table 1. Adjusted Odds Ratios (aORs) [a] indicating the association of CUD with a psychiatric disorder National Epidemiologic Survey on Alcohol and Related Conditions (NESARC) 2001–2002 and NESARC-III 2012–2013.

	Any 12-Month Cannabis Use Disorder		Any Lifetime Cannabis Use Disorder	
	NESARC aOR (95% CI) [b]	NESARC-III aOR (95% CI)	NESARC aOR (95% CI)	NESARC-III aOR (95% CI)
Any other substance use disorder	– [c]	9.3 (7.70–11.21)	–	14.5 (11.95–17.60)
Alcohol use disorder	7.8 (6.21–9.89)	6.0 (5.10–6.97)	10.3 (9.15–11.66)	7.8 (6.95–8.74)
Any other drug use disorder	–	9.0 (6.65–12.19)	–	10.0 (8.56–11.76)
Nicotine use disorder	–	6.2 (5.24–7.34)	–	6.6 (5.79–7.64)
Nicotine dependence	5.1 (4.19–6.31)	–	5.2 (4.67–5.79)	–
Any mood disorder	2.9 (2.28–3.60)	3.8 (3.10–4.56)	2.9 (2.63–3.26)	3.3 (2.94–3.73)
Major Depressive Disorder	1.8 (1.29–2.52)	2.8 (2.33–3.41)	1.9 (1.69–2.14)	2.6 (2.26–2.95)
Bipolar I	3.1 (1.77–5.48)	5.0 (3.65–6.75)	2.5 (2.08–3.10)	3.8 (3.10–4.59)
Bipolar II	4.3 (3.02–6.14)	2.7 (1.10–6.62)	4.3 (3.59–5.08)	2.8 (1.51–5.23)
Dysthymia	1.9 (1.09–3.28)	–	2.3 (1.71–2.95)	–
Any anxiety disorder	2.4 (1.90–3.15)	2.8 (2.24–3.39)	2.4 (2.19–2.73)	2.9 (2.54–3.31)
Panic Disorder	–	3.3 (2.50–4.48)	–	3.2 (2.66–3.76)
Panic with agoraphobia	4.9 (2.86–8.36)	–	3.9 (2.84–5.34)	–
Panic without agoraphobia	2.6 (1.59–4.09)	–	2.7 (2.23–3.20)	–
Agoraphobia	–	2.6 (1.64–4.06)	–	2.9 (2.25–3.79)
Social Phobia	2.4 (1.61–3.57)	2.3 (1.61–3.27)	2.4 (1.98–2.78)	2.7 (2.22–3.40)
Specific Phobia	2.2 (1.60–3.04)	1.7 (1.28–2.29)	2.2 (1.92–2.52)	2.1 (1.73–2.46)
Generalized Anxiety Disorder	4.3 (2.75–6.70)	3.7 (2.79–5.02)	2.7 (2.25–3.19)	3.2 (2.75–3.74)
Post-Traumatic Stress Disorder	–	4.3 (3.26–5.64)	–	3.8 (3.15–4.67)
Any personality disorder	3.9 (3.18–4.66)	4.8 (3.96–5.75)	3.2 (2.87–3.55)	4.7 (4.18–5.28)
Antisocial	6.0 (4.66–7.79)	3.8 (3.05–4.75)	6.7 (5.70–7.92)	4.7 (4.07–5.34)
Avoidant	2.6 (1.80–3.85)	–	2.7 (2.10–3.37)	–
Dependent	7.2 (3.96–13.07)	–	3.6 (2.24–5.86)	–
Obsessive-Compulsive	2.5 (1.92–3.31)	–	2.1 (1.84–2.42)	–
Paranoid	2.9 (2.13–3.86)	–	2.7 (2.32–3.22)	–
Histrionic	4.1 (2.92–5.84)	–	3.2 (2.59–3.83)	–
Schizoid	2.7 (1.98–3.77)	–	2.5 (2.08–3.07)	–
Schizotypal	–	4.4 (3.60–5.46)	–	4.0 (3.46–4.72)
Borderline	–	5.0 (4.13–6.10)	–	4.5 (3.96–5.19)

[a] ORs were controlled for sex, race/ethnicity, age, marital status, education, household income, urbanicity, and region at both time points.
[b] CI: Confidence Interval. [c] Due to the use of DSM-IV to measure psychiatric disorders in the NESARC, and DSM-5 to measure the same disorders in NESARC-III, not every diagnosis matched up. Thus, diagnoses not in one paper are indicated by '–'.

Although there is less information on CUD and rates of other specific SUDs in the NSDUH, trend data allow for identification of potential patterns of polysubstance use. NSDUH data show that when cannabis is used for the first time prior to alcohol or cigarettes, youth are more likely to later show heavy patterns of cannabis use and develop CUD. [53]. Consistent with NESARC, NSDUH data show strong associations between CUD symptoms and concurrent nicotine dependence, and that concurrent cannabis and cigarette use is associated with a greater number of CUD symptoms compared to non-cigarette smokers [54]. Furthermore, both cannabis users and those with CUD are significantly less likely to quit smoking cigarettes than non-users [55]. Data also show that in adolescents, concurrent use of cannabis and tobacco is more common (5.4%) than use of either cannabis or tobacco only (2.2% and 3.9%, respectively) [56]. However, data for those over the age of 18 show that tobacco use only is more prevalent (24.0%) than co-use (5.2%) or use of cannabis only (2.3%). Analysis of adult data also shows that co-use of cannabis and tobacco is increasing over time [57], although the adolescent trend data do not report a significant increase in co-use over time [56]. Future studies of NSDUH data should identify cannabis use, CUD, and potential co-use patterns of cocaine, sedatives, stimulants, club drugs, opioids, heroin, and 'other' drugs. The causal role of cannabis as a "gateway drug" to other illicit substance use is unclear. Some studies show the onset of cannabis use prior to other substances [42,58,59]. For example, a 25-year longitudinal study found a strong association between adolescent use of cannabis and later other drug use, and that the odds of later other illicit drug use increased as cannabis was used more frequently (at least weekly versus at least monthly or less than monthly) [60].

Because both medical cannabis and prescribed opioids are now legal for patients experiencing chronic pain in many locations, understanding how these two substances are used concurrently is a high priority. The comorbidity of CUD and opioid use disorder (OUD) has been shown in national data, indicating that cannabis use is associated with greater non-medical opioid use in pain patients (aOR 2.99) [61], and in the general population [52]. This is consistent with some findings in veteran samples, revealing that a CUD diagnosis is strongly associated with greater opioid prescription fills [62], although another study has shown the opposite: that co-occurring CUD and OUD are associated with less prescription fills than in veteran patients with OUD alone [63]. Also, recent data analyzing daily self-report of drug use among problematic substance users show that regardless of pain level, on days where non-medical opioids were used, the odds that cannabis was used on the same day were around double (aOR 1.86) [64].

Moreover, cannabis remains the most commonly used drug among those who drink alcohol [2]. Therefore, studies determining how changes in the legal status in cannabis will impact the simultaneous use of alcohol are needed, as well as the frequency and severity of alcohol use disorder (AUD) and CUD. The presence of any CUD significantly increases odds of a co-occurring AUD [28,40], and over half of those with a past-year CUD have a comorbid AUD [40], suggesting the risk of simultaneous use. Numerous studies report the simultaneous use of alcohol and cannabis among adolescents [65–67]. Data from the National Alcohol Survey (NAS) show that simultaneous use of cannabis and alcohol is associated with greater quantities of alcohol use, elevated risk of drunk driving, alcohol-related social problems, and harm to self [68]. Further studies have identified potential risks of co-use of alcohol and cannabis. One review identified that individuals who co-use alcohol and cannabis experience more alcohol-related problems than those who use alcohol alone [69], and similarly reported findings regarding elevated risk of drunk driving when both alcohol and cannabis are used [69]. Because of these risks, and given that the presence of more than one SUD is associated with poorer prognosis than one SUD alone [70], additional clinical research is necessary to identify effective intervention strategies for individuals experiencing problematic co-use of alcohol and cannabis.

3.2. CUD and Psychotic Disorders

Psychotic disorders are rare in the general population [71,72] and their lifetime prevalence varies somewhat across studies. However, the substantial burden of psychotic disorders on the individuals afflicted, their caretakers, and economic costs to society as a whole is clear [72]. While the nature of the relationship between cannabis use and psychosis has been debated, reviews and meta-analyses indicate that cannabis use may be one of the causal factors in the risk for incidence and poor prognosis of psychosis [16,73]. Different lines of evidence suggest that the relationship may be causal, including timing, order, dose–response relationship, and studies ruling out potential confounders. Cannabis use is associated with treated psychotic disorders [73–80]. THC is the component that increases risk [79,81–86]. Most of these studies addressed cannabis use rather than cannabis use disorders. For example, a 6-country study showed strong associations of cannabis frequency and THC potency with first-episode psychosis (OR 4.8) [75].

Reviews and meta-analyses of prospective studies show that previous cannabis use predicts treated first-episode psychosis [73,74,79,87]. Studies addressing potential reverse causation either ruled it out [88–90] or found bi-directionality, i.e., partial causality [91,92]. In addition, among patients with psychotic disorders, cannabis is among the most widely abused substances [93–95]. While in general, substance use disorders predict psychosis relapse [96], meta-analyses specifically focused on cannabis show that continued cannabis use among patients with psychotic disorders predicts psychotic symptom severity, worse functioning and greater risk of relapse (defined as hospitalization) [80,97]. This may be due to the potential for cannabis to directly exacerbate psychosis symptoms [80] or to adverse effects on antipsychotic medication adherence [97,98].

Numerous studies have addressed a dose–response relationship between cannabis and psychosis in terms of frequency of use, THC potency, or both. A systematic review (2007) [99] and a 2016 meta-analysis [100] found that greater frequency of cannabis use was associated with greater risk for psychosis. The odds of psychosis were significantly greater among those using high-potency cannabis compared to low-potency users [101]. We re-computed the ORs in this paper [101] within frequency strata, finding that ORs for the risk for psychosis by THC potency remained strong and significant within all frequency levels (OR = 3.9–4.7). Moreover, high- but not low-potency cannabis use predicts poor antipsychotic medication adherence [102]. Additional reports also indicate increased risk for psychosis from products with higher THC potency. One such study utilizing Danish health records linked an increase in cannabis-induced psychosis since 2006 to an increase in both frequency of use and THC concentration over time [77]. A recent study using NESARC and NESARC-III data showed that participants reporting that a doctor or other health professional told them they had schizophrenia or a psychotic episode were more likely to be frequent cannabis users and have a current CUD diagnosis than other participants [103].

On the other hand, meta-analyses have shown that cannabis use is associated with better cognitive function in patients with schizophrenia, for example, one meta-analysis that found that patients with schizophrenia who reported a history of using cannabis performed better on visual and working memory tasks than those who did not [104]. However, these data were limited and the findings have not always been replicated with larger pooled samples [105]. Additionally, much of the literature focuses on the relationship of cannabis use to psychosis. Data remain limited on the role and severity of CUD in relation to psychotic disorders. Thus, studies are needed in order to better understand the role of cannabis and CUD in the incidence, course and cognition of psychotic disorders.

Many issues remain unresolved about the relationship between cannabis use and psychotic disorders. Because of the serious, chronic and impairing nature of psychotic disorders such as schizophrenia and schizo-affective disorders, research on mechanisms of the effect of cannabis on psychosis and how that may differ across population subgroups is a highly important area of ongoing research.

3.3. CUD and Mood Disorders

Numerous studies indicate a higher prevalence of mood disorders among those with a CUD compared to others in the general population [28,40,106–109]. Specifically, NESARC data show higher levels of major depressive disorder (MDD), bipolar I, bipolar II, and DSM-IV dysthymia in those with both a past-year and lifetime CUD, with strongest odds ratios (ORs) reported for major depression (OR 1.9 lifetime, 1.8 past-year) and bipolar I (OR 2.5 lifetime, 3.1 past-year) [40]. These findings are consistent with a later analysis using data from the NESARC-III, indicating associations between DSM-5 CUD and MDD, bipolar I, and bipolar II, with a stronger association for bipolar I than bipolar II (past-year OR: 5.0 vs. 2.7, lifetime OR: 3.8 vs. 2.8) [28].

Furthermore, a three-year follow-up study of NESARC participants found that a CUD diagnosis was associated with later severity of MDD. Specifically, both baseline cannabis use and CUD predicted a greater number of MDD symptoms three years later, compared to nonusers [110]. There was no significant difference between groups in overall MDD remission rate or quality of life at three-year follow-up, but cannabis users were more likely to experience some specific symptoms, including anhedonia, sleep problems, changes in body weight, and psychomotor agitation or retardation at follow up. These depressive symptoms have substantial overlap with symptoms of DSM-5 cannabis withdrawal syndrome (CWS) [111] (see Table 2), and are commonly reported symptoms among patients entering psychiatric or primary care. CWS is present in ~12% of frequent cannabis users [112], is associated with major depression, and can cause significant impairment [113,114]. Due to the overlap in symptoms, frequent cannabis users who are unaware of the existence of cannabis withdrawal could mistake its symptoms for those of depression, and continue using cannabis in an effort to self-medicate the symptoms, although prospective studies show that among psychiatric patients with depression, cannabis use predicts a worse course over time [115,116].

Table 2. DSM-5 Major Depressive Disorder criteria, and overlapping cannabis withdrawal symptoms.

DSM-5 MDD Criteria and Overlapping Symptoms in CWD.	DSM-5 Major Depressive Disorder	DSM-5 Cannabis Withdrawal Syndrome
Depressed mood—indicated by subjective report or observation by others (in children and adolescents, can be irritable mood).	✓	✓
Loss of interest or pleasure in almost all activities—indicated by subjective report or observation by others.	✓	
Significant unintentional weight loss/gain or decrease/increase in appetite	✓	✓
Sleep disturbance (insomnia or hypersomnia).	✓	✓
Psychomotor changes (agitation or retardation) severe enough to be observable by others.	✓	✓
Tiredness, fatigue, or low energy, or decreased efficiency with which routine tasks are completed.	✓	✓
A sense of worthlessness or excessive, inappropriate, or delusional guilt (not merely self-reproach or guilt about being sick).	✓	
Impaired ability to think, concentrate, or make decisions—indicated by subjective report or observation by others.	✓	
Recurrent thoughts of death (not just fear of dying), suicidal ideation, or suicide attempts.	✓	

Analyses of NSDUH data also indicate associations between cannabis use and depressive episodes [44,49,50,109]. Using data from 728,691 participants from 2002–2012 in the National Survey on Drug Use and Health (NSDUH), both daily and non-daily cannabis use was more than twice as prevalent in those with past-year MDD compared to those without MDD (past 30-day use: 18.94% vs. 8.67% in 2017, $p < 001$) [117]. Additionally, participants with MDD perceive cannabis as less risky compared to those without, and while perception of risk decreased in those with MDD and those without MDD from 2002 to 2017, the decrease was significantly greater in those with MDD than in others (OR 0.90 vs. 0.93, $p < 001$) [117]. Finally, data from the National Health and Nutrition Examination Survey (NHANES) have shown that the strength of the association between cannabis use and depression has increased over time, and that participants with MDD were more likely to experience daily or near-daily cannabis use than those without [118], consistent with the prior NSDUH findings.

While causality cannot be inferred from these cross-sectional studies, twin modeling has evaluated whether CUD changes the risk of the development of MDD. One study analyzing 565 monozygotic twin pairs and 640 dizygotic twin pairs (total n = 2410) found that among the monozygotic pairs that included 1 twin with CUD and 1 twin without CUD the twin with CUD was significantly more likely to have MDD (46.0%) than their co-twin without CUD (28.12%) [119]. These results are consistent with a meta-analysis of longitudinal data, finding cannabis users at an increased risk for developing depression [120] compared to non-users. However, whether these findings are due to causality or shared risk factors remains unclear. In addition, studies that can clarify contradictory evidence of the role of gender in cannabis use and the risk of developing depression [121,122] are also needed.

Three NESARC studies have evaluated the relationship of CUD and bipolar disorders [28,40,123]. All studies consistently showed associations between bipolar I and bipolar II with CUD, with comparatively stronger association of bipolar I with CUD (Table 1). However, these results may not be unique to cannabis use specifically, as prior research has shown higher prevalence of SUDs in people with bipolar I than any other psychiatric diagnosis [124,125]. Additional analyses have shown that individuals with bipolar disorder and a co-occurring CUD are at an elevated risk for having another concurrent SUD, as well as antisocial personality disorder, in comparison to those with bipolar disorder and no CUD [123]. A recent meta-analysis of 53 studies of bipolar disorder patients (51,756 pooled participants) found that around 20% of the samples qualified for lifetime CUD, higher than general population estimates [126]. Cumulatively, these findings provide strong evidence of the association of CUD with bipolar disorders. Additionally, current experimental data show that among individuals with bipolar I, the presence of an SUD was not a predictor of time to recovery from depression, although SUD presence was associated with a greater likelihood of switching from depression to a manic, mixed, or hypomanic state [127]. However, this study did not assess cannabis use or CUD specifically.

3.4. CUD and Anxiety Disorders

Anxiety disorders are the most prevalent mental illness in the United States, impacting over 30% of adults in their lifetime [128]. The prevalence of these disorders increases the importance of understanding their relationship to cannabis use, and CUD.

When taken in high doses, THC can cause symptoms of anxiety, as well as panic attacks [129,130], suggesting the potential to exacerbate anxiety disorders such as panic disorder and generalized anxiety. However, cannabidiol (CBD) has been shown to reduce symptoms of anxiety [131], showing a possible complementary effect [132]. Emerging evidence suggests cannabis as a treatment for anxiety disorders, particularly post-traumatic stress disorder (PTSD), specifically, one systematic review that identified therapeutic benefit of medical cannabis for PTSD symptoms, including internalizing symptoms and nightmares [133]. However, a recent longitudinal study among a veteran population with PTSD who also used non-medical opioids found that cannabis use had no significant impact on PTSD symptoms at follow-up [134]. Dose may play a role in the way cannabis impacts PTSD symptoms acutely and long-term, since at low doses, THC has been shown to reduce stress-induced corticosterone release and amygdala activity in the brain, thus aiding in PTSD stress symptoms [135]. However, this is complicated by potential adverse effects of long-term cannabis use, such as the potential for downregulation of cannabinoid 1 receptors [135]. Because this can impair the stress mechanisms in individuals with PTSD, this opens the potential for long-term negative impacts of cannabis use on PTSD symptoms. Nonetheless, interpretation of findings from prospective studies is complicated by the potential for long-term adverse effects such as the later development of CUD [136], highlighting the need for the monitoring of medical cannabis use among clinical populations. In particular, NESARC data have shown that those with PTSD are significantly more likely to develop CUD compared to those without (9.4% vs. 2.2%) [41].

There is some evidence from NESARC data that while social anxiety disorder and CUD may not be as strongly associated as other anxiety disorders, SAD may be a predictor of cannabis dependence [137]. This could be due to the use of cannabis as a coping mechanism in social situations [138]. Furthermore, SAD and a co-occurring CUD can lead to a poorer prognosis of SAD symptoms long term [137].

Both the NESARC and NESARC-III have established comorbidity of CUD and anxiety disorders, including panic disorder with agoraphobia, generalized anxiety disorder (GAD) and PTSD [28,40]. However, the directionality of effect between cannabis use, CUD, and anxiety disorders remains unclear. While one study based on retrospective information obtained in adulthood suggested that the onset of an anxiety disorder occurs prior to first onset of cannabis dependence symptoms [139], numerous other prospective studies have illustrated the risk of adolescent cannabis use on the later development of an anxiety disorder [140,141]. In particular, one of these studies involving adolescents found an association between daily use of cannabis in mid-teens, and the presence of an anxiety disorder at age 29 (aOR 2.5) [141]. However, in general, the role of cannabis in the etiology, prognosis, and treatment of anxiety disorders remains unclear, and additional research is needed to clarify these issues.

3.5. CUD and Personality Disorders

Individuals with personality disorders think and behave in a way that deviates from cultural expectations and that causes distress [111]. Personality disorders can impact an individual over an extended period of time, affecting concepts of identity, control of emotional responses, and relationships with other people [111]. DSM-5 identifies 10 personality disorders. NESARC data show associations between current (past-year) CUD and a personality disorders (OR 2.6–7.2), with strongest associations reported between CUD and dependent or antisocial personality disorder [40]. These associations between current CUD and a personality disorder have also been established in NESARC-III (OR 3.8–5.0), reporting stronger ORs of CUD and borderline or antisocial personality disorder in comparison to schizotypal personality disorder. Furthermore, a NESARC analysis of 5196 participants with a personality disorder found that 9% of the sample reported past-year cannabis use, with the highest proportion of cannabis users in those with a Cluster B personality disorder (antisocial; borderline; histrionic; narcissistic) compared to Cluster A (paranoid; schizoid; schizotypal), or Cluster C (avoidant; dependent; antisocial) [43]. These findings support an emerging line of evidence that personality disorder traits (i.e., interpersonal reactivity, an RDoC construct) could partially explain the variance in associations between specific personality disorders and CUD [142], and that cannabis may be used as a way to self-medicate. Cannabis use among those with a personality disorder was associated with an increased rate of other SUDs three years later [43]. However, there were no strong associations between cannabis use and other later psychiatric disorders, suggesting that cannabis users with a personality disorder may only be at significantly elevated risk for additional SUDs. Additional longitudinal research is lacking on the long-term outcomes of cannabis use and use disorder among those with a concurrent personality disorder.

Individuals with any personality disorder are significantly more likely to have a past year CUD than those without (OR 3.8–5.0) [28]. NESARC-III data show that borderline personality disorder has the strongest association, compared to antisocial and schizotypal [28], and these findings are consistent with a twin study [143], as well as numerous other studies [144,145]. However, the specific mechanisms behind CUD and co-occurring personality disorders are yet to be understood. A twin study in the Norwegian general population found that genetics may play a role in cannabis use, cannabis use disorder and some personality disorder traits, but not others [143]. Genetic and environmental correlations between personality disorder traits and cannabis use suggest that genetic risk in borderline and antisocial personality disorder traits accounted for significant variance in cannabis use, however not for schizoid or dependent personality disorder traits [143]. Conversely, schizoid and dependent traits were associated with lower levels of cannabis use [143]. Thus, much remains to be clarified about the relationship of cannabis use and cannabis use disorders to personality disorders.

4. Discussion

Due to the rapidly changing legal status of cannabis, the review aims to summarize the potential risks of frequent cannabis use by synthesizing the recent literature reporting on cannabis use, CUD, and comorbid psychopathologies. Although cannabis is increasingly perceived as a harmless substance, empirical evidence suggests considerable potential for adverse effects, including an increased risk for a host of concurrent psychiatric illnesses. Identifying these risks is more relevant now than ever, in light of the rapidly changing legal status of medicinal and recreational cannabis. While a large body of research ties cannabis use and CUD to elevated risks of other psychiatric illness, analyses of the specificities of these associations have produced mixed findings. Extensive evidence links both past-year and lifetime cannabis use and CUD with other substance use, with the strongest associations for alcohol use compared to other illicit drugs. Although directionality is implied that cannabis could be one potential "gateway" to later use of other substances, the role of cannabis as the causal factor in other illicit drug use remains to be clarified, due to the potential effect of common pre-existing risk factors for both cannabis and other substances. Nonetheless, the clear association of cannabis use with later illicit drug use suggests the need for appropriate intervention strategies for those at risk of developing a CUD, in order to diminish later SUD risk. Furthermore, risk of concurrent CUD and OUD should be considered in clinical contexts. American Medical Association (AMA) guidelines currently state that regular use of cannabinoids should not be a reason to suspend medication use in treatment of addiction involving opioids [146]. At the same time, given that states increasingly permit legal medical and recreational cannabis use, the potential has increased for opioids and cannabinoids to be misused concurrently. Thus, due to the risk for co-occurring CUD with other SUDs, clinicians should carefully evaluate the appropriate psychosocial treatment.

Strong evidence also links cannabis use and psychosis, with additional lines of evidence suggesting that cannabis could potentially be a causal factor in later psychosis. However, the complexities of genetic and additional environmental risk factors complicate this relationship, and the role of cannabis use in cognition of those with schizophrenia has generated inconsistent findings. Thus, further longitudinal research which takes into account confounds will aid in delineating this relationship.

National data suggest that cannabis use and CUD are associated with mood disorders, particularly depression and bipolar I. Twin study models show potential directionality between cannabis use and later depression, however replicated results on larger samples are necessary in order to make firmer conclusions. Furthermore, cannabis use and CUD are higher in those with bipolar disorder than the general population, but little research exists regarding the course of this comorbidity, and inconsistent findings regarding elevated risk factors have been reported [139–141]. Much more remains to be clarified about the nature of cannabis use among those with bipolar disorders, and about the impact of such use on the course and prognosis of bipolar disorders. Nonetheless, proportionally higher rates of frequent cannabis use and CUD among those with a mood disorder underscores the clinical importance of cannabis abuse screenings concurrently with mood disorder screenings.

Similarly, CUD is associated with both anxiety disorders and personality disorders, yet evidence regarding the specific role of cannabis in the course of these disorders is limited. More specifically, the role of genetic in risk of CUD among individuals with a personality disorder is complex and not well understood, and more definitive evidence of the relationship of cannabis use with personality disorders could help guide clinical practice. Furthermore, while some data show potential therapeutic benefit of medical cannabis for individuals with PTSD, these results are complicated by a potential increased risk for abuse of cannabis as well as potential long-term harms [41]. Therefore, the increased risk of CUD should be recognized in clinical settings, in conjunction with any potential therapeutic benefits of cannabis for anxiety. The lack of evidence between CUD and co-occurring PTSD is noted in particular, since as of 2020, PTSD is a qualifying condition for medical cannabis approval in 26 states [147]. Thus, additional experimental data and clinical trials investigating the use of cannabis among PTSD patients are needed in order to provide more conclusive evidence of the acute and long-term effects. Similar clinical data are needed for other psychiatric diagnoses qualifying as a condition for medical cannabis approval, for example bipolar disorder, ADHD, and anorexia.

Considering rapidly changing state laws regarding the legality of cannabis, the current disconnect between the cannabis industry, public opinion, and scientific literature is striking. Cannabis is a $13.6 billion industry [148–150], with millions spent yearly on lobbying to increase legalization [151,152]. Bearing in mind the potential for poorer prognosis among those with psychiatric comorbidities, if they also use cannabis or have a CUD [36], public and provider education on the current evidence regarding cannabis use, CUD, and a co-occurring disorder is essential to properly guide clinical practice, policy, and decisions of the general public about whether to use cannabis or not.

5. Conclusions and Future Directions

Overall, beginning with the Epidemiologic Catchment Area study in the 1980s and accumulating to today, a large body of literature indicates substantial associations between frequent cannabis use, CUD, and additional psychiatric illnesses. Considerable evidence indicates that state medical cannabis laws increase cannabis use and use disorder in adult populations [20,153,154], consistent with evidence indicating that state recreational laws increase adult non-medical cannabis use and CUD [155]. Because of the elevated risk of CUD and co-occurring mental illness, this time of changing cannabis legislation is a critical time to highlight the increased need for effective prevention and treatment strategies for the co-occurrence of CUD with other substance and psychiatric disorders.

One proposed future direction to aid in clarifying the relationship between cannabis use, CUD, and comorbid psychiatric illness is a greater level of standardization of cannabis use definitions in empirical research. Since the frequency of use, potency of cannabis products, and severity of CUD are linked to stronger associations with a comorbid psychiatric diagnosis [28], and cannabis potency is increasing internationally, better measures of the amounts of cannabis consumed could help to elucidate outcomes. Because of this, awareness of THC to CBD ratios as well as amounts of each could help play a role in deciphering mixed findings. However, no standardized, scientifically valid and widely used measure of cannabis exposure exists thus far, a critical gap in the existing body of literature. Creating measures of cannabis exposure faces several challenges, such as a lack of a standard unit to measure cannabis consumption that are analogous to the standard drink units and measures of binge drinking for alcohol consumption. Recent articles have noted the difficulties in measuring cannabis consumption patterns, which are further complicated by inaccuracies in cannabis product labels [156], which have drawn attention to the need for further standardization measures [157] that can be used for clinical as well as research purposes.

The strengths of this narrative review are noted. First, this review aimed to synthesize recent studies regarding cannabis use, CUD, and co-occurring disorders to bring together what is known and identify gaps in the literature in one summation. We believe that by organizing the current literature this way, we are also able to identify points of controversy in the field, for example studies showing opposite results regarding the role that cannabis plays in cognitive function among individuals with schizophrenia [104,105]. This underscores the complex nature of cannabis, and that further research is necessary in order to identify its role for most comorbidities. Limitations of this review are also present. By adopting the narrative review methodology, no quantitative meta-analysis of results or systematic search according to an official guide was conducted, leaving opportunity for this to be done in a future study. Second, the complex dose-dependent effects of cannabinoids on the brain is an additional point to consider when discussing the associations of cannabis use with other psychopathologies. Thus, an updated review of the major compounds found in cannabis and their relationship with co-occurring disorders is also needed.

Finally, given the extent of comorbidity of cannabis use, CUD, and other comorbid substance and psychiatric illnesses, greater guidance is needed for clinicians in terms of education about potential risks, methods of assessment and monitoring, and the most effective treatment strategies among patients with cannabis use or CUD and substance use or psychiatric disorders. For patients with comorbid substance use disorders, clinician guidance is needed to determine which substances merit treatment focus when more than one is involved (the most common case), and how to prioritize that focus when more than one substance is involved. For patients with cannabis use or CUD and psychiatric disorders, guidance may be needed on modifications in behavioral treatments and/or medication strategies.

Author Contributions: Conceptualization, D.H. and C.W.; initial literature search, C.W.; writing—original draft preparation, C.W. and D.H.; writing—review and editing, D.H. and C.W.; supervision, D.H. All authors have read and agreed to the published version of the manuscript.

Funding: This research received no external funding

Institutional Review Board Statement: Not applicable.

Informed Consent Statement: Not applicable.

Data Availability Statement: Data sharing not applicable.

Conflicts of Interest: The authors declare no conflict of interest.

References

1. National Institute on Drug Abuse. Marijuana Research Report. July 2020. Available online: https://www.drugabuse.gov/download/1380/marijuana-research-report.pdf (accessed on 11 August 2020).
2. Substance Abuse Center for Behavioral Health Statistics and Quality. Results from the 2018 National Survey on Drug Use and Health: Detailed Tables. 2019. Available online: https://www.samhsa.gov/data/report/2018-nsduh-detailed-tables (accessed on 11 August 2020).
3. DISA Global Solutions. Map of Marijuana Legality by State. July 2020. Available online: https://disa.com/map-of-marijuana-legality-by-state (accessed on 11 August 2020).
4. United Nations Office on Drug and Crime. World Drug Report 2019: Executive Summary. 2019. Available online: https://wdr.unodc.org/wdr2019/prelaunch/WDR19_Booklet_1_EXECUTIVE_SUMMARY.pdf (accessed on 11 August 2020).
5. Home Office of the Government of the United Kingdom, Seizures of Drugs in England and Wales, Financial Year Ending 2019 Second Edition. 2019. Available online: https://assets.publishing.service.gov.uk/government/uploads/system/uploads/attachment_data/file/870323/seizures-drugs-mar2019-hosb3119.pdf (accessed on 11 August 2020).
6. European Monitoring Centre for Drugs and Drug Addiction. Cannabis Legalisation in Europe: An Overview. March 2017. Available online: https://www.emcdda.europa.eu/system/files/publications/4135/TD0217210ENN.pdf (accessed on 11 August 2020).
7. European Monitoring Centre for Drugs and Drug Addiction. Cannabis Policy: Status and Recent Developments. 2016. Available online: https://www.emcdda.europa.eu/publications/topic-overviews/cannabis-policy/html_en (accessed on 11 August 2020).
8. Piontek, D.; Kraus, L.; Bjarnason, T.; Demetrovics, Z.; Ramstedt, M. Individual and country-level effects of cannabis-related perceptions on cannabis use. A multilevel study among adolescents in 32 European countries. *J. Adolesc. Health* **2013**, *52*, 473–479. [CrossRef]
9. Carliner, H.; Brown, Q.L.; Sarvet, A.L.; Hasin, D.S. Cannabis use, attitudes, and legal status in the U.S.: A review. *Prev. Med.* **2017**, *104*, 13–23. [CrossRef] [PubMed]
10. Hall, W.; Degenhardt, L. The adverse health effects of chronic cannabis use. *Drug Test. Anal.* **2014**, *6*, 39–45. [CrossRef] [PubMed]
11. Camchong, J.; Lim, K.O.; Kumra, S. Adverse Effects of Cannabis on Adolescent Brain Development: A Longitudinal Study. *Cereb. Cortex.* **2017**, *27*, 1922–1930. [CrossRef] [PubMed]
12. Ashton, J.C. Is Cannabis Harmless? Focus on Brain Function. *Curr. Drug Res. Rev.* **2019**, *11*, 33–39. [CrossRef]
13. Hasin, D.S. US Epidemiology of Cannabis Use and Associated Problems. *Neuropsychopharmacology* **2018**, *43*, 195–212. [CrossRef]
14. Hasin, D.S.; Saha, T.D.; Kerridge, B.T.; Goldstein, R.B.; Chou, S.P.; Zhang, H.; Jung, J.; Pickering, R.P.; Ruan, W.J.; Smith, S.M.; et al. Prevalence of Marijuana Use Disorders in the United States Between 2001–2002 and 2012–2013. *JAMA Psychiatry* **2015**, *72*, 1235–1242. [CrossRef]
15. Chandra, S.; Radwan, M.M.; Majumdar, C.G.; Church, J.C.; Freeman, T.P.; ElSohly, M.A. New trends in cannabis potency in USA and Europe during the last decade (2008–2017). *Eur. Arch. Psychiatry Clin. Neurosci.* **2019**, *269*, 5–15. [CrossRef]
16. Murray, R.M.; Hall, W. Will Legalization and Commercialization of Cannabis Use Increase the Incidence and Prevalence of Psychosis? *JAMA Psychiatry* **2020**, *77*, 777–778. [CrossRef]

17. Freeman, T.P.; van der Pol, P.; Kuijpers, W.; Wisselink, J.; Das, R.K.; Rigter, S.; van Laar, M.; Griffiths, P.; Swift, W.; Niesink, R.; et al. Changes in cannabis potency and first-time admissions to drug treatment: A 16-year study in the Netherlands. *Psychol. Med.* **2018**, *48*, 2346–2352. [CrossRef]
18. Freeman, T.P.; Groshkova, T.; Cunningham, A.; Sedefov, R.; Griffiths, P.; Lynskey, M.T. Increasing potency and price of cannabis in Europe, 2006–2016. *Addiction* **2019**, *114*, 1015–1023. [CrossRef] [PubMed]
19. Wagner, F.A.; Anthony, J.C. Male-female differences in the risk of progression from first use to dependence upon cannabis, cocaine, and alcohol. *Drug Alcohol. Depend.* **2007**, *86*, 191–198. [CrossRef] [PubMed]
20. Hasin, D.S.; Sarvet, A.L.; Cerda, M.; Keyes, K.M.; Stohl, M.; Galea, S.; Wall, M.M. US Adult Illicit Cannabis Use, Cannabis Use Disorder, and Medical Marijuana Laws: 1991–1992 to 2012–2013. *JAMA Psychiatry* **2017**, *74*, 579–588. [CrossRef] [PubMed]
21. Butterworth, P.; Slade, T.; Degenhardt, L. Factors associated with the timing and onset of cannabis use and cannabis use disorder: Results from the 2007 Australian National Survey of Mental Health and Well-Being. *Drug Alcohol. Rev.* **2014**, *33*, 555–5. [CrossRef]
22. Weiss, S.R.B.; Wargo, E.M. Commentary: Navigating the complexities of marijuana. *Prev. Med.* **2017**, *104*, 10–12. [CrossRef]
23. Hasin, D.; Endicott, J.; Lewis, C. Alcohol and drug abuse in patients with affective syndromes. *Compr. Psychiatry* **1985**, *26*, 283–2. [CrossRef]
24. Regier, D.A.; Farmer, M.E.; Rae, D.S.; Locke, B.Z.; Keith, S.J.; Judd, L.L.; Goodwin, F.K. Comorbidity of mental disorders with alcohol and other drug abuse. Results from the Epidemiologic Catchment Area (ECA) Study. *JAMA* **1990**, *264*, 2511–25. [CrossRef]
25. Cohen, P.; Cohen, J. The clinician's illusion. *Arch. Gen. Psychiatry* **1984**, *41*, 1178–1182. [CrossRef]
26. Conway, K.P.; Compton, W.; Stinson, F.S.; Grant, B.F. Lifetime comorbidity of DSM-IV mood and anxiety disorders and specific drug use disorders: Results from the National Epidemiologic Survey on Alcohol and Related Conditions. *J. Clin. Psychiatry* **2006**, *67*, 247–257. [CrossRef]
27. Hasin, D.S.; Sarvet, A.L.; Meyers, J.L.; Saha, T.D.; Ruan, W.J.; Stohl, M.; Grant, B.F. Epidemiology of Adult DSM-5 Major Depressive Disorder and Its Specifiers in the United States. *JAMA Psychiatry* **2018**, *75*, 336–346. [CrossRef]
28. Hasin, D.S.; Kerridge, B.T.; Saha, T.D.; Huang, B.; Pickering, R.; Smith, S.M.; Jung, J.; Zhang, H.; Grant, B.F. Prevalence and Correlates of DSM-5 Cannabis Use Disorder, 2012–2013: Findings from the National Epidemiologic Survey on Alcohol and Related Conditions-III. *Am. J. Psychiatry* **2016**, *173*, 588–599. [CrossRef] [PubMed]
29. Hasin, D.S.; Grant, B.F. The National Epidemiologic Survey on Alcohol and Related Conditions (NESARC) Waves 1 and 2: Review and summary of findings. *Soc. Psychiatry Psychiatr. Epidemiol.* **2015**, *50*, 1609–1640. [CrossRef] [PubMed]
30. Hasin, D.S.; Greenstein, E.; Aivadyan, C.; Stohl, M.; Aharonovich, E.; Saha, T.; Goldstein, R.; Nunes, E.V.; Jung, J.; Zhang, H.; et al. The Alcohol Use Disorder and Associated Disabilities Interview Schedule-5 (AUDADIS-5): Procedural validity of substance use disorders modules through clinical re-appraisal in a general population sample. *Drug Alcohol. Depend.* **2015**, *148*, 40–. [CrossRef] [PubMed]
31. Grant, B.F.; Saha, T.D.; Ruan, W.J.; Goldstein, R.B.; Chou, S.P.; Jung, J.; Zhang, H.; Smith, S.M.; Pickering, R.P.; Huang, B.; et al. Epidemiology of DSM-5 Drug Use Disorder: Results From the National Epidemiologic Survey on Alcohol and Related Conditions-III. *JAMA Psychiatry* **2016**, *73*, 39–47. [CrossRef] [PubMed]
32. Grant, B.F.; Stinson, F.S.; Dawson, D.A.; Chou, S.P.; Ruan, W.J.; Pickering, R.P. Co-occurrence of 12-month alcohol and drug use disorders and personality disorders in the United States: Results from the National Epidemiologic Survey on Alcohol and Related Conditions. *Arch. Gen. Psychiatry* **2004**, *61*, 361–368. [CrossRef]
33. Hasin, D.S.; Grant, B.F. Major depression in 6050 former drinkers: Association with past alcohol dependence. *Arch. Gen. Psychiatry* **2002**, *59*, 794–800. [CrossRef] [PubMed]
34. Grant, B.F.; Stinson, F.S.; Dawson, D.A.; Chou, S.P.; Dufour, M.C.; Compton, W.; Pickering, R.P.; Kaplan, K. Prevalence and co-occurrence of substance use disorders and independent mood and anxiety disorders: Results from the National Epidemiologic Survey on Alcohol and Related Conditions. *Arch. Gen. Psychiatry* **2004**, *61*, 807–816. [CrossRef]
35. Compton, W.M.; Thomas, Y.F.; Stinson, F.S.; Grant, B.F. Prevalence, correlates, disability, and comorbidity of DSM-IV drug abuse and dependence in the United States: Results from the national epidemiologic survey on alcohol and related conditions. *Arch. Gen. Psychiatry* **2007**, *64*, 566–576. [CrossRef]
36. Makovski, T.T.; Schmitz, S.; Zeegers, M.P.; Stranges, S.; van den Akker, M. Multimorbidity and quality of life: Systematic literature review and meta-analysis. *Ageing Res. Rev.* **2019**, *53*, 100903. [CrossRef] [PubMed]
37. Cougle, J.R.; Hakes, J.K.; Macatee, R.J.; Chavarria, J.; Zvolensky, M.J. Quality of life and risk of psychiatric disorders among regular users of alcohol, nicotine, and cannabis: An analysis of the National Epidemiological Survey on Alcohol and Related Conditions (NESARC). *J. Psychiatr. Res.* **2015**, *66–67*, 135–141. [CrossRef]
38. Skodol, A.E. Impact of personality pathology on psychosocial functioning. *Curr. Opin. Psychol.* **2018**, *21*, 33–38. [CrossRef] [PubMed]
39. Fortin, M.; Bravo, G.; Hudon, C.; Lapointe, L.; Almirall, J.; Dubois, M.F.; Vanasse, A. Relationship between multimorbidity and health-related quality of life of patients in primary care. *Qual. Life Res.* **2006**, *15*, 83–91. [CrossRef] [PubMed]
40. Stinson, F.S.; Ruan, W.J.; Pickering, R.; Grant, B.F. Cannabis use disorders in the USA: Prevalence, correlates and co-morbidity. *Psychol. Med.* **2006**, *36*, 1447–1460. [CrossRef] [PubMed]

41. Bilevicius, E.; Sommer, J.L.; Asmundson, G.J.G.; El-Gabalawy, R. Associations of PTSD, chronic pain, and their comorbidity on cannabis use disorder: Results from an American nationally representative study. *Depress. Anxiety* **2019**, *36*, 1036–1046. [CrossRef]
42. Hayley, A.C.; Stough, C.; Downey, L.A. DSM-5 cannabis use disorder, substance use and DSM-5 specific substance-use disorders: Evaluating comorbidity in a population-based sample. *Eur. Neuropsychopharmacol.* **2017**, *27*, 732–743. [CrossRef]
43. Shalit, N.; Rehm, J.; Lev-Ran, S. The association between cannabis use and psychiatric comorbidity in people with personality disorders: A population-based longitudinal study. *Psychiatry Res.* **2019**, *278*, 70–77. [CrossRef]
44. Pacek, L.R.; Weinberger, A.H.; Zhu, J.; Goodwin, R.D. Rapid increase in the prevalence of cannabis use among people with depression in the United States, 2005–2017: The role of differentially changing risk perceptions. *Addiction* **2020**, *115*, 935–943. [CrossRef]
45. National Center for Biotechnology Information. PubMed User Guide. 2020. Available online: https://pubmed.ncbi.nlm.nih.gov/help/#:~{}:text=Last%20Update%3A%20March%2031%2C%202020.&text=PubMed%20comprises%20over%2030%20million,science%20journals%2C%20and%20online%20books (accessed on 10 December 2020).
46. Grant, B.F.; Dawson, D.A. Introduction to the National Epidemiologic Survey on Alcohol and Related Conditions. Available online: https://pubs.niaaa.nih.gov/publications/arh29-2/74-78.htm (accessed on 11 August 2020).
47. National Institute on Alcohol Abuse and Alcoholism. National Epidemiologic Survey on Alcohol and Related Conditions-III (NESARC-III). Available online: https://www.niaaa.nih.gov/research/nesarc-iii (accessed on 11 August 2020).
48. Substance Abuse and Mental Health Services Administration. NSDUH: About the Survey. Available online: https://nsduhweb.rti.org/respweb/about_nsduh.html (accessed on 11 August 2020).
49. Gukasyan, N.; Strain, E.C. Relationship between cannabis use frequency and major depressive disorder in adolescents: Findings from the National Survey on Drug Use and Health 2012–2017. *Drug Alcohol. Depend.* **2020**, *208*, 107867. [CrossRef]
50. Weinberger, A.H.; Zhu, J.; Lee, J.; Anastasiou, E.; Copeland, J.; Goodwin, R.D. Cannabis use among youth in the United States, 2004–2016: Faster rate of increase among youth with depression. *Drug Alcohol. Depend.* **2020**, *209*, 107894. [CrossRef]
51. Carra, G.; Bartoli, F.; Riboldi, I.; Trotta, G.; Crocamo, C. Poverty matters: Cannabis use among people with serious mental illness: Findings from the United States survey on drug use and health, 2015. *Int. J. Soc. Psychiatry* **2018**, *64*, 656–659. [CrossRef]
52. Liang, D.; Wallace, M.S.; Shi, Y. Medical and non-medical cannabis use and risk of prescription opioid use disorder: Findings from propensity score matching. *Drug Alcohol. Rev.* **2019**, *38*, 597–605. [CrossRef] [PubMed]
53. Fairman, B.J.; Furr-Holden, C.D.; Johnson, R.M. When Marijuana Is Used before Cigarettes or Alcohol: Demographic Predictors and Associations with Heavy Use, Cannabis Use Disorder, and Other Drug-related Outcomes. *Prev. Sci.* **2019**, *20*, 225–233. [CrossRef] [PubMed]
54. Dierker, L.; Braymiller, J.; Rose, J.; Goodwin, R.; Selya, A. Nicotine dependence predicts cannabis use disorder symptoms among adolescents and young adults. *Drug Alcohol. Depend.* **2018**, *187*, 212–220. [CrossRef] [PubMed]
55. Weinberger, A.H.; Pacek, L.R.; Wall, M.M.; Gbedemah, M.; Lee, J.; Goodwin, R.D. Cigarette smoking quit ratios among adults in the USA with cannabis use and cannabis use disorders, 2002–2016. *Tob. Control* **2020**, *29*, 74–80. [CrossRef]
56. Schauer, G.L.; Peters, E.N. Correlates and trends in youth co-use of marijuana and tobacco in the United States, 2005–2014. *Drug Alcohol. Depend.* **2018**, *185*, 238–244. [CrossRef]
57. Schauer, G.L.; Berg, C.J.; Kegler, M.C.; Donovan, D.M.; Windle, M. Assessing the overlap between tobacco and marijuana: Trends in patterns of co-use of tobacco and marijuana in adults from 2003–2012. *Addict. Behav.* **2015**, *49*, 26–32. [CrossRef]
58. Silins, E.; Horwood, L.J.; Patton, G.C.; Fergusson, D.M.; Olsson, C.A.; Hutchinson, D.M.; Spry, E.; Toumbourou, J.W.; Degenhardt, L.; Swift, W.; et al. Young adult sequelae of adolescent cannabis use: An integrative analysis. *Lancet Psychiatry* **2014**, *1*, 286–293. [CrossRef]
59. Secades-Villa, R.; Garcia-Rodriguez, O.; Jin, C.J.; Wang, S.; Blanco, C. Probability and predictors of the cannabis gateway effect: A national study. *Int. J. Drug Policy* **2015**, *26*, 135–142. [CrossRef]
60. Fergusson, D.M.; Boden, J.M.; Horwood, L.J. Cannabis use and other illicit drug use: Testing the cannabis gateway hypothesis. *Addiction* **2006**, *101*, 556–569. [CrossRef]
61. Olfson, M.; Wall, M.M.; Liu, S.M.; Blanco, C. Cannabis Use and Risk of Prescription Opioid Use Disorder in the United States. *Am. J. Psychiatry* **2018**, *175*, 47–53. [CrossRef]
62. Hefner, K.; Sofuoglu, M.; Rosenheck, R. Concomitant cannabis abuse/dependence in patients treated with opioids for non-cancer pain. *Am. J. Addict.* **2015**, *24*, 538–545. [CrossRef] [PubMed]
63. De Aquino, J.P.; Sofuoglu, M.; Stefanovics, E.; Rosenheck, R. Adverse Consequences of Co-Occurring Opioid Use Disorder and Cannabis Use Disorder Compared to Opioid Use Disorder Only. *Am. J. Drug Alcohol. Abuse* **2019**, *45*, 527–537. [CrossRef] [PubMed]
64. Gorfinkel, L.; Stohl, M.; Greenstein, E.; Aharonovich, E.; Olfson, M.; Hasin, D. Is cannabis substituted for non-medical opioids? Using daily measurements to assess the strength of the association between cannabis and opioid use. *Addiction* **2020**, in press.
65. Briere, F.N.; Fallu, J.S.; Descheneaux, A.; Janosz, M. Predictors and consequences of simultaneous alcohol and cannabis use in adolescents. *Addict. Behav.* **2011**, *36*, 785–788. [CrossRef]
66. Terry-McElrath, Y.M.; O'Malley, P.M.; Johnston, L.D. Alcohol and marijuana use patterns associated with unsafe driving among U.S. high school seniors: High use frequency, concurrent use, and simultaneous use. *J. Stud. Alcohol. Drugs* **2014**, *75*, 378–389. [CrossRef] [PubMed]

67. Martin, C.S.; Kaczynski, N.A.; Maisto, S.A.; Tarter, R.E. Polydrug use in adolescent drinkers with and without DSM-IV alcohol abuse and dependence. *Alcohol. Clin. Exp. Res.* **1996**, *20*, 1099–1108. [CrossRef] [PubMed]
68. Subbaraman, M.S.; Kerr, W.C. Simultaneous versus concurrent use of alcohol and cannabis in the National Alcohol Survey. *Alcohol. Clin. Exp. Res.* **2015**, *39*, 872–879. [CrossRef] [PubMed]
69. Yurasek, A.M.; Aston, E.R.; Metrik, J. Co-use of Alcohol and Cannabis: A Review. *Curr. Addict. Rep.* **2017**, *4*, 184–193. [CrossRef]
70. Dutra, L.; Stathopoulou, G.; Basden, S.L.; Leyro, T.M.; Powers, M.B.; Otto, M.W. A meta-analytic review of psychosocial interventions for substance use disorders. *Am. J. Psychiatry* **2008**, *165*, 179–187. [CrossRef]
71. Chang, W.C.; Wong, C.S.M.; Chen, E.Y.H.; Lam, L.C.W.; Chan, W.C.; Ng, R.M.K.; Hung, S.F.; Cheung, E.F.C.; Sham, P.C.; Chiu, H.F.K.; et al. Lifetime Prevalence and Correlates of Schizophrenia-Spectrum, Affective, and Other Non-affective Psychotic Disorders in the Chinese Adult Population. *Schizophr. Bull.* **2017**, *43*, 1280–1290. [CrossRef]
72. Rossler, W.; Salize, H.J.; van Os, J.; Riecher-Rossler, A. Size of burden of schizophrenia and psychotic disorders. *Eur. Neuropsychopharmacol.* **2005**, *15*, 399–409. [CrossRef] [PubMed]
73. Sideli, L.; Quigley, H.; la Cascia, C.; Murray, R.M. Cannabis Use and the Risk for Psychosis and Affective Disorders. *J. Dual. Diagn.* **2020**, *16*, 22–42. [CrossRef] [PubMed]
74. Brown, A.S. The environment and susceptibility to schizophrenia. *Prog. Neurobiol.* **2011**, *93*, 23–58. [CrossRef] [PubMed]
75. Di Forti, M.; Quattrone, D.; Freeman, T.P.; Tripoli, G.; Gayer-Anderson, C.; Quigley, H.; Rodriguez, V.; Jongsma, H.E.; Ferraro, L.; la Cascia, C.; et al. The contribution of cannabis use to variation in the incidence of psychotic disorder across Europe (EU-GEI): A multicentre case-control study. *Lancet Psychiatry* **2019**, *6*, 427–436. [CrossRef]
76. Boydell, J.; van Os, J.; Caspi, A.; Kennedy, N.; Giouroukou, E.; Fearon, P.; Farrell, M.; Murray, R.M. Trends in cannabis use prior to first presentation with schizophrenia, in South-East London between 1965 and 1999. *Psychol. Med.* **2006**, *36*, 1441–1446. [CrossRef]
77. Hjorthoj, C.; Larsen, M.O.; Starzer, M.S.K.; Nordentoft, M. Annual incidence of cannabis-induced psychosis, other substance induced psychoses and dually diagnosed schizophrenia and cannabis use disorder in Denmark from 1994 to 2016. *Psychol. Med.* **2019**, 1–6. [CrossRef]
78. Goncalves-Pinho, M.; Braganca, M.; Freitas, A. Psychotic disorders hospitalizations associated with cannabis abuse or dependence: A nationwide big data analysis. *Int. J. Methods Psychiatr. Res.* **2020**, *29*, e1813. [CrossRef]
79. Murray, R.M.; Englund, A.; Abi-Dargham, A.; Lewis, D.A.; di Forti, M.; Davies, C.; Sherif, M.; McGuire, P.; D'Souza, D.C. Cannabis-associated psychosis: Neural substrate and clinical impact. *Neuropharmacology* **2017**, *124*, 89–104. [CrossRef]
80. Schoeler, T.; Monk, A.; Sami, M.B.; Klamerus, E.; Foglia, E.; Brown, R.; Camuri, G.; Altamura, A.C.; Murray, R.; Bhattacharyya, S. Continued versus discontinued cannabis use in patients with psychosis: A systematic review and meta-analysis. *Lancet Psychiatry* **2016**, *3*, 215–225. [CrossRef]
81. D'Souza, D.C.; Radhakrishnan, R.; Sherif, M.; Cortes-Briones, J.; Cahill, J.; Gupta, S.; Skosnik, P.D.; Ranganathan, M. Cannabinoids and Psychosis. *Curr. Pharm. Des.* **2016**, *22*, 6380–6391.
82. Hindley, G.; Beck, K.; Borgan, F.; Ginestet, C.E.; McCutcheon, R.; Kleinloog, D.; Ganesh, S.; Radhakrishnan, R.; D'Souza, D.C.; Howes, O.D. Psychiatric symptoms caused by cannabis constituents: A systematic review and meta-analysis. *Lancet Psychiatry* **2020**, *7*, 344–353. [CrossRef]
83. Di Forti, M.; Morgan, C.; Selten, J.P.; Lynskey, M.; Murray, R.M. High-potency cannabis and incident psychosis: Correcting the causal assumption—Authors' reply. *Lancet Psychiatry* **2019**, *6*, 466–467. [CrossRef]
84. Gayer-Anderson, C.; Jongsma, H.E.; di Forti, M.; Quattrone, D.; Velthorst, E.; de Haan, L.; Selten, J.P.; Szoke, A.; Llorca, P.M.; Tortelli, A.; et al. The EUropean Network of National Schizophrenia Networks Studying Gene-Environment Interactions (EU-GEI): Incidence and First-Episode Case-Control Programme. *Soc. Psychiatry Psychiatr. Epidemiol.* **2020**, *55*, 645–657. [CrossRef] [PubMed]
85. Belbasis, L.; Kohler, C.A.; Stefanis, N.; Stubbs, B.; van Os, J.; Vieta, E.; Seeman, M.V.; Arango, C.; Carvalho, A.F.; Evangelou, E. Risk factors and peripheral biomarkers for schizophrenia spectrum disorders: An umbrella review of meta-analyses. *Acta Psychiatr. Scand.* **2018**, *137*, 88–97. [CrossRef]
86. Ganesh, S.; Cortes-Briones, J.; Ranganathan, M.; Radhakrishnan, R.; Skosnik, P.D.; D'Souza, D.C. Psychosis-relevant effects of intravenous delta-9-tetrahydrocannabinol—A mega analysis of individual participant-data from human laboratory studies. *Int. J. Neuropsychopharmacol.* **2020**, *23*, 559–570. [CrossRef]
87. Henquet, C.; Murray, R.; Linszen, D.; van Os, J. The environment and schizophrenia: The role of cannabis use. *Schizophr. Bull.* **2005**, *31*, 608–612. [CrossRef]
88. van Os, J.; Bak, M.; Hanssen, M.; Bijl, R.V.; de Graaf, R.; Verdoux, H. Cannabis use and psychosis: A longitudinal population-based study. *Am. J. Epidemiol* **2002**, *156*, 319–327. [CrossRef]
89. Arseneault, L.; Cannon, M.; Poulton, R.; Murray, R.; Caspi, A.; Moffitt, T.E. Cannabis use in adolescence and risk for adult psychosis: Longitudinal prospective study. *BMJ* **2002**, *325*, 1212–1213. [CrossRef]
90. Power, R.A.; Verweij, K.J.; Zuhair, M.; Montgomery, G.W.; Henders, A.K.; Heath, A.C.; Madden, P.A.; Medland, S.E.; Wray, N.R.; Martin, N.G. Genetic predisposition to schizophrenia associated with increased use of cannabis. *Mol. Psychiatry* **2014**, *19*, 1201–1204. [CrossRef]
91. Fergusson, D.M.; Horwood, L.J.; Ridder, E.M. Tests of causal linkages between cannabis use and psychotic symptoms. *Addiction* **2005**, *100*, 354–366. [CrossRef]

92. Van Os, J.; Sham, P. Gene-Environment Interactions. In *The Epidemiology of Schizophrenia*; Murray, R.M., Stilo, S.A., Eds.; Cambridge University Press: Cambridge, UK, 2003; pp. 235–254.
93. Alisauskiene, R.; Loberg, E.M.; Gjestad, R.; Kroken, R.A.; Jorgensen, H.A.; Johnsen, E. The influence of substance use on the effectiveness of antipsychotic medication: A prospective, pragmatic study. *Nord. J. Psychiatry* **2019**, *73*, 281–287. [CrossRef] [PubMed]
94. Brunette, M.F.; Mueser, K.T.; Babbin, S.; Meyer-Kalos, P.; Rosenheck, R.; Correll, C.U.; Cather, C.; Robinson, D.G.; Schooler, N.R.; Penn, D.L.; et al. Demographic and clinical correlates of substance use disorders in first episode psychosis. *Schizophr. Res.* **2018**, *194*, 4–12. [CrossRef] [PubMed]
95. Margolis, A.; Rosca, P.; Kurs, R.; Sznitman, S.R.; Grinshpoon, A. Routine Drug Screening for Patients in the Emergency Department of a State Psychiatric Hospital: A Naturalistic Cohort Study. *J. Dual Diagn.* **2016**, *12*, 218–226. [CrossRef] [PubMed]
96. Alvarez-Jimenez, M.; Priede, A.; Hetrick, S.E.; Bendall, S.; Killackey, E.; Parker, A.G.; McGorry, P.D.; Gleeson, J.F. Risk factors for relapse following treatment for first episode psychosis: A systematic review and meta-analysis of longitudinal studies. *Schizophr. Res.* **2012**, *139*, 116–128. [CrossRef] [PubMed]
97. Foglia, E.; Schoeler, T.; Klamerus, E.; Morgan, K.; Bhattacharyya, S. Cannabis use and adherence to antipsychotic medication: A systematic review and meta-analysis. *Psychol. Med.* **2017**, *47*, 1691–1705. [CrossRef]
98. Schoeler, T.; Petros, N.; di Forti, M.; Klamerus, E.; Foglia, E.; Murray, R.; Bhattacharyya, S. Poor medication adherence and risk of relapse associated with continued cannabis use in patients with first-episode psychosis: A prospective analysis. *Lancet Psychiatry* **2017**, *4*, 627–633. [CrossRef]
99. Moore, T.H.; Zammit, S.; Lingford-Hughes, A.; Barnes, T.R.; Jones, P.B.; Burke, M.; Lewis, G. Cannabis use and risk of psychotic or affective mental health outcomes: A systematic review. *Lancet* **2007**, *370*, 319–328. [CrossRef]
100. Marconi, A.; di Forti, M.; Lewis, C.M.; Murray, R.M.; Vassos, E. Meta-analysis of the Association Between the Level of Cannabis Use and Risk of Psychosis. *Schizophr. Bull.* **2016**, *42*, 1262–1269. [CrossRef]
101. Di Forti, M.; Marconi, A.; Carra, E.; Fraietta, S.; Trotta, A.; Bonomo, M.; Bianconi, F.; Gardner-Sood, P.; O'Connor, J.; Russo, M.; et al. Proportion of patients in south London with first-episode psychosis attributable to use of high potency cannabis: A case-control study. *Lancet Psychiatry* **2015**, *2*, 233–238. [CrossRef]
102. Schoeler, T.; Petros, N.; di Forti, M.; Klamerus, E.; Foglia, E.; Murray, R.; Bhattacharyya, S. Effect of continued cannabis use on medication adherence in the first two years following onset of psychosis. *Psychiatry Res.* **2017**, *255*, 36–41. [CrossRef]
103. Livne, O.; Shmulewitz, D.; Sarvet, A.; Hasin, D. Association of cannabis use-related predictor variables and self-reported psychotic disorders: US adults, 2001–2002 and 2012–2013. *medRxiv* **2020**. [CrossRef]
104. Yucel, M.; Bora, E.; Lubman, D.I.; Solowij, N.; Brewer, W.J.; Cotton, S.M.; Conus, P.; Takagi, M.J.; Fornito, A.; Wood, S.J.; et al. The impact of cannabis use on cognitive functioning in patients with schizophrenia: A meta-analysis of existing findings and new data in a first-episode sample. *Schizophr. Bull.* **2012**, *38*, 316–330. [CrossRef] [PubMed]
105. Schoeler, T.; Kambeitz, J.; Behlke, I.; Murray, R.; Bhattacharyya, S. The effects of cannabis on memory function in users with and without a psychotic disorder: Findings from a combined meta-analysis. *Psychol. Med.* **2016**, *46*, 177–188. [CrossRef]
106. Worley, M.J.; Trim, R.S.; Roesch, S.C.; Mrnak-Meyer, J.; Tate, S.R.; Brown, S.A. Comorbid depression and substance use disorder: Longitudinal associations between symptoms in a controlled trial. *J. Subst. Abuse Treat.* **2012**, *43*, 291–302. [CrossRef] [PubMed]
107. Sarvet, A.L.; Hasin, D. The natural history of substance use disorders. *Curr. Opin. Psychiatry* **2016**, *29*, 250–257. [CrossRef] [PubMed]
108. Davis, L.; Uezato, A.; Newell, J.M.; Frazier, E. Major depression and comorbid substance use disorders. *Curr. Opin. Psychiatry* **2008**, *21*, 14–18. [CrossRef]
109. Carra, G.; Bartoli, F.; Crocamo, C. Trends of major depressive episode among people with cannabis use: Findings from the National Survey on Drug Use and Health 2006–2015. *Subst. Abuse* **2019**, *40*, 178–184. [CrossRef]
110. Feingold, D.; Rehm, J.; Lev-Ran, S. Cannabis use and the course and outcome of major depressive disorder: A population based longitudinal study. *Psychiatry Res.* **2017**, *251*, 225–234. [CrossRef]
111. American Psychiatric Association. *Diagnostic and Statistical Manual of Mental Disorders*, 5th ed.; American Psychiatric Association: Arlington, VA, USA, 2013.
112. Livne, O.; Shmulewitz, D.; Lev-Ran, S.; Hasin, D.S. DSM-5 cannabis withdrawal syndrome: Demographic and clinical correlates in U.S. adults. *Drug Alcohol. Depend.* **2019**, *195*, 170–177. [CrossRef]
113. Hasin, D.S.; Keyes, K.M.; Alderson, D.; Wang, S.; Aharonovich, E.; Grant, B.F. Cannabis withdrawal in the United States: Results from NESARC. *J. Clin. Psychiatry* **2008**, *69*, 1354–1363. [CrossRef]
114. Cornelius, J.R.; Chung, T.; Martin, C.; Wood, D.S.; Clark, D.B. Cannabis withdrawal is common among treatment-seeking adolescents with cannabis dependence and major depression, and is associated with rapid relapse to dependence. *Addict. Behav.* **2008**, *33*, 1500–1505. [CrossRef] [PubMed]
115. Bahorik, A.L.; Leibowitz, A.; Sterling, S.A.; Travis, A.; Weisner, C.; Satre, D.D. Patterns of marijuana use among psychiatry patients with depression and its impact on recovery. *J. Affect. Disord.* **2017**, *213*, 168–171. [CrossRef] [PubMed]
116. Bahorik, A.L.; Sterling, S.A.; Campbell, C.I.; Weisner, C.; Ramo, D.; Satre, D.D. Medical and non-medical marijuana use in depression: Longitudinal associations with suicidal ideation, everyday functioning, and psychiatry service utilization. *J. Affect. Disord.* **2018**, *241*, 8–14. [CrossRef] [PubMed]

117. Pacek, L.R.; Mauro, P.M.; Martins, S.S. Perceived risk of regular cannabis use in the United States from 2002 to 2012: Difference by sex, age, and race/ethnicity. *Drug Alcohol. Depend.* **2015**, *149*, 232–244. [CrossRef] [PubMed]
118. Gorfinkel, L.R.; Stohl, M.; Hasin, D. Association of Depression With Past-Month Cannabis Use Among US Adults Aged 20 to Years, 2005 to 2016. *JAMA Netw. Open* **2020**, *3*, e2013802. [CrossRef]
119. Smolkina, M.; Morley, K.I.; Rijsdijk, F.; Agrawal, A.; Bergin, J.E.; Nelson, E.C.; Statham, D.; Martin, N.G.; Lynskey, M.T. Cannabis and Depression: A Twin Model Approach to Co-morbidity. *Behav. Genet.* **2017**, *47*, 394–404. [CrossRef]
120. Lev-Ran, S.; Roerecke, M.; le Foll, B.; George, T.P.; McKenzie, K.; Rehm, J. The association between cannabis use and depression: A systematic review and meta-analysis of longitudinal studies. *Psychol. Med.* **2014**, *44*, 797–810. [CrossRef]
121. Lai, H.M.; Sitharthan, T. Exploration of the comorbidity of cannabis use disorders and mental health disorders among inpatients presenting to all hospitals in New South Wales, Australia. *Am. J. Drug Alcohol. Abuse* **2012**, *38*, 567–574. [CrossRef]
122. Crane, N.A.; Langenecker, S.A.; Mermelstein, R.J. Gender differences in the associations among marijuana use, cigarette use, and symptoms of depression during adolescence and young adulthood. *Addict. Behav.* **2015**, *49*, 33–39. [CrossRef]
123. Lev-Ran, S.; le Foll, B.; McKenzie, K.; George, T.P.; Rehm, J. Bipolar disorder and co-occurring cannabis use disorders: Characteristics, co-morbidities and clinical correlates. *Psychiatry Res.* **2013**, *209*, 459–465. [CrossRef]
124. McElroy, S.L.; Altshuler, L.L.; Suppes, T.; Keck, P.E., Jr.; Frye, M.A.; Denicoff, K.D.; Nolen, W.A.; Kupka, R.W.; Leverich, G.; Rochussen, J.R.; et al. Axis I psychiatric comorbidity and its relationship to historical illness variables in 288 patients with bipolar disorder. *Am. J. Psychiatry* **2001**, *158*, 420–426. [CrossRef] [PubMed]
125. Krishnan, K.R. Psychiatric and medical comorbidities of bipolar disorder. *Psychosom. Med.* **2005**, *67*, 1–8. [CrossRef] [PubMed]
126. Pinto, J.V.; Medeiros, L.S.; da Rosa, G.S.; de Oliveira, C.E.S.; Crippa, J.A.S.; Passos, I.C.; Kauer-Sant'Anna, M. The prevalence and clinical correlates of cannabis use and cannabis use disorder among patients with bipolar disorder: A systematic review with meta-analysis and meta-regression. *Neurosci. Biobehav. Rev.* **2019**, *101*, 78–84. [CrossRef] [PubMed]
127. Ostacher, M.J.; Perlis, R.H.; Nierenberg, A.A.; Calabrese, J.; Stange, J.P.; Salloum, I.; Weiss, R.D.; Sachs, G.S.; Investigators, S. Impact of substance use disorders on recovery from episodes of depression in bipolar disorder patients: Prospective data from the Systematic Treatment Enhancement Program for Bipolar Disorder (STEP-BD). *Am. J. Psychiatry* **2010**, *167*, 289–297. [CrossRef]
128. National Institute of Mental Health. Prevalence of Any Anxiety Disorder Among Adults. November 2017. Available online: https://www.nimh.nih.gov/health/statistics/any-anxiety-disorder.shtml. (accessed on 11 August 2020).
129. Hall, W.; Solowij, N. Adverse effects of cannabis. *Lancet* **1998**, *352*, 1611–1616. [CrossRef]
130. Tournier, M.; Sorbara, F.; Gindre, C.; Swendsen, J.D.; Verdoux, H. Cannabis use and anxiety in daily life: A naturalistic investigation in a non-clinical population. *Psychiatry Res.* **2003**, *118*, 1–8. [CrossRef]
131. Sharpe, L.; Sinclair, J.; Kramer, A.; de Manincor, M.; Sarris, J. Cannabis, a cause for anxiety? A critical appraisal of the anxiogenic and anxiolytic properties. *J. Transl. Med.* **2020**, *18*, 374. [CrossRef]
132. Bhattacharyya, S.; Morrison, P.D.; Fusar-Poli, P.; Martin-Santos, R.; Borgwardt, S.; Winton-Brown, T.; Nosarti, C.; O' Carroll, C.M.; Seal, M.; Allen, P.; et al. Opposite effects of delta-9-tetrahydrocannabinol and cannabidiol on human brain function and psychopathology. *Neuropsychopharmacology* **2010**, *35*, 764–774. [CrossRef]
133. Orsolini, L.; Chiappini, S.; Volpe, U.; Berardis, D.; Latini, R.; Papanti, G.D.; Corkery, A.J.M. Use of Medicinal Cannabis and Synthetic Cannabinoids in Post-Traumatic Stress Disorder (PTSD): A Systematic Review. *Medicina* **2019**, *55*, 525. [CrossRef]
134. De Aquino, J.P.; Sofuoglu, M.; Stefanovics, E.A.; Rosenheck, R.A. Impact of cannabis on non-medical opioid use and symptoms of posttraumatic stress disorder: A nationwide longitudinal VA study. *Am. J. Drug Alcohol. Abuse* **2020**, *46*, 1–11. [CrossRef]
135. Hill, M.N.; Campolongo, P.; Yehuda, R.; Patel, S. Integrating Endocannabinoid Signaling and Cannabinoids into the Biology and Treatment of Posttraumatic Stress Disorder. *Neuropsychopharmacology* **2018**, *43*, 80–102. [CrossRef]
136. Metrik, J.; Stevens, A.K.; Gunn, R.L.; Borsari, B.; Jackson, K.M. Cannabis use and posttraumatic stress disorder: Prospective evidence from a longitudinal study of veterans. *Psychol. Med.* **2020**, 1–11. [CrossRef] [PubMed]
137. Buckner, J.D.; Heimberg, R.G.; Schneier, F.R.; Liu, S.M.; Wang, S.; Blanco, C. The relationship between cannabis use disorder and social anxiety disorder in the National Epidemiological Study of Alcohol and Related Conditions (NESARC). *Drug Alcohol. Depend.* **2012**, *124*, 128–134. [CrossRef] [PubMed]
138. Buckner, J.D.; Zvolensky, M.J. Cannabis and related impairment: The unique roles of cannabis use to cope with social anxiety and social avoidance. *Am. J. Addict.* **2014**, *23*, 598–603. [CrossRef] [PubMed]
139. Agosti, V.; Nunes, E.; Levin, F. Rates of psychiatric comorbidity among U.S. residents with lifetime cannabis dependence. *Am. J. Drug Alcohol. Abuse* **2002**, *28*, 643–652. [CrossRef]
140. Wittchen, H.U.; Frohlich, C.; Behrendt, S.; Gunther, A.; Rehm, J.; Zimmermann, P.; Lieb, R.; Perkonigg, A. Cannabis use and cannabis use disorders and their relationship to mental disorders: A 10-year prospective-longitudinal community study in adolescents. *Drug Alcohol. Depend.* **2007**, *88* (Suppl. 1), S60–S70. [CrossRef]
141. Degenhardt, L.; Coffey, C.; Romaniuk, H.; Swift, W.; Carlin, J.B.; Hall, W.D.; Patton, G.C. The persistence of the association between adolescent cannabis use and common mental disorders into young adulthood. *Addiction* **2013**, *108*, 124–133. [CrossRef]
142. Chabrol, H.; Melioli, T.; Goutaudier, N. Association between personality disorders traits and problematic cannabis use in adolescents. *Subst. Use Misuse* **2015**, *50*, 552–556. [CrossRef]
143. Gillespie, N.A.; Aggen, S.H.; Neale, M.C.; Knudsen, G.P.; Krueger, R.F.; South, S.C.; Czajkowski, N.; Nesvag, R.; Ystrom, E.; Kendler, K.S.; et al. Associations between personality disorders and cannabis use and cannabis use disorder: A population-based twin study. *Addiction* **2018**, *113*, 1488–1498. [CrossRef]

144. Raynal, P.; Chabrol, H. Association between schizotypal and borderline personality disorder traits, and cannabis use in young adults. *Addict. Behav.* **2016**, *60*, 144–147. [CrossRef]
145. Vest, N.A.; Murphy, K.T.; Tragesser, S.L. Borderline personality disorder features and drinking, cannabis, and prescription opioid motives: Differential associations across substance and sex. *Addict. Behav.* **2018**, *87*, 46–54. [CrossRef] [PubMed]
146. American Medical Association. The National Practice Guideline for the Use of Medications in the Treatment of Addiction Involving Opioid Use. 2015. Available online: https://newmexico.networkofcare.org/content/client/1446/2.6_17_AsamNationalPracticeGuidelines.pdf (accessed on 10 December 2020).
147. ProCon. *Legal Medical Marijuana States and DC*; Encyclopaedia Britannica: Chicago, IL, USA, 2020.
148. Moon, A.; Prentice, C. High Tech, High Finance and High Times for U.S. Pot Industry. In *Reuters*; Thomson Reuters Corporation: London, UK, 2017.
149. Dsouza, D. The Future of the Marijuana Industry in America. In *Investopedia*; IAC Media Company: New York, NY, USA, 2020.
150. Evans, P. 8 Incredible Facts about the Booming US Marijuana Industry. In *Business Insider*; Insider Inc.: New York, NY, USA, 2019.
151. Center for Responsive Politics. Industry Profile: Marijuana. Available online: https://www.opensecrets.org/federal-lobbying/industries/summary?cycle=2019&id=N09 (accessed on 11 August 2020).
152. Branfalt, T.G. Cannabis Industry Spent $11M on Federal Lobbying in 2019. 2020. Available online: https://www.ganjapreneur.com/cannabis-industry-spent-11m-on-federal-lobbying-in-2019/ (accessed on 11 August 2020).
153. Wen, H.; Hockenberry, J.M.; Cummings, J.R. The effect of medical marijuana laws on adolescent and adult use of marijuana, alcohol, and other substances. *J. Health Econ.* **2015**, *42*, 64–80. [CrossRef] [PubMed]
154. Martins, S.S.; Mauro, C.M.; Santaella-Tenorio, J.; Kim, J.H.; Cerda, M.; Keyes, K.M.; Hasin, D.S.; Galea, S.; Wall, M. State-level medical marijuana laws, marijuana use and perceived availability of marijuana among the general U.S. population. *Drug Alcohol. Depend.* **2016**, *169*, 26–32. [CrossRef] [PubMed]
155. Cerda, M.; Mauro, C.; Hamilton, A.; Levy, N.S.; Santaella-Tenorio, J.; Hasin, D.; Wall, M.M.; Keyes, K.M.; Martins, S.S. Association Between Recreational Marijuana Legalization in the United States and Changes in Marijuana Use and Cannabis Use Disorder From 2008 to 2016. *JAMA Psychiatry* **2020**, *77*, 165–171. [CrossRef] [PubMed]
156. Bonn-Miller, M.O.; Loflin, M.J.E.; Thomas, B.F.; Marcu, J.P.; Hyke, T.; Vandrey, R. Labeling Accuracy of Cannabidiol Extracts Sold Online. *JAMA* **2017**, *318*, 1708–1709. [CrossRef] [PubMed]
157. Loflin, M.J.E.; Kiluk, B.D.; Huestis, M.A.; Aklin, W.M.; Budney, A.J.; Carroll, K.M.; D'Souza, D.C.; Dworkin, R.H.; Gray, K.M.; Hasin, D.S.; et al. The state of clinical outcome assessments for cannabis use disorder clinical trials: A review and research agenda. *Drug Alcohol. Depend.* **2020**, *212*, 107993. [CrossRef]

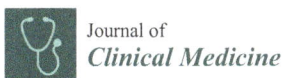

Article

Health-Related Quality of Life in Male Patients under Treatment for Substance Use Disorders with and without Major Depressive Disorder: Influence in Clinical Course at One-Year Follow-Up

Julia E. Marquez-Arrico [1], José Francisco Navarro [2] and Ana Adan [1,3,*]

1. Department of Clinical Psychology and Psychobiology, School of Psychology, University of Barcelona, Passeig de la Vall d'Hebrón 171, 08035 Barcelona, Spain; jmarquez@ub.edu
2. Department of Psychobiology, School of Psychology, University of Málaga, Campus de Teatinos s/n, 29071 Málaga, Spain; navahuma@uma.es
3. Institute of Neurosciences, University of Barcelona, 08035 Barcelona, Spain
* Correspondence: aadan@ub.edu; Tel.: +34-933-125-060

Received: 29 July 2020; Accepted: 23 September 2020; Published: 26 September 2020

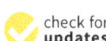

Abstract: Health-related quality of life (HRQoL) assessment has interest as an indicator of degree of affectation and prognosis in mental disorders. HRQoL is impaired in both Substance Use Disorder (SUD) and Major Depressive Disorder (MDD), two conditions highly prevalent, although less studied when both are coexisting (SUD + MDD). Hence, we decided to explore HRQoL with the SF-36 survey in a sample of 123 SUD and 114 SUD + MDD patients (51 symptomatic and 63 asymptomatic of depressive symptoms) under treatment. We performed analyses to examine HRQoL among groups, and its predictive value at 3-, 6- and 12-month follow-ups through regression models. Patients with SUD + MDD had worse HRQoL than SUD patients and population norms. For Mental Health, Vitality, and General Health dimensions, lower scores were observed for SUD + MDD regardless the presence/absence of depressive symptoms. For Physical Functioning and Health Change, depressive symptomatology and not the comorbidity of SUD + MDD diagnoses explained HRQoL limitations. At 3-, 6- and 12-month follow-ups we observed two predictors of relapses, General Health for asymptomatic SUD + MDD, and Physical Functioning for SUD. Improving HRQoL in SUD + MDD may be targeted during patient's treatment; future studies should explore the influence of HRQoL on patient's prognosis taking into account the presence/absence of depressive symptomatology.

Keywords: health-related quality of life; substance use disorder; dual disorders; major depressive disorder; dual depression; relapses

1. Introduction

Health-related quality of life (HRQoL) is one of the constructs with more interest in recent years as an indicator of treatment results in patients with different mental disorders. These include substance use disorder (SUD), severe mental disorders, and comorbidity among them, known as dual disorders [1–3]. Both from the field of research and from clinical practice, different indicators of success of the treatment or recovery of the patient are currently being investigated, beyond the simple reduction of psychiatric symptoms and withdrawal from substance use [4,5]. There are different published studies that explain the relevance of certain variables that function as indicators of the patient's prognosis [6–8], among which is quality of life [8,9]. Undoubtedly, having indicators at the start of treatment that report a poor clinical evolution can be key for adjusting the intervention to the specific needs of each patient [10,11].

The HRQoL is a multidimensional construct of special relevance since it reports the effects that the disorder has on the patient's daily functioning, the degree of involvement generated by the disorder, and the subjective perception of the limitations that they experience in their daily life [12,13]. In this way, the HRQoL study provides important guidance for establishing treatment goals and knowing the degree of functional recovery of the patient beyond the reduction of symptoms, which is always a goal for therapeutic intervention [3,14].

Several studies indicate that patients with dual disorders have a worse HRQoL compared to patients with only one diagnosis [12,15,16]. Comorbidity between an SUD and a mental disorder has been consistently associated with worse quality of life in different domains. However, most of the studies carried out to date are cross-sectional and they have been developed with reduced sample sizes of dual disorder patients without considering the possible effect of the symptomatology from the comorbid mental disorder. It has been found that patients with dual disorders exhibit worse physical functioning and vitality [12,17]; thus, they experience, for example, daily limitations in their physical activities and they tend to be worn-out every day. Dual disorder has been also linked to worse mental health, in some cases with symptoms such as depression, anxiety, nervousness, and frequent insomnia [14,17,18] and to greater limitations in social functioning [14,18,19] as compared with patients who are only diagnosed with SUD. For example, patients may demonstrate problems when they have to attend to social meetings or family reunions due to their health. Therefore, previous studies point out clearly that dual disorders are linked to several limitations that affect patients' daily cognitive and social functioning; however, no study has assessed the specific limitations considering psychiatric diagnosis as a differentiating variable.

If the most prevalent diagnoses of severe mental disorder in patients with dual disorders are considered, it is found that major depressive disorder (MDD) is one of the most frequently diagnosed conditions [19–22]. MDD is also associated with a worse quality of life [23–25]. MDD patients show worse HRQoL compared to the normal population, highlighting their low scores in the domains of social functioning [25–27], vitality, mental health, and emotional role [27–29]. Both the nature of the affective symptoms of MDD and the limitations generated by the disorders, at the cognitive and social levels, are consistently linked to a loss of quality of life [29].

More specifically, if the presence of a comorbid SUD and MDD is analyzed, a special severity is seen in this type of patient. This coexistence of diagnoses is related to more frequent depressive episodes [30] and of greater severity [31], a high risk of suicide [32], a worse prognosis in relation to addiction [33], and significant problems at the socioeconomic level [34]. For all these reasons, the study of the characteristics of patients with dual depression (SUD + MDD) and their HRQoL is of special interest, since it can provide valuable data on their adherence to treatment, prognosis and/or recovery [3,9,35,36]. The exploration of the influence of SUD vs. SUD + MDD on HRQoL is also of great interest due to its theoretical and clinical implications, since it could provide data on which HRQoL dimensions are especially affected by each of these conditions.

One of the most widely used instruments in mental health to study HRQoL is the Ware-Sherbourne SF-36 survey [37]. The SF-36 reports dimensional data for eight primary scales: Physical Functioning, Role-Physical, Role-Emotional, Social Functioning, Mental Health, General Health, Bodily Pain, and Vitality. It also provides a self-perceived item measuring changes in general health over the last year (Health Change item). This instrument has provided significant data when evaluating HRQoL in patients with SUD [38–40], MDD [13,41], as well as with dual pathology [5,42]. It is an instrument that can be used as an indicator of the evolution of the patient with SUD and, in addition, it has been shown to be sensitive to the presence of the diagnosis of MDD, having even suggested that it may be useful as a screening instrument [26,43].

Despite the data regarding HRQoL, which have revealed a negative impact on SUD, MDD, and comorbidity (SUD + MDD), very few studies have analyzed this topic. Most of the studies published to date have focused on the presence of SUD or MDD comorbidly to an organic pathology, but very few studies have used HRQoL in patients with SUD and MDD as the main diagnostic condition, or comorbidity between them. Furthermore, none of those studies have assessed the predictive role of HRQoL throughout the course of patient's treatment for either SUD or MDD. The study of patients with SUD vs. SUD + MDD can extend the knowledge about dual depression and its specific therapeutic needs, as well as informing about possible targeted treatment that consider the patient's subjective perspective and their insights. All these data could provide a subjective complementary perspective to clinicians, which also results in information that could be used to enhance the effectiveness of health care.

Furthermore, these studies use cross-sectional designs and only describe the dimensions of HRQoL without exploring its possible predictive role throughout the course of patient treatment. In the present study, we propose to analyze the differences in HRQoL in a sample of patients with SUD compared to patients with SUD + MDD (we expect to observe poorer HRQoL in patients with SUD + MDD than in SUD). Moreover, we intend to elucidate the possible predictive value of HRQoL at 3, 6, and 12 months of follow-up. In addition, we will explore differences and possible relationships based on the presence/absence of depressive symptoms in patients with SUD and MDD in order to identify their contribution both in the dimensions of quality of life and in the evolution during one year of follow-up. This study aims to provide data that encourage the adoption of an integrated recovery-oriented model that considers wider outcomes than abstinence as the main goal of treatment [1,15,18].

2. Experimental Section

2.1. Participants

A total of 237 voluntary patients were recruited and assigned to two groups according to their clinical diagnoses: SUD (N = 123) and SUD + MDD (N = 114; dual disorder condition). This study was a multicenter research, with participants from different public and private clinical centers specialized in SUD and mental health with inpatient and outpatient programs. Among these centers there were therapeutic communities, addiction treatment units, hospital's mental health units, and community addictions centers, which are mostly addressed to men. The inclusion criteria followed for this study were: (1) male gender (based on the greater prevalence of men in SUD and dual disorder diagnoses, and also due to their larger presence in our clinical centers); (2) aged 19 to 55 years; (3) a current diagnosis of SUD, including those with addiction in early remission according to DSM-5 criteria (abstinence period from 3 to 12 months, without relapses in the last 3 months); (4) a diagnosis of MDD for the dual disorder condition established according to DSM-5 criteria [44]; (5) currently under treatment for their MDD, but in a clinically stable condition. All patients in our sample were in treatment programs for their corresponding diagnoses and had obtained negative results in all their abstinence urine analyses. Patients within the SUD group did not have history of previous MDD. On the other hand, the exclusion criteria followed were: (1) Meeting DSM-5 criteria for a current substance-induced disorder; (2) meeting DSM-5 criteria for any current diagnosis different than SUD or MDD; (3) psychiatric condition due to medical disease; (4) unstable or uncontrolled symptomatology (i.e., withdrawal); (5) inability to complete study interviews or instruments.

2.2. Procedure

In the first place, patients were screened in their respective treatment centers by their treating psychiatrist and/or psychologist who followed the inclusion/exclusion criteria. These patients passed through and extensive assessment and evaluation protocol at the beginning of their treatment (since they are part of a larger study) in each of their centers, which includes discarding substance-induced mood disorders and confirming their diagnosis (in our case the SUD and the MDD). Once the patients agreed to participate, they were provided and signed an informed consent. A post graduate psychologist from our research group assessed the patients individually and also collected the follow up data at 3, 6, and 12 months. For the follow-up a structured 21-item questionnaire was used, specifically designed for our study. The main variables registered during follow-ups were relapses (presence/absence), patients' treatment status ("in treatment," "drop-out" when the patient abandoned treatment against medical advice, and "discharged" when the patient left treatment because it has achieved therapeutic goals and professionals are advising treatment to finish), suicide attempts (yes/no), number of medical appointments attended, and need for medical assistance (yes/no). None of the participants were compensated for their participation and the only benefit they obtained was a report of their results.

The assessment protocol was approved by the Research Committee of the University of Barcelona (IRB00003099) and is part of a wider research project. The present study complies with the tenets of the Declaration of Helsinki.

2.3. Measures

2.3.1. Sociodemographic and Clinical Variables

We designed a structured interview specifically for our study to conduct with each patient in order to assess variables such as age, civil status, years of schooling, social situation, and living arrangements, among others. This interview was also employed to collect data on diagnosis according to DSM-5 criteria, personal/family psychiatric and medical records, history of suicide attempts, and SUD/MDD age of onset. In addition, the structured clinical interview for DSM-IV-TR Axis I Disorders (SCID-I) was administered to collect other clinical variables, such as medication prescribed, hospitalizations, type and number of drugs used, and abstinence period, as well as to confirm patients' diagnoses. The SCID-I for DSM-IV-TR was used since the corresponding Spanish version for the DSM-5 was not available at the time of conducting the present study.

We used the drug abuse screening test (DAST-20) in its Spanish version [45] to obtain a measure of the SUD characteristics in the SUD and SUD + MDD groups. The DAST-20 provides a total severity score ranging from 0 to 20 (1–5 low; 6–10 intermediate; 11–15 substantial; 16–20 severe), with higher scores indicating that a more intensive therapeutic intervention was recommended. Regarding psychiatric symptoms, depressive symptoms in patients with SUD + MDD group were measured with the Spanish version of the 17-item Hamilton depression rating scale [46], its cut-off points being: 0–7, no current depression (asymptomatic condition); 8–13, low; 14–18, mild; 19–22, severe; and >23, very severe depressive symptoms. Following these criteria confirmed by clinical professionals' opinion, patients in the SUD + MDD group were classified in subgroups as asymptomatic (Hamilton from 0 to 7) and symptomatic (Hamilton from 8 up to 23). Moreover, the patient's motivation and social behavior were assessed, as an additional measure of the MDD, with the Social Adaption Self-evaluation Scale (SASS) [47]. The instrument consists of 21 items, with a range from 0 to 60, considering a score of less than 25 as social maladjustment, between 35 and 52 as normal, and those higher than 55 indicating an over-adaptation.

2.3.2. Health-Related Quality of Life

For a measure of HRQoL we used the SF-36 survey in its Spanish version [48]. The SF-36 is a 36-item measure of HRQoL and consists of eight primary components: Physical Functioning (performing all physical daily activities from dressing and bathing to the most vigorous ones and its limitations due to health), Role Physical (reports the existence of problems in working and other daily activities due to health), Role Emotional (reports the existence of problems in working and other daily activities due to emotional problems), Social Functioning (measures the interference with normal social activities due to physical or emotional problems), Mental Health (reports the existence of nervousness and depression), General Health (evaluates personal health and the belief about how it is going to progress in the future), Bodily Pain (measures the existence of severe and extremely limiting pain), and Vitality (refers to the level of feeling tired and worn out all the time). Scores in the SF-36 range from 0 to 100, where a higher score indicates a better HRQoL and lesser limitations. This instrument includes an additional self-perceived item measuring changes in general health over the last year (Health Change item). The questionnaire also provides two secondary composite standardized scales using T scores (with a mean of 50 and standard deviation of 10): the Physical Health Component Summary and the Mental Health Component Summary. There are Spanish normative data for the scores of the primary scales of the SF-36 in the general population [48], which we will use to compare the groups of patients in our study.

2.3.3. Statistical Analysis

Firstly, descriptive statistics (frequencies, means, and standard errors) were obtained for the sociodemographic and clinical variables for the SUD and SUD + MDD groups, as well as for the clinical characteristics of MDD in symptomatic and asymptomatic patients SUD + MDD. The possible differences in such variables among groups were explored by univariate analyses of variance (ANOVA) for continuous data. Nonparametric tests were conducted with Chi-Square statistic calculated according to the type of variable analyzed and the comparison groups.

For exploring HRQoL dimensions, we first performed multivariate analyses of covariance (MANCOVA) introducing the SF-36 dimensions as dependent variables, and the group (SUD and SUD + MDD) as the independent variable, in order to detect differences in HRQoL. We also considered treatment modality and the main substance of dependence as possible interaction factors for HRQoL in these variance analyses. A secondary MANCOVA was performed considering, in this case, the SUD group and two SUD + MDD subgroups depending on their symptomatic or asymptomatic condition. Thus, for this secondary MANCOVA, post-hoc comparisons were adjusted by Bonferroni's correction so as to identify the role of depressive symptoms in HRQoL for the SUD, symptomatic SUD + MDD, and asymptomatic SUD + MDD groups. In all the variance analyses, age was considered as a covariate to control its possible effect, given that our groups differed significantly in this variable, with the SUD + MDD patients being older on average.

The predictive value of HRQoL at 3, 6, and 12 months of follow-ups was explored through logistic regression coefficients and linear regressions depending on the type of variable. Variables were dummy coded (1 = yes/0 = no) in the case of categorical variables such as presence of relapses, treatment status (in treatment, discharged, drop-out), and suicide attempts; the quantity of medical consultations attended was treated as a continuous variable. Logistic regression coefficients and their standard errors were back-transformed to generate odds-ratios (ORs) and their 95% confidence intervals. An attrition analysis was performed so as to explore the possible baseline differences among the participants who completed or abandoned our study for sociodemographic and clinical variables. All statistical analyses were carried out using the SPSS/PC+ statistics package (version 17.0, SPSS Inc., Chicago, IL, USA), and tests were two-tailed with the type I error set at 5%.

3. Results

3.1. Results in Sociodemographic and Clinical Variables

The participants in our sample had a mean age of 39.35 years ($SD = 8.69$), with patients with SUD + MDD being older than patients with SUD ($p < 0.001$). As we can see in Table 1, the patients in the sample were mostly single or divorced/separated, with no significant differences between groups in the marital status variable. Regarding the level of studies, the average years of schooling (10.95 years; $SD = 2.64$) places our sample below the level of secondary education in Spain, without significant differences according to diagnosis. On the other hand, regarding the economic situation, significant differences between groups were observed. While in the SUD + MDD group there is a high percentage of disability pension and, to a lesser extent, unemployment, in the group with SUD the conditions of being working or unemployed as well as without economic income are predominant ($p < 0.001$).

Table 1. Sociodemographic and clinical data for the two groups. Means and standard deviation or percentages, and statistical contrasts.

	SUD + MDD (N = 114)	SUD (N = 123)	Statistical Contrast
Sociodemographic Data			
Age (years)	41.55 ± 8.64	37.32 ± 8.27	$t_{(235)} = 3.83$ ***
Marital status			$\chi^2_{(4)} = 9.77$
Single	46.4%	56.6%	
Stable partner	6.3%	7.4%	
Married	8.9%	13.9%	
Separated/divorced	35.7%	22.2%	
Widower	2.7%	0%	
Years of schooling	11.17 ± 2.84	10.75 ± 2.43	$t_{(235)} = 1.23$
Economic situation			$\chi^2_{(4)} = 30.02$ ***
Active	10.7%	28.7%	
Unemployed	25.9%	28.7%	
Disability pension	44.6%	14.8%	
Sick leave (due SUD treatment)	8.9%	10.7%	
No income	9.8%	17.2%	
Medical and Psychiatric Data			
Medical disease comorbidity [a]	50%	31%	$\chi^2_{(6)} = 14.98$ **
Hypercholesterolemia	9.5%	2.4%	
Respiratory system disease	10.7%	8.2%	
Hepatitis	8.0%	7.4%	
Diabetes	3.6%	1.6%	
Hypertension	6.3%	2.5%	
HIV	4.5%	5.7%	
Other	2.5%	6.3%	
Daily number of medications	2.94 ± 1.63	0.83 ± 1.27	$t_{(235)} = 10.97$ ***
Type of medication prescribed [a]			
Antidepressants	71.0%	18.9%	$\chi^2_{(1)} = 63.93$ ***
Anxiolytics	42.4%	9.8%	$\chi^2_{(1)} = 33.16$ ***
Mood Stabilizers	42.6%	13.9%	$\chi^2_{(1)} = 25.96$ ***
Disulfiram	26.2%	15.2%	$\chi^2_{(1)} = 4.45$
Other	28.7%	13.9%	$\chi^2_{(1)} = 25.78$ ***
History of suicide attempt	46.4%	19.0%	$\chi^2_{(1)} = 21.72$ **
Number of lifetime suicidal attempts	1.06 ± 2.08	0.32 ± 0.77	$t_{(235)} = 3.65$ ***
SUD-Related Data			
Quantity of substance used [a]	2.69 ± 1.48	2.56 ± 1.64	$t_{(235)} = 0.66$
Substance of use [a]			
Alcohol	83.0%	72.1%	$\chi^2_{(1)} = 3.96$
Cocaine	76.8%	86.9%	$\chi^2_{(1)} = 5.27$
Cannabis	42.9%	39.3%	$\chi^2_{(1)} = 0.98$
Hallucinogens	19.6%	18.9%	$\chi^2_{(1)} = 0.23$
Opioids	18.8%	16.4%	$\chi^2_{(1)} = 0.22$
Sedatives	14.3%	6.6%	$\chi^2_{(1)} = 3.78$
DAST-20	13.10 ± 4.40	12.73 ± 3.78	$t_{(235)} = 0.65$
Main substance of dependence			$\chi^2_{(4)} = 7.88$
Alcohol	12.5%	10.4%	
Cocaine	11.5%	12.4%	
Alcohol and cocaine	34.9%	34.4%	
Alcohol and sedatives	2.7%	1.8%	
Polydrug use	38.4%	41.0%	
Mean abstinence period (months)	9.95 ± 5.65	7.52 ± 2.93	$t_{(235)} = 1.40$
Substance use disorder age onset (years)	21.56 ± 9.71	20.63 ± 7.70	$t_{(235)} = 0.81$
Years of substance use disorder	19.10 ± 10.69	15.93 ± 9.32	$t_{(235)} = 2.44$

SUD + MDD: Substance use disorder with comorbid depression; SUD: Substance use disorder; DAST-20: Drug Abuse Screening Test; HDRS: Hamilton Depression Rating Scale; [a] Percentages will not equal 100 as each participant may be in more than one category at the same time; ** $p < 0.01$; *** $p \leq 0.001$.

In relation to clinical characteristics, a greater presence of medical illness and medication use was observed in the SUD + MDD group compared to the SUD group ($p < 0.001$); antidepressants were the drugs most used by both groups. On the other hand, the history of suicide attempts and the number of them was higher in the group with SUD + MDD ($p < 0.001$).

Likewise, regarding the clinical characteristics of the SUD group, no differences were observed between groups in the substance of consumption, the most prevalent being alcohol, cocaine, and cannabis in both groups. Results on the DAST-20 scale indicate that both SUD + MDD and SUD patients have a substantial need for treatment (mean 12.92; SD = 4.09), without significant differences between groups. There were also no differences in the DAST-20 scale considering the presence/absence of depressive symptoms for patients in the SUD + MDD group. The mean of months of abstinence in the total sample was 8.73 months (SD = 3.40) without significant differences between diagnostic groups. There were also no differences between groups in the variable age of onset of SUD, nor in the years of its duration.

Regarding depressive psychiatric symptoms (see Table 2), the SUD + MDD group was subdivided according to the score on the Hamilton scale in asymptomatic (scores ≤ 7; N = 63; 44.7%) and symptomatic patients (scores ≥ 8; N = 51; 55.3%). The consideration of the presence of symptoms did not provide significant differences either in the age of onset of depression or in the years of its duration. Likewise, the data on the SASS scale of social adaptation did not show differences between asymptomatic and symptomatic SUD + MDD patients, and in both cases the scores were in the normal range.

Table 2. Clinical measures (means and standard deviation) for de dual disorder group with Substance Use Disorder and Major Depressive Disorder according to the presence/absence of depressive symptoms.

	Symptomatic SUD + MDD (N = 51)	Asymptomatic SUD + MDD (N = 63)	Statistical Contrast
Major depressive disorder age onset (years)	28.65 ± 9.35	30.16 ±8.78	$t = 0.865$
Years of major depressive disorder	13.96 ±9.46	10.50 ± 7.93	$t = -2.60$
Hamilton Depression Rating Scale	12.39 ± 4.78	4.03 ± 3.08	$t = -7.48$ ***
Social Adaption Self-evaluation Scale	34.80 ± 8.21	38.43 ± 7.51	$t = -1.45$

SUD + MDD: Substance use disorder with comorbid depression. *** $p < 0.001$.

3.2. Results in Health-Related Quality of Life for the SUD and SUD + MDD Groups

The analysis between groups considering the presence/absence of comorbid MDD (SUD + MDD vs. SUD groups) is presented in Table 3. Significant differences were observed in the dimensions of Physical Functioning ($p = 0.036$), Social Functioning ($p = 0.022$), Role Emotional ($p = 0.012$), Mental Health ($p < 0.001$), Vitality ($p = 0.001$), and General Health ($p < 0.001$), as well as for the Health Change item ($p = 0.001$). In all cases, the SUD + MDD group exhibited lower scores compared to the SUD group. Treatment modality (the highest contrast for the Vitality dimension: $F_{(2,235)} = 1.795$; $p = 0.636$; $\eta p^2 = 0.005$) and the main substance of dependence (the highest contrast for Mental Health dimension: $F_{(2,235)} = 2.471$; $p = 0.520$; $\eta p^2 = 0.008$) did not provide significant results either for the main effects for HRQoL or in the interaction between groups.

The analysis of the differences among the groups considering the presence/absence of depressive symptoms in the SUD + MDD group (symptomatic vs. asymptomatic subgroups, see Table 4), indicated that the lowest scores in the Physical Functioning and Health Change dimensions observed in the SUD + MDD group were explained by those symptomatic patients ($p < 0.001$ in all cases), since the scores of the asymptomatic SUD + MDD patients did not differ from those of the SUD group. On the other hand, in the Mental Health, Vitality, and General Health dimensions, the lowest scores of patients with SUD + MDD compared to the SUD group were observed regardless of the presence/absence of depressive symptoms ($p < 0.001$ in all cases). In this second analysis, the differences in the Social Functioning and Role Emotional dimensions obtained by not considering the depressive symptoms in SUD + MDD have disappeared.

Table 3. Health-related quality of life results according to the diagnosis. First multivariate analyses of covariance (MANCOVA) analysis with descriptive statistics (mean and standard error), normative data, F, and eta square (ηp^2) tests.

SF-36 Dimensions	SUD + MDD (N = 114)	SUD (N = 123)	$F_{(2,235)}$	ηp^2
Physical Functioning	88.34 ± 1.35	92.36 ± 1.30	4.443 *	0.019
Social Functioning	70.50 ± 2.50	78.65 ± 2.40	5.334 *	0.022
Role Physical	77.42 ± 3.25	77.20 ± 3.12	0.002	0.001
Role Emotional	53.07 ± 3.72	66.39 ± 3.57	6.471 *	0.027
Mental Health	52.29 ± 1.59	65.65 ± 1.53	35.458 ***	0.133
Vitality	50.36 ± 1.73	66.61 ± 1.66	44.550 ***	0.161
Bodily Pain	72.34 ± 2.53	76.68 ± 2.44	1.479	0.006
General Health	62.84 ± 1.75	73.42 ± 1.68	18.436 ***	0.074
Health Change item	77.50 ± 2.21	90.64 ± 2.12	17.849 ***	0.071
Physical Composite Scale	60.19 ± 1.54	61.39 ± 1.48	0.305	0.001
Mental Composite Scale	42.71 ± 1.63	51.60 ± 1.56	14.961 ***	0.061

SF-36: The Short Form Health Survey; SUD + MDD: Substance Use Disorder with comorbid Major Depression Disorder; SUD: Substance Use Disorder; * $p < 0.05$; *** $p \leq 0.001$.

Regarding the composite scales, the comparison between the SUD + MDD and SUD groups indicates differences only in the Mental Health Component scale ($p < 0.001$), with the SUD + MDD group having the lowest score (see Table 3). The difference in Mental Health Component is observed regardless of the presence/absence of depressive symptoms for patients in the SUD + MDD group (see Table 4).

3.3. Population Values in the SF-36 and Scores Obtained in the SUD and SUD + MDD Groups

The comparison of the scores of our patients with respect to the population data (see Figure 1), allows us to add that both groups (SUD and SUD + MDD) present scores below the expected average in the dimensions of Role Physical, Role Emotional Mental Health, Vitality, and Bodily Pain of SF-36, although the impact is greater in the SUD + MDD group. Furthermore, both in the SUD group and in the SUD + MDD group, the values are similar to those of the general population in Physical Functioning. Considering the scales of Social Functioning and General Health of HRQoL, the SUD group shows adequate values, while in the case of the SUD + MDD group these are lower.

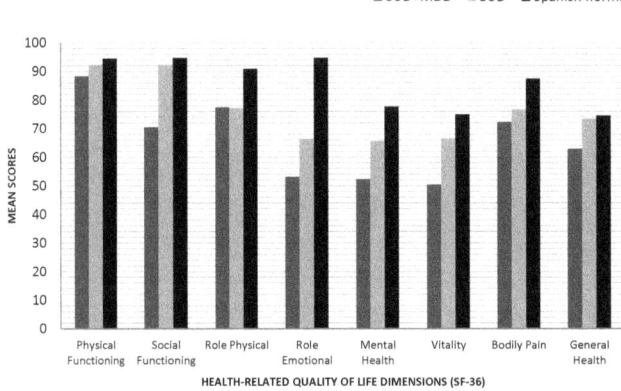

Figure 1. Mean scores in health-related quality of life dimensions (SF-36) according to the diagnosis, comparison with Spanish normative data from healthy individuals. SF-36: The Short Form Health Survey; SUD + MDD: Substance Use Disorder with comorbid Major Depression Disorder; SUD: Substance Use Disorder.

Table 4. Health-related quality of life results according to the diagnosis and presence/absence of depressive symptoms. Second MANCOA analysis with descriptive statistics (mean and standard error), normative data, F, and eta square (ηp^2) tests.

SF-36 Dimensions	SUD + MDD Symptomatic (N = 51)	SUD + MDD Asymptomatic (N = 63)	SUD (N = 123)	F	ηp^2	Contrasts
Physical Functioning	83.42 ± 1.98	92.02 ± 1.77	92.36 ± 1.30	7.230 ***	0.059	SUD and SUD + MDD asymptomatic > SUD + MDD symptomatic
Social Functioning	70.41 ± 3.74	70.58 ± 3.35	78.65 ± 2.40	2.656	0.022	
Role Physical	71.60 ± 4.81	82.07 ± 4.31	77.20 ± 3.12	1.331	0.011	
Role Emotional	52.18 ± 5.55	53.78 ± 4.97	66.39 ± 3.57	3.246	0.027	
Mental Health	49.03 ± 2.36	54.90 ± 2.11	65.65 ± 1.53	19.662 ***	0.145	SUD > SUD + MDD symptomatic/asymptomatic
Vitality	48.42 ± 2.57	51.91 ± 2.30	66.61 ± 1.66	22.800 ***	0.165	SUD > SUD + MDD symptomatic/asymptomatic
Bodily Pain	68.63 ± 3.77	75.30 ± 3.37	76.68 ± 2.44	1.625	0.014	
General Health	62.86 ± 2.61	62.83 ± 2.34	73.42 ± 1.68	9.178 ***	0.074	SUD > SUD + MDD symptomatic/asymptomatic
Health Change item	83.78 ± 3.25	72.49 ± 2.91	77.50 ± 2.21	12.547 ***	0.098	SUD and SUD + MDD asymptomatic > SUD + MDD symptomatic
Physical Composite Scale	59.37 ± 2.30	60.84 ± 2.06	61.40 ± 1.48	0.26	0.002	
Mental Composite Scale	42.77 ± 2.43	42.67 ± 2.18	51.60 ± 1.57	7.449 ***	0.176	SUD > SUD + MDD symptomatic/asymptomatic

SF-36: The Short Form Health Survey; SUD + MDD: Substance Use Disorder with comorbid Major Depression Disorder; SUD: Substance Use Disorder; *** $p \leq 0.001$.

The HRQoL analysis, evaluating the presence/absence of depressive symptoms in the SUD + MDD group (see Figure 2), allows us to clarify that symptomatic patients obtain the lowest scores in Physical Functioning, Role Physical, Mental Health, Vitality, and Bodily Pain compared to population data. Finally, in the case of the Social Functioning dimension, SUD + MDD patients, both symptomatic and asymptomatic, show lower scores compared to normative data.

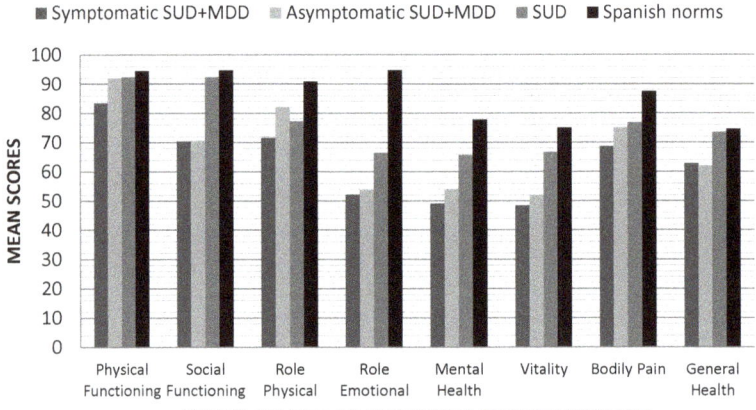

Figure 2. Mean scores in health-related quality of life dimensions (SF-36) according to the diagnosis and considering the presence of depressive symptomatology in dual depressed patients compared with the Spanish normative data in healthy individuals. SF-36: The Short Form Health Survey; SUD + MDD: Substance Use Disorder with comorbid Major Depression Disorder; SUD: Substance Use Disorder.

3.4. Predictive Value of Health-Related Quality of Life Dimensions at 3, 6, and 12 Months of Follow-Up

At 3 months of follow-up, we observed that some dimensions of the SF-36 have a predictive value for both the SUD and the asymptomatic SUD + MDD groups (see Table 5). The asymptomatic patients with SUD + MDD who were still on treatment were those with lower scores on Emotional Role ($p = 0.008$). The presence of relapses as early as three months is associated in SUD patients with a lower score in Physical Functioning ($p = 0.009$) and in asymptomatic patients with SUD + MDD with high scores in General Health dimension ($p = 0.026$). Furthermore, the score in the Vitality dimension was negatively linked to the number of medical consultations in asymptomatic SUD + MDD ($p = 0.001$) and with the need for medical care in the SUD group ($p = 0.033$). Finally, at three months of follow-up, no quality of life dimension provided significant relationships with the variables studied for symptomatic patients in the SUD + MDD group.

As shown in Table 5, at 6 months of follow-up we observed that high scores in the Bodily Pain dimension were related to having been discharged from the treatment in patients with SUD ($p = 0.023$); thus, the patients with the highest scores received the highest number of medical discharges. On the one hand, high scores in Vitality were related to being under treatment in symptomatic patients with SUD + MDD ($p = 0.023$), while lower scores were related to the need for medical care in SUD patients ($p = 0.008$). On the other hand, the lower the Physical Functioning score the more frequent was the presence of relapses in the SUD group ($p = 0.034$); and the lower the General Health score, the greater the number of medical visits required by patients in the asymptomatic group with SUD + MDD ($p < 0.001$).

Finally, at 12 months of follow-up (see Table 5), the Emotional Role dimension was associated with having been discharged from the treatment in patients with SUD ($p = 0.025$), while the high scores in the Vitality dimension were linked with continuing treatment in symptomatic patients with SUD + MDD ($p = 0.015$). Likewise, the lower the score in the Bodily Pain dimension, the more frequent was the dropping-out treatment for patients in the symptomatic SUD + MDD group ($p = 0.012$). On the other hand, low scores in Physical Functioning were linked to the presence of relapses in the SUD group ($p = 0.038$). In patients of the asymptomatic SUD + MDD group, high General Health scores were associated with the presence of relapses ($p = 0.010$) and with a lower need for medical consultations ($p = 0.002$).

Table 5. Results from the logistic and linear regression models for health-related quality of life dimensions and follow-up data at 3, 6, and 12 months for the groups.

SF-36 Dimensions	Follow-Up Data Variables at 3 Months	SUD + MDD Symptomatic (N = 51)	SUD + MDD Asymptomatic (N = 63)	SUD (N = 123)
Role Emotional	Being at treatment		OR = 0.979 * β = −0.022	
Physical Functioning	Relapses			OR = 0.957 ** β = −0.044
General Health	Relapses		OR = 1.028 * β = 0.028	
Vitality	Quantity of medical consultations		R^2 = 0.261 *** β = −0.527	
Vitality	Need for medical assistance			OR = 0.949 * β = −0.052
	Follow-up Data Variables at 6 Months	SUD + MDD Symptomatic (N = 51)	SUD + MDD Asymptomatic (N = 63)	SUD (N = 123)
Bodily Pain	Discharge from treatment			OR = 1.023 * β = 0.022
Vitality	Being in treatment	OR = 1.046 * β = 0.045		
Physical Functioning	Relapses			OR = 0.965 * β = −0.036
General Health	Quantity of medical consultations		R^2 = 0.304 *** β = −0.570	
Vitality	Need for medical assistance			OR = 0.915 ** β = −0.089
	Follow-up Data Variables at 12 Months	SUD + MDD Symptomatic (N = 40)	SUD + MDD Asymptomatic (N = 45)	SUD (N = 87)
Role Emotional	Discharge from treatment			OR = 1.014 * β = 0.014
Vitality	Being in treatment	OR = 1.064 * β = 0.062		
Bodily Pain	Drop-out treatment	OR = 0.959 ** β = −0.042		
Physical Functioning	Relapses			OR = 0.958 * β = −0.042
General Health	Relapses		OR = 1.035** β = 0.035	
General Health	Quantity of medical consultations		R^2 = 0.262** β = −0.535	

SF-36: The Short Form Health Survey; SUD + MDD: Substance Use Disorder with comorbid Major Depression Disorder; SUD: Substance Use Disorder; * $p \leq 0.05$; ** $p < 0.01$; *** $p < 0.001$.

In all follow-up analyses (3, 6, and 12 months), treatment modality and the main substance of dependence did not work as interaction factors for none of the groups ($p > 0.752$ for ORs and $p > 0.358$ for lineral regressions).

Regarding follow-up data, we observed that no subject was lost from our study at 3 and 6 months of follow-ups, but at 12 months follow-up 65 patients were missed (29 with SUD + MDD and 36 with SUD). We did not find any significant differences between those subjects who completed the study nor for those who were in treatment and those who drop-out/were discharged ($p > 0.274$) (see Tables 6 and 7).

Table 6. Attrition analysis for sociodemographic and clinical variables between patients who had/did not had follow-up data at 12-months. Means and standard deviation or percentages, and statistical contrasts.

	With 12-Months Follow-Up Baseline Data (N = 172)	Without 12-Months Follow-Up Baseline Data (N = 65)	Statistical Contrasts
Sociodemographic Data			
Age (years)	39.55 ± 8.69	38.00 ± 8.74	$t_{(235)} = 0.91$
Marital status			$\chi^2_{(4)} = 8.44$
Single	57%	56%	
Stable partner	7.4%	6.3%	
Married	12.3%	13.7%	
Separated/divorced	21.8%	24.0%	
Widower	1.5%	0%	
Years of schooling	10.92 ± 2.59	11.13 ± 2.95	$t_{(235)} = -0.41$
Economic situation			$\chi^2_{(4)} = 6.69$
Active	21.6%	23.3%	
Unemployed	25.0%	27.0%	
Disability pension	29.4%	26.7%	
Sick leave (due SUD treatment)	9.3%	13.3	
No income	14.7%	9.7%	
Medical and Psychiatric Data			
Medical disease comorbidity [a]	33.3%	30.1%	$\chi^2_{(6)} = 6.18$
Hypercholesterolemia	3.4%	2.3%	
Respiratory system disease	10.5%	8.8%	
Hepatitis	8.4%	10.0%	
Diabetes	2.9%	1.9%	
Hypertension	4.9%	6.3%	
HIV	4.9%	6.7%	
Other	11.3%	14.2%	
Daily number of medications	1.90 ± 1.84	1.21 ± 1.29	$t_{(235)} = 10.97$ ***
Type of medication prescribed [a]			
Antidepressants	43.7%	39.3%	$\chi^2_{(1)} = 1.78$
Anxiolytics	26.6%	23.9%	$\chi^2_{(1)} = 1.26$
Mood Stabilizers	12.9%	10.7%	$\chi^2_{(1)} = 5.66$
Disulfiram	10.2%	12.5%	$\chi^2_{(1)} = 0.99$
Other	13.5%	14.8%	$\chi^2_{(1)} = 1.69$
History of suicide attempt	32.0%	33.3%	$\chi^2_{(1)} = 2.91$
Number of lifetime suicidal attempts	0.68 ± 1.65	0.63 ± 1.00	$t_{(235)} = 0.165$
SUD Related Data			
Quantity of substance used [a]	2.58 ± 1.55	2.90 ± 1.78	$t_{(235)} = -1.04$
Substance of use [a]			
Alcohol	80.3%	83.7%	$\chi^2_{(1)} = 3.14$
Cocaine	82.4%	80%	$\chi^2_{(1)} = 5.98$
Cannabis	40.1%	43.3%	$\chi^2_{(1)} = 0.76$
Hallucinogens	19.6%	16.7%	$\chi^2_{(1)} = 0.14$
Opioids	17.9%	18.1%	$\chi^2_{(1)} = 0.41$
Sedatives	5.6%	8.3%	$\chi^2_{(1)} = 4.39$
DAST-20	13.59 ± 4.16	14.48 ± 3.43	$t_{(235)} = 1.20$
Main substance of dependence			
Alcohol	10.3%	8.7%	
Cocaine	10.8%	9.3%	
Alcohol and cocaine	29.7%	33.3%	
Alcohol and sedatives	1.5%	2.3%	
Polydrug use	39.7%	40.0%	
Mean abstinence period (months)	8.67 ± 4.41	7.20 ± 4.03	$t_{(235)} = 0.68$

Table 6. Cont.

	With 12-Months Follow-Up Baseline Data (N = 172)	Without 12-Months Follow-Up Baseline Data (N = 65)	Statistical Contrasts
Substance use disorder age onset (years)	21.45 ± 9.02	18.53 ± 6.08	$t_{(235)} = 1.71$
Years of substance use disorder	17.34 ± 10.16	18.26 ± 9.93	$t_{(235)} = -0.47$

SUD + MDD: Substance use disorder with comorbid depression; SUD: Substance use disorder; DAST-20: Drug Screening Test; HDRS: Hamilton Depression Rating Scale; [a] Percentages will not equal 100 as each participant may be in more than one category at the same time.

Table 7. Clinical measures (means and standard deviation) for de dual disorder group with Substance Use Disorder and Major Depressive Disorder with/without follow-up data at 12 months.

	SUD + MDD with 12-Months Follow-Up Baseline Data (N = 85)	SUD + MDD without 12-Months Follow-Up Baseline Data (N = 29)	Statistical Contrasts
Major depressive disorder age onset (years)	29.77 ± 9.23	27.71 ± 7.99	$t = 0.86$
Years of major depressive disorder	12.39 ± 8.70	10.82 ± 9.59	$t = 0.69$
Hamilton Depression Rating Scale	9.72 ± 5.80	10.50 ± 5.82	$t = -0.47$
Social Adaption Self-evaluation Scale	35.56 ± 7.19	36.30 ± 10.87	$t = -0.286$

SUD + MDD: Substance use disorder with comorbid depression.

4. Discussion

In this study we aimed to analyze the differences in HRQoL between two groups with SUD considering the presence/absence of a MDD comorbid diagnosis, as well as its relationship with follow-up data during 12 months. Our main findings point out that patients with SUD + MDD have more limitations in their quality of life due to health than patients with SUD and no comorbidity. Therefore, dual depressed patients have poorer Physical Functioning, Social Functioning, Mental Health, and General Health; they also experience fewer positive health changes in the last 12 months (Health Change Item). When the presence of depressive symptoms was controlled for patients with SUD + MDD we observed that these were only relevant for the limitations in Physical Functioning and Health Change Item; depressive symptoms were not explaining the majority of the primary outcomes observed whereas the comorbidity of SUD + MDD itself did. The different dimensions of the SF-36 seem to have a greater predictive value for asymptomatic SUD + MDD and SUD patients than for symptomatic SUD + MDD patients.

The results obtained at the sociodemographic level indicate that our sample is similar to that described in previous studies carried out in patients with a dual disorder [15,17], with patients in the group with dual depression being mostly pensioners due to illness, while patients who did not show psychiatric comorbidity were either working or on sick leave due to the SUD. Regarding the clinical characteristics linked to the SUD, we highlight that the main substances of use are in line with the previous data [5,16], with alcohol, cocaine, and cannabis being the most prevalent in both groups. Furthermore, the age of onset of SUD in dual depressive patients was earlier than the age of diagnosis of depression, and alcohol was the most prevalent substance in this group. All this points to the possibility that the addictive disorder may have relevance in the development of depressive mental pathology, being consistent with research that has documented the relationship between alcohol dependence and the development of depression [4,49].

In relation to the results in HRQoL considering comorbidity and the presence/absence of depressive symptoms, it should be noted that dual depressive patients with symptoms are those who report worse Physical Functioning and, therefore, have more limitations in their daily life, for example with walking, making physical efforts, climbing stairs, and carrying groceries. This observation is similar to that of published data [28] and suggests that depressive symptoms are related to physical limitations in the development of the patient's daily life. The main clinical implication of this finding is that SUD + MDD patients, who are very frequently encouraged to increase their daily activity levels (using an evidenced-based therapeutic approach), may need more time for their progressive behavioral activation considering their physical limitations. Likewise, when we compare the groups with population values, it is observed that the presence of depressive symptoms is the differential aspect in this quality of life dimension, since dual asymptomatic depressive patients and SUD show scores very similar to those of the normative data. Based on the results of our study (the first one to address the impact of depressive symptoms in HRQoL of dual depression) it is worth noting the need for therapeutic approaches to improve physical functioning, especially for symptomatic patients with SUD + MDD.

On the other hand, in line with previous findings [26], we found that SUD + MDD comorbidity was linked to a worse quality of life as a result of Mental Health, regardless of whether the patient was symptomatic or asymptomatic. The comorbidity between depression and SUD is related to limitations in the patient's daily life as a result of nervousness, insomnia, and low mood, without the need to experience depressive symptoms at that time. Although the SUD group also reported worse Mental Health compared to population data, it was the SUD + MDD group that showed the greatest limitations in this dimension of HRQoL. Therefore, regardless of the mood of the patient with SUD + MDD at the time the treatment is being carried out, it is a type of patient with whom it would be necessary to use specific techniques aimed at managing anxious and affective symptoms. A clinical implication of this finding is that the SF-36 and its Mental Health dimension seems to be sensitive to the existence of a MDD and it might be used as a screening instrument in addiction's treatment centers; this observation also adds evidence to previous findings [26,43] about HRQoL as an indicator of mood disorders.

The dual disorder group was the one that showed a lower energy level, more tiredness and exhaustion (Vitality dimension), not being explained by the presence of active symptoms of the MDD. This observation is consistent with previous work [25,29] and, although the SUD group also presented worse Vitality, regarding the normative data, poorer quality of life resulting from a low Vitality was especially linked to SUD + MDD comorbidity. Thus, it may be important to include strategies in treatment programs that help SUD patients to increase their energy levels (such as physical exercise, outdoor activities) [50,51], and this seems especially necessary with SUD + MDD patients. Moreover, as dual depressed patients present insomnia very frequently (according to the Mental Health dimension), they could specially benefit from strategies focused on improving their sleep quality, prioritizing a behavioral approach, but the consideration of a pharmacological treatment is also necessary. All these actions could result in better wakefulness and circadian rhythm adjustment [50]. In addition, the results in the General Health dimension indicated a worse perception by patients with SUD + MDD, not being related to whether they were symptomatic or asymptomatic, as compared to SUD patients and the population mean. Therefore, the existence of the diagnosis of depression comorbid to the SUD is linked to a perception of the patient that they can become ill easily, or that their health is going to worsen, and the emotional affective state of the moment would not be modulating this perception. An approach with cognitive-behavioral techniques in the context of a comprehensive treatment of SUD + MDD patients developing positive thoughts regarding their General Health could be very beneficial. Thus, treatment could be especially focused on cognitive-restructuring and cognitive therapy so as to adjust patients' perception to their actual mood symptoms and clinical evolution.

Finally, we found that the perception of the Health Change experienced in the last year was higher in patients with SUD and asymptomatic patients SUD + MDD, compared to symptomatic SUD + MDD. This observation is consistent with previous findings that directly related the reduction of depressive symptoms during treatment with a significant improvement in HRQoL [52]. Our data add evidence to the need of integrated treatments models for dual depressed patients addressed to improve patient's mood and their affective symptoms, instead of treatments that especially aim to achieve abstinence and prevent relapses. Future studies should further explore the specific influence of depressive symptoms on the recovery of the patient with dual disorder. In sum, our results confirm previous observations regarding the complications presented by patients with dual disorders as a diagnostic entity [1,12,14] and provide evidence regarding the need for a global therapeutic approach for patients with dual depression, beyond the mere approach to the typical affective symptoms of MDD.

Predictive Value of HRQoL Dimensions

Regarding the predictive value of the HRQoL dimensions, we observed that different dimensions are related to different variables at the follow-up points. It seems that the different aspects of HRQoL have a diverse role at prognosis and this role is not so consistent for symptomatic patients SUD + MDD patients. At 3 months of follow-up, we highlight that no dimension was shown to be related to the evolution of symptomatic SUD + MDD patients. However, in asymptomatic MDD patients, we observed that the greater the problems generated by the emotional state (Role Emotional), the greater the probability that the patient was continuing under treatment; in this case, experiencing daily difficulties resulting from emotional state was associated with therapeutic adherence. Future studies may explore if these patients could be experiencing an important emotional support from their therapeutic teams which helps bonding them and keeps them on track with treatment. Relapses at 3 months were related to two different quality of life dimensions depending on whether the patient was asymptomatic SUD + MDD or a patient with SUD. Thus, in patients with SUD, worse physical function (limitations in daily physical activities) was associated with a greater probability of having relapses throughout the year of follow-up (3, 6, and 12 months); these data are in agreement with published studies that associate the use of maladaptive coping strategies with a higher probability of relapse in patients with dual disorders [6,51]. Future studies should deepen this relationship and investigate whether the presence of physical problems in SUD reduces the patient's motivation to maintain abstinence or whether consumption works as a strategy to cope with these daily limitations. On the other hand, in asymptomatic patients with SUD + MDD, better General Health is associated with a greater presence of relapses. This finding points to the study of the role that the perception of a better general health state plays in the non-compliance with the treatment guidelines and in the possible exposure to risk situations that induce relapses. Therefore, asymptomatic SUD + MDD patients under treatment and better General Health from the SF-36 may be considered as higher risk to relapse patients; emphasizing relapse prevention strategies with them could be especially relevant.

At 6 months of evolution of the patient under treatment for the SUD, it should be noted that a lower presence of Bodily Pain symptoms increased the probability of being discharged from the treatment in those diagnosed with SUD. Thus, it was more probable for patients with SUD and no pain or no limitations due to pain to achieve therapeutic goals significantly so as to be discharged from their treatment center. In contrast, no HRQoL dimension showed predictive value with discharge from treatment in patients with SUD + MDD. The Vitality dimension exhibited different relationships with the evolution of the patient according to his diagnosis. Thus, symptomatic SUD + MDD patients who experienced greater Vitality had a greater probability of continuing treatment at the 6-month follow-up. Future studies should deepen into whether the fact of feeling more energetic and less tired represents a factor in favor of motivation for change or therapeutic adherence. In patients with SUD, greater tiredness and exhaustion (lower vitality) was associated with a greater frequency of needing medical assistance at 6 months of follow-up. Therefore, our data add support to previous works [4,12–14] and shows the need of future studies that explore if a higher need of medical services in SUD patients is related to dysphoric feelings, such as tiredness, or whether it is due to other health-associated variables. The improvement of this quality of life dimension in patients with SUD may be a key aspect in order to reduce the patient's need to require medical care resources different from those already received for the addictive disorder and may promote the reincorporation to the working world.

At 12 months of follow-up, we observed that the lower the limitations caused by their emotional state (greater Role Emotional) in patients with SUD, the greater the probability that they had been discharged from the treatment. In other words, patients with SUD and without problems at work or other daily activities as a result of emotional problems have a good prognosis as they were more likely to achieve treatment goals as to be discharged. Hence, specific interventions to improve the emotional state of the SUD patient could benefit the success of the treatment. On the other hand, in symptomatic patients with SUD + MDD, it was observed that having a higher energy level (greater Vitality) increased the probability that they were still receiving treatment for SUD at one year of follow-up, while the experience of limitations as a result of physical pain (minor Bodily Pain) increased the probability of treatment discontinuation (drop-out). In the latter case, future research could assess the influence of physical pain on the motivation of the symptomatic patient with SUD + MDD to stay adhered to the treatment for SUD. Finally, we also observed at one year of follow-up in asymptomatic patients with SUD + MDD that the probability of relapse increased as the state of General Health was better, while in SUD patients we again found that the greater the physical limitations in daily functioning (Physical Functioning) the higher the probability of relapse. In this way, it is observed that the different dimensions in HRQoL point to possible lines of therapeutic intervention in patients with SUD and, taking into account the psychiatric comorbidity with MDD, they contribute aspects of great clinical interest for the future based on the presence/absence of depressive symptoms.

The present study has several strengths and some possible limitations. We highlight as a strong point that this is the first work that analyzes HRQoL in a sample of patients with SUD + MDD, evaluating their symptomatic or asymptomatic depressive state, and comparing them with a group of patients with only SUD diagnosis, as well as with population data. In addition, other strong points of our study are that we have explored the predictive role of the different dimensions of HRQoL at 3, 6, and 12 months of follow-ups and provided data with clinical utility for the management of the patient under treatment for SUD. As possible limitations, we can point out that our sample is made up of only men, thus limiting the generalization of results to male patients in treatment for SUD. The data on the dimensions of HRQoL come from a self-reported questionnaire, thus being subjective data resulting from the individual perception of each patient. Future studies should overcome these limitations and confirm our findings with complementary objective measurements that increase knowledge at both theoretical and applied levels.

5. Conclusions

Patients with SUD + MDD comorbidity show a worse HRQoL as compared to patients with SUD and existing population data. In the Mental Health, Vitality, and General Health dimensions, the worst quality of life is observed regardless of whether the patient with SUD + MDD is symptomatic or asymptomatic, while in the Physical Functioning dimension, as well as in the Health Change dimension, it is the presence of depressive symptoms that seems to explain the worse quality of life and not the psychiatric comorbidity. The analysis of the HRQoL dimensions must consider whether the patient with SUD + MDD is symptomatic/asymptomatic for a better interpretation of the results and their integration in the treatment.

In relation to the possible influence of HRQoL on the evolution of the patient at 3, 6, and 12 months of follow-up, a differential analysis is also essential, considering the depressive psychiatric comorbidity and the symptomatic/asymptomatic affective state of the patient. Thus, we did not observe relapse predictors in patients with symptomatic SUD + MDD in any of the follow-ups, while we found predictive value in all measurements throughout the year of follow-up (3, 6, and 12 months) for relapses, in General Health for asymptomatic patients with SUD + MDD and in Physical Functioning for SUD. The different dimensions of the SF-36 seem to have a greater predictive value for asymptomatic SUD + MDD and SUD patients than for symptomatic SUD + MDD patients. Future studies should deepen this line of research, as well as assess the influence of specific interventions aimed at improving the different dimensions of HRQoL in patients under treatment for SUD, with and without depressive comorbidity.

Author Contributions: Conceptualization, A.A.; methodology, A.A. and J.F.N.; formal analysis, J.E.M.-A. and A.A.; investigation, J.E.M.-A. and A.A.; funding acquisition, A.A.; writing—original draft preparation, all authors.; writing—review and editing, all authors. All authors have read and agreed to the published version of the manuscript.

Funding: This research was funded by the Spanish Ministry of Economy, Industry and Competitiveness (PSI2015-65026-MINECO/FEDER/UE), the Generalitat de Catalunya (2017SGR-748), and the Spanish Ministry of Economy and Business (PSI2017-90806-REDT).

Acknowledgments: We thank the Gressol Man Project Foundation in Catalonia, ATRA group, Mental Health of Vall Hebron Hospital, Addiction's Division of the Maresme Health Consortium, Sin Consumir, Dianova Association Spain, Ayuda a los Toxicómanos Association (A.A.T.), and the Centro de Higiene Mental Les Corts Association for providing the sample of the study.

Conflicts of Interest: The authors declare no conflict of interest.

References

1. Juel, A.; Kristiansen, C.B.; Madsen, N.J.; Munk-Jørgensen, P.; Hjorth, P. Interventions to improve lifestyle and quality-of-life in patients with concurrent mental illness and substance use. *Nord. J. Psychiatry* **2016**, *41*, 1–8.
2. Abdel-Baki, A.; Ouellet-Plamondon, C.; Salvat, É.; Grar, K.; Potvin, S. Symptomatic and functional outcomes of substance use disorder persistence 2 years after admission to a first-episode psychosis program. *Psychiatry Res.* **2017**, *247*, 113–119. [CrossRef] [PubMed]
3. Worley, J. Recovery in substance use disorders: What to know to inform practice. *Issues Ment. Health Nurs.* **2016**, *2840*, 1–12. [CrossRef] [PubMed]
4. Ibáñez, C.; Cáceresa, J.; Brucher, R.; Seijas, D. Trastornos del ánimo y trastornos por uso de sustancias: Una comorbilidad compleja y frecuente. *Rev. Médica Clínica Las Condes* **2020**, *31*, 174–182. [CrossRef]
5. Daigre, C.; Perea-Ortueta, M.; Berenguer, M.; Esculies, O.; Sorribes-Puertas, M.; Palma-Alvarez, R.; Martínez-Luna, N.; Ramos-Quiroga, J.A.; Grau-López, L. Psychiatric factors affecting recovery after a long term treatment program for substance use disorder. *Psychiatry Res.* **2019**, *276*, 283–289. [CrossRef]
6. Marquez-Arrico, J.E.; Río-Martínez, L.; Navarro, J.; Prat, G.; Forero, D.; Adan, A. Coping strategies in male patients under treatment for substance use disorders and/or severe mental illness: Influence in clinical course at one-year follow-up. *J. Clin. Med.* **2019**, *8*, 1972. [CrossRef]
7. De Moura, A.; Pinto, R.; Ferros, L.; Jongenelen, I.; Negreiros, J. Efficacy indicators of four methods in outpatient addiction treatment. *Arch. Clin. Psychiatry* **2017**, *44*, 117–121. [CrossRef]
8. Aguiar, P.; Neto, D.; Lambaz, R.; Chick, J.; Ferrinho, P. Prognostic factors during outpatient treatment for alcohol dependence: Cohort study with 6 months of treatment follow-up. *Alcohol Alcohol.* **2012**, *47*, 702–710. [CrossRef]
9. Laudet, A.B. The case for considering quality of life in addiction research and clinical practice. *Addict. Sci. Clin. Pract.* **2011**, *6*, 44–55.
10. Hansebout, R.R.; Cornacchi, S.D.; Haines, T.; Goldsmith, C. How to use article about prognosis. *Contin. Med. Educ.* **2009**, *52*, 328–336.
11. Croft, P.; Altman, D.G.; Deeks, J.J.; Dunn, K.M.; Hay, A.D.; Hemingway, H.; LeResche, L.; Peat, G.; Perel, P.; Petersen, S.E.; et al. The science of clinical practice: Disease diagnosis or patient prognosis? Evidence about "what is likely to happen" should shape clinical practice. *BMC Med.* **2015**, *13*, 20. [CrossRef]
12. Díaz-Morán, S.; Palma-Álvarez, R.F.; Grau-López, L.; Daigre, C.; Barral, C.; Ros-Cucurull, E.; Casas, M.; Roncero, C. Self-perceived quality of life in cocaine dependents with or without dual diagnosis. *Salud Ment.* **2015**, *38*, 397–402. [CrossRef]
13. Saarijärvi, S.; Salminen, J.K.; Toikka, T.; Raitasalo, R. Health-related quality of life among patients with major depression. *Nord. J. Psychiatry* **2002**, *56*, 261–264. [CrossRef] [PubMed]
14. Lozano, Ó.M.; Rojas, A.J.; Calderón, F.F. Psychiatric comorbidity and severity of dependence on substance users: How it impacts on their health-related quality of life? *J. Ment. Health* **2017**, *26*, 119–126. [CrossRef] [PubMed]
15. Adan, A.; Marquez-Arrico, J.E.; Gilchrist, G. Comparison of health-related quality of life among men with different co-existing severe mental disorders in treatment for substance use. *Health Qual. Life Outcomes* **2017**, *15*, 209. [CrossRef] [PubMed]
16. Marquez-Arrico, J.E.; Río-Martínez, L.; Navarro, J.F.; Prat, G.; Adan, A. Personality profile and clinical correlates of patients with substance use disorder with and without comorbid depression under treatment. *Front. Psychiatry* **2019**, *9*, 764. [CrossRef]
17. Benaiges, I.; Prat, G.; Adan, A. Health-related quality of life in patients with dual diagnosis: Clinical correlates. *Health Qual. Life Outcomes* **2012**, *10*, 106. [CrossRef]

18. Astals, M.; Domingo-salvany, A.; Buenaventura, C.C.; Tato, J.; Vazquez, J.M.; Martín-Santos, R.; Torrens, M. Impact of substance dependence and dual diagnosis on the quality of life of heroin users seeking. *Subst. Use Misuse* **2009**, *43*, 612–632. [CrossRef]
19. Lai, H.M.X.; Cleary, M.; Sitharthan, T.; Hunt, G.E. Prevalence of comorbid substance use, anxiety and mood disorders in epidemiological surveys, 1990–2014: A systematic review and meta-analysis. *Drug Alcohol Depend.* **2015**, *154*, 1–13. [CrossRef]
20. Arya, S.; Singh, P.; Gupta, R. Psychiatric comorbidity and quality of life in patients with alcohol dependence syndrome. *Indian J. Soc. Psychiatry* **2017**, *33*, 336–341. [CrossRef]
21. Brook, J.S.; Zhang, C.; Rubenstone, E.; Primack, B.A.; Brook, D.W. Comorbid trajectories of substance use as predictors of antisocial personality disorder, major depressive episode, and generalized anxiety disorder. *Addict. Behav.* **2016**, *62*, 114–121. [CrossRef] [PubMed]
22. Davis, L.; Uezato, A.; Newell, J.M.; Frazier, E. Major depression and comorbid substance use disorders. *Curr. Opin. Psychiatry* **2008**, *21*, 14–18. [CrossRef]
23. Tang, A.L.; Thomas, S.J.; Larkin, T. Cortisol, oxytocin, and quality of life in major depressive disorder. *Qual. Life Res.* **2019**, *28*, 2919–2928. [CrossRef]
24. Giammanco, M.D.; Gitto, L. Coping, uncertainty and health-related quality of life as determinants of anxiety and depression on a sample of hospitalized cardiac patients in Southern Italy. *Qual. Life Res.* **2016**, *25*, 2941–2956. [CrossRef]
25. Kristjánsdóttir, J.; Olsson, G.I.; Sundelin, C.; Naessen, T. Could SF-36 be used as a screening instrument for depression in a Swedish youth population? *Scand. J. Caring Sci.* **2011**, *25*, 262–268. [CrossRef] [PubMed]
26. ten Doesschate, M.C.; Koeter, M.W.J.; Bockting, C.L.H.; Schene, A.H. Health related quality of life in recurrent depression: A comparison with a general population sample. *J. Affect. Disord.* **2010**, *120*, 126–132. [CrossRef]
27. Lin, C.H.; Yen, Y.C.; Chen, M.C.; Chen, C.C. Depression and pain impair daily functioning and quality of life in patients with major depressive disorder. *J. Affect. Disord.* **2014**, *166*, 173–178. [CrossRef]
28. Cho, Y.; Lee, J.K.; Kim, D.H.; Park, J.H.; Choi, M.; Kim, H.J.; Nam, M.J.; Lee, K.U.; Han, K.; Park, Y.G. Factors associated with quality of life in patients with depression: A nationwide population-based study. *PLoS ONE* **2019**, *14*, e0219455. [CrossRef] [PubMed]
29. Shumye, S.; Belayneh, Z.; Mengistu, N. Health related quality of life and its correlates among people with depression attending outpatient department in Ethiopia: A cross sectional study. *Health Qual. Life Outcomes* **2019**, *17*, 1–9. [CrossRef]
30. Torrens, M.; Gilchrist, G.; Domingo-Salvany, A. Psychiatric comorbidity in illicit drug users: Substance-induced versus independent disorders. *Drug Alcohol Depend.* **2011**, *113*, 147–156. [CrossRef]
31. Boschloo, L.; van den Brink, W.; Penninx, B.W.J.H.; Wall, M.M.; Hasin, D.S. Alcohol-use disorder severity predicts first-incidence of depressive disorders. *Psychol. Med.* **2012**, *42*, 695–703. [CrossRef] [PubMed]
32. Aharonovich, E.; Liu, X. Suicide attempts in substance abusers: Effects of major depression in relation to substance use disorders. *Am. J. Psychiatry* **2002**, *159*, 1600–1602. [CrossRef] [PubMed]
33. Samet, S.; Fenton, M.C.; Nunes, E.; Greenstein, E.; Aharonovich, E.; Hasin, D. Effects of independent and substance-induced major depressive disorder on remission and relapse of alcohol, cocaine and heroin dependence. *Addiction* **2013**, *108*, 115–123. [CrossRef]
34. Dagher, R.K.; Green, K.M. Does depression and substance abuse co-morbidity affect socioeconomic status? Evidence from a prospective study of urban African Americans. *Psychiatry Res.* **2014**, *30*, 115–121. [CrossRef]
35. Green, C.A.; Yarborough, M.T.; Polen, M.R.; Janoff, S.L.; Yarborough, B.J.H. Dual recovery among people with serious mental illnesses and substance problems: A qualitative analysis. *J. Dual Diagn.* **2015**, *11*, 33–41. [CrossRef]
36. Garner, B.R.; Scott, C.K.; Dennis, M.L.; Funk, R.R. The relationship between recovery and health-related quality of life. *J. Subst. Abus. Treat.* **2014**, *47*, 293–298. [CrossRef]
37. Ware, J.E.; Sherbourne, C.D. The MOS 36-item short-form health survey (SF-36). I. Conceptual framework and item selection. *Med. Care* **1992**, *30*, 473–483. [CrossRef]
38. Tiffany, S.T.; Friedman, L.; Greenfield, S.F.; Hasin, D.S.; Jackson, R. Beyond drug use: A systematic consideration of other outcomes in evaluations of treatments for substance use disorders. *Addiction* **2012**, *107*, 709–718. [CrossRef]
39. Torrens, M. Quality of life as a means of assessing outcome in opioid dependence treatment. *Heroin Addict. Relat. Clin. Probl.* **2008**, *11*, 33–36.

40. Griffin, M.L.; Bennett, H.E.; Fitzmaurice, G.M.; Hill, K.P.; Provost, S.E.; Weiss, R.D. Health-related quality of life among prescription opioid-dependent patients: Results from a multi-site study. *Am. J. Addict.* **2015**, *24*, 308–314. [CrossRef]
41. Silveira, E.; Taft, C.; Sundh, V.; Waern, M.; Palsson, S.; Steen, B. Performance of the SF-36 Health Survey in screening for depressive and anxiety disorders in an elderly female Swedish population. *Qual. Life Res.* **2005**, *14*, 1263–1274. [CrossRef] [PubMed]
42. Teoh Bing Fei, J.; Yee, A.; Habil, M.H. Bin Psychiatric comorbidity among patients on methadone maintenance therapy and its influence on quality of life. *Am. J. Addict.* **2016**, *25*, 49–55. [CrossRef] [PubMed]
43. Aydemir, O.; Ergün, H.; Soygür, H.; Kesebir, S.; Tulunay, C. Quality of life in major depressive disorder: A cross-sectional study. *Turk. J. Psychiatry* **2009**, *20*, 205–212. [CrossRef]
44. American Psychiatric Association. *Manual Diagnóstico y Estadístico de los Trastornos Mentales: DSM-5*; Editorial Médica Panamericana: Madrid, Spain, 2014; ISBN 9788498358100.
45. Gálvez, B.P.; Fernández, L.G. Validación española del drug abuse screening test (DAST-20 y DAST-10). *Salud y Drogas* **2010**, *10*, 35–50.
46. Lobo, A.; Chamorro, L.; Luque, A.; Dal-ré, R.; Badia, X.; Baró, E. Validación de las versiones en español de la Montgomery-Asberg Depression Rating Scale y la Hamilton Anxiety Rating Scale para la evaluación de la depresión y de la ansiedad. *Med. Clin.* **2002**, *118*, 493–499. [CrossRef]
47. Bobes, J.; González, M.P.; Bascarán, M.T.; Corominas, A.; Adan, A.; Sánchez, J.; Such, P. Validación de la versión española de la Escala de Adaptación Social en depresivos. *Actas Esp. Psiquiatr.* **1999**, *27*, 71–80.
48. Alonso, J.; Regidor, E.; Barrio, G.; Prieto, L. Valores poblacionales de referencia de la versión española del Cuestionario de Salud SF-36. *Med. Clin.* **1998**, *36*, 1–10.
49. Boden, J.M.; Fergusson, D.M. Alcohol and depression. *Addiction* **2011**, *106*, 906–914. [CrossRef]
50. Adan, A. A cronobiological approach to addiction. *J. Subst. Use* **2013**, *18*, 171–183. [CrossRef]
51. Mangione, K.K.; Miller, A.H.; Naughton, I.V. Cochrane Review: Improving physical function and training in older adults. *Phys. Ther.* **2010**, *90*, 1711–1715. [CrossRef]
52. Cao, Y.; Li, W.; Shen, J.; Malison, R.T.; Zhang, Y. Health-related quality of life and symptom severity in Chinese patients with major depressive disorder. *Asia-Pac. Psychiatry* **2013**, *5*, 276–283. [CrossRef] [PubMed]

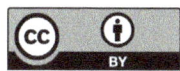

© 2020 by the authors. Licensee MDPI, Basel, Switzerland. This article is an open access article distributed under the terms and conditions of the Creative Commons Attribution (CC BY) license (http://creativecommons.org/licenses/by/4.0/).

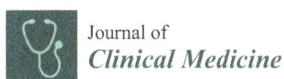

Article

Alcohol Induced Depression: Clinical, Biological and Genetic Features

Adriana Farré [1,2,3], **Judit Tirado** [2], **Nino Spataro** [4], **María Alías-Ferri** [2,3], **Marta Torrens** [1,2,3] **and Francina Fonseca** [1,2,3,*]

1. Institut de Neuropsiquiatria i Addiccions (INAD), Hospital del Mar, 08003 Barcelona, Spain; AFarre@parcdesalutmar.cat (A.F.); mtorrens@parcdesalutmar.cat (M.T.)
2. Grup de Recerca en Addiccions, Institut Hospital del Mar d'Investigacions Mèdiques (IMIM), 08003 Barcelona, Spain; jtirado@imim.es (J.T.); malias@imim.es (M.A.-F.)
3. Psychiatry Department, Universitat Autònoma de Barcelona, Cerdanyola del Valles, 08193 Barcelona, Spain
4. Genetics Laboratory, UDIAT-Centre Diagnòstic, Parc Taulí Hospital Universitari, Institut d'Investigació i Innovació Parc Taulí I3PT, 08208 Sabadell, Spain; nspataro@tauli.cat
* Correspondence: ffonseca@parcdesalutmar.cat

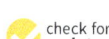

Received: 2 July 2020; Accepted: 12 August 2020; Published: 18 August 2020

Abstract: Background: In clinical practice, there is the need to have clinical and biological markers to identify induced depression. The objective was to investigate clinical, biological and genetic differences between Primary Major Depression (Primary MD) and Alcohol Induced MD (AI-MD). Methods: Patients, of both genders, were recruited from psychiatric hospitalisation units. The PRISM instrument was used to establish the diagnoses. Data on socio-demographic/family history, clinical scales for depression, anxiety, personality and stressful life events were recorded. A blood test was performed analysing biochemical parameters and a Genome Wide Association Study (GWAS) to identify genetic markers associated with AI-MD. Results: A total of 80 patients were included (47 Primary MD and 33 AI-MD). The AI-MD group presented more medical comorbidities and less family history of depression. There were differences in traumatic life events, with higher scores in the AI-MD (14.21 ± 11.35 vs. 9.30 ± 7.38; $p = 0.021$). DSM-5 criteria were different between groups with higher prevalence of weight changes and less anhedonia, difficulties in concentration and suicidal thoughts in the AI-MD. None of the genetic variants reached significance beyond multiple testing thresholds; however, some suggestive variants were observed. Conclusions: This study has found clinical and biological features that may help physicians to identify AI-MD and improve its therapeutic approach.

Keywords: primary major depression; alcohol use disorder; alcohol induced major depression; biomarkers; comorbidity; clinical characteristics; GWAS

---

1. Introduction

Major Depression (MD) and alcohol use disorders (AUD) are two of the more prevalent mental health disorders in the general population and constitute a major health burden worldwide [1,2]. Clinical [3–7] and epidemiological [8–12] studies show that MD and Alcohol Use Disorder (AUD) frequently co-occur. A systematic review of longitudinal or cross-sectional epidemiological studies found that the presence of either disorder doubled the risk of the second disorder [13], meaning that patients with MD are twice as likely to develop an AUD and vice versa [14].

Diagnosis and treatment of the commonly co-occurring AUD and depressive disorders implies many challenges [15]. Diagnosis is particularly challenging because, as described in other substances with addiction liability, the acute and chronic effects related to alcohol consumption/withdrawal can mimic depressive symptoms. In this sense, MD associated to any SUD has been recognized by both, DSM and ICD classifications for a long time (DSM-IV, IV-TR and DSM-5; ICD-10, ICD-11). The need to differentiate between primary and substance-induced mood disorders has been long-established due to their prevalence and important treatment implications (see systematic reviews published by Schuckit in 2006, Nunes and Levin 2004, Torrens et al., 2005) [16–18]. In particular, the differentiation among independent depression or alcohol-induced depression has been extensively studied in terms of characteristics, prognosis, suicide risk and relapse risk among others [11,13,19–26]. Given the available knowledge, it can thus be stated that induced depressive episodes can be as or more serious than primary or independent ones, both in terms of relapse to substance use [3,27] and in the severity of depressive symptomatology [21,28], including risk of suicide [19,22]. This difference may be especially relevant for treatment management [18,23]. In the case of alcohol, each type of depressive episode could be considered as two different diseases since Primary MD patients' present greater familial risk to develop a primary episode, while this association is not present for the induced episodes [29].

It is has been enough established that depressed patients exhibited elevated levels of C Reactive Protein (CRP) and a significant decrease in their Thyroid-stimulating hormone (TSH) levels, directly related with hypothyroidism [30,31]. Alcohol abuse is a major cause of abnormal liver function and liver enzyme activities are important screening tools for detecting liver disease [32]. Other biomarkers such as cholesterol and triglycerides were previously associated with depression and alcohol use disorder. Although with controversial results, metabolic syndrome, especially lipid dysregulation have been found in primary depression [33,34]; furthermore, alcohol consumption has been related with a tendency towards hypertrigliceridemia [35].

Furthermore, MD and AUD are complex disorders which encompass multiple genetic and environmental factors [30]. Both AUD and MD have substantial genetic contributions with heritability estimates of 50–60% for AUD [31] and 30–40% for MD [32]. Increased familial recurrence risk and heritability have been associated with earlier-onset and recurrent depression [33–35] as well as greater depression severity or impairment [36,37].

Common genetic factors that influence the co-occurrence of MD and AUD have been sought in family, twin, and adoption studies [36–43]. GWASs have reported genome-wide significant findings for AUD [44,45] and MD [46–50]. However, no consistent findings have been reported for comorbid AUD and MD [51,52]. Discovering the genetic component of shared liability presents an opportunity to clarify the aetiology of both disorders [51]. Evidence suggests that genetic influences underlying psychiatric and substance use disorders might differ across ancestry groups. In a recent report from Zhou et al. [52], a single genome-wide significant variant was detected, located in the SEMA3A gene. The variant was only common enough to be tested in the African American sample; however, nearby variants in the European American sample that occurred with sufficient frequency to test showed no evidence of association [52].

Given the high prevalence and related negative impact of the comorbidity between AUD and Induced Major Depressions (I-MD), the need to distinguish between co-morbid conditions (i.e., independent psychiatric problems) and conditions where psychiatric symptoms are secondary to substance use has become crucial for clinicians working with substance use disorder patients. As far as we know, there are no studies that characterize Induced Major Depressions (I-MD) from a clinical ad biological perspective to differentiate them from Primary Major Depression (Primary MD). The objective of the present study was to investigate clinical, biological and genetic differences between Primary MD and AI-MD.

2. Material and Methods

2.1. Design

This is a cross-sectional study comparing two different phenotypes of MD: The Primary MD and the AI-MD.

2.2. Participants and Recruitment

From November 2015 to October 2017, a total of 111 patients were assessed for eligibility. Participants were recruited from detoxification, dual diagnosis and acute psychiatric units from the Neuropsychiatry and Addiction Institute of Parc de Salut Mar in Barcelona (PSMAR). Both Primary MD and AI-MD diagnoses were done according to DSM-IV-TR criteria [53]. Inclusion criteria included both genders, aged between 18 and 65 years and of Caucasian origin. Exclusion criteria for both groups were: language barrier or intellectual difficulties that limited the understanding of evaluations, history of pathological conditions or any kind of somatic disorder or disease that the investigator considered unsuitable for the study, other concomitant psychiatric disorder in axis I and any diagnosis of substance use disorder (current or life-time, except nicotine use disorder) (DSM-IV-TR) in the MD group; in the AI-MD group, any other diagnosis of substance use disorder than alcohol use disorder or nicotine use disorder (DSM-IV-TR). Participants from the AI-MD group recruited in the detoxification unit were included in the study at the end of their admission (mean days of admission 13); all of them were under pharmacological treatment of their alcohol abstinence syndrome and also, all participants had punctuations in the Revised Clinical Institute Withdrawal Assessment for Alcohol Scale (CIWA-Ar) below 10 at the inclusion.

2.3. Measures

2.3.1. Clinical Assessments

Participants were evaluated using the Spanish version of the Psychiatric Research Interview for Substance and Mental Diseases (PRISM) [54,55] according to "Diagnostic and Statistical Manual of Mental Disorders-4th Edition-Text Revision" (DSM-IV-TR) criteria [53], including a protocol of a family history of depression. In addition, the validated Spanish version of the following instruments were used: severity of depression was assessed using the Spanish validated version of the "Hamilton Depression rating Scale (HAM-D)" [56], the Spanish validated version of the "Beck Depression Inventory (BDI)" [57] and the Spanish validated version of the "Scale for Suicide Ideation (SSI)" [58]. Anxiety severity was evaluated with the Spanish validated version of the "Hamilton Anxiety rating Scale (HAM-A)" [59] and the Spanish validated version of "State-Trait Anxiety Inventory (STAI-R)" [60]. Personality was assessed with the Spanish validated version of the "Temperament and Character Inventory (TCI)" of Cloninger [61]. Traumatic and stressful life events were evaluated with the Spanish validated version of the "Life Stressor Checklist-Revised" (LSC-R) [62].

2.3.2. Blood Samples

A total of 20 mL of blood sample was collected from each participant. From the total, 10 mL was used to conduct a blood test, assessing the levels of C Reactive Protein (CRP), Thyroid-stimulating hormone (TSH), liver function (bilirubin, alanine transaminase (ALT), aspartate transaminase (AST), alkaline phosphatase (ALP), and gamma-glutamyl transpeptidase (GGT)) and lipids (triglycerides and cholesterol). The other 10mL of blood sample was collected to perform the GWAS analysis.

2.4. Procedure

The study was approved by the Ethical and Clinical Research Committee of the institution (CEIC number: 2015/6012/I). Written informed consent was obtained from each subject after they received a complete description of the study and had been given the chance to discuss any questions or issues before the start. Study participants were reimbursed with 20 euros for their participation in the study. Participation in this study consisted in one visit of approximately 3 h, where participants were interviewed and blood samples were collected. Genetic samples were adequately stored under professional biobanking procedures until the end of the recruitment period and then prepared for analysis. Blood samples were analysed by the Hospital del Mar (Laboratori de Referència de Catalunya). Genetic samples were adequately stored by UPF-CompOmics under professional biobanking procedures until the end of the recruitment period. Afterwards, biological samples were provided to the Genomics Core Facility service at the National Genotyping Center (CeGen) for sample preparation. Finally, genetic data from CeGen were shared with UPF-CompOmics for analysis.

2.5. Data Analysis

2.5.1. Clinical and Blood Tests

Analysis of clinical and blood test data were performed using SPSS Version 23 (IBM SPSS Statistics for Windows (IBM Corp., Armonk, NY, USA). Frequencies, percentages, mean and standard deviations (SD) were calculated. Analysis of the relationship between variables was performed through Chi-Square for dichotomous variables and T-Test (independent samples) for continuous variables. A 5% or lower p-value (i.e., <0.05) was considered statistically significant.

2.5.2. Genetic Data

- Genotyping procedure

The protocol used in the processing of this platform is detailed in the user guide "Axiom™ 2.0 Assay Manual Workflow", available at www.thermofisher.com. In summary, the total genomic DNA was amplified and fragmented up to 25–125 bp. These fragments were purified and re-suspended in the hybridization solution that was transferred to the GeneTitan Instrument to follow its fully automated processing (hybridization in the array plates, staining, washing and scanning). The raw images were automatically processed and the genotypes were obtained by applying the Axiom algorithm, available through the Axiom Analysis Suite software (version, 4.0. Affymetrix, Inc.; Santa Clara, CA, USA, www.thermofisher.com).

- Association analysis

For the association analysis, we used a whole genome association analysis toolset called Plink. We performed 3 different tests separately: (i) basic allelic chi-square; (ii) Fisher's exact test and (iii) logistic regression to test for differences between the individuals affected by Primary MD and the individuals affected by AI-MD.

Apart from testing each single variant, a covariates analysis was also conducted into the logistic model. A total of 16 different covariates were included in the analysis, all of them related with clinical features considered relevant for depression heritability. These covariates were: gender, age, birth date, race, depression family history, alcohol family history, SUD family history, depression age of onset, severity of depression (HAM-D, BECK and SSI), anxiety scales (HAM-A, STAI-R and STAI-E), number of suicide attempts and live events scale (LSC-R).

3. Results

A total of 111 patients were assessed for eligibility. Twenty of them met at least one of the exclusion criteria and eleven refused to participate. A total of 80 participants were included in the study, 47 with Primary MD and 33 with an AI-MD diagnosis.

3.1. Clinical

Clinical results included socio-demographic/family history and the results of the different clinical scales for clinical assessment of depression severity, anxiety severity, personality and traumatic and stressful life events.

3.1.1. Socio-Demographic/Family History

No significant differences were found between the two groups in terms of main sociodemographic characteristics (Table 1); although, subjects with Primary MD had a higher education level in comparison with participants in the AI-MD group. Regarding medical comorbidities, a significant difference was found ($p = 0.026$) with more subjects from the AI-MD group (54.5%) reporting this condition in comparison to Primary MD participants (29.8%). The majority of comorbidities included any hepatic disease and lipid metabolism disorders.

There were no significant differences with respect to hospitalization due to medical comorbidities. Most of the participants reported to be in pharmacological treatment with antidepressants without differences between Primary MD and AI-MD group (100% vs. 96.7% respectively; $p = 0.37$). Almost 80% of Primary MD participants provided information on history of depression in family members with differences between groups ($p = 0.042$). In contrast, a higher percentage of AI-MD participants reported alcohol and substance use disorders in their family history. Fifty-three percent of AI-MD patients and 28.3% of Primary MD group of patients reported a family history of alcohol use ($p = 0.033$). Finally, differences were also found for a family history of other substance use disorders (31.3% of AI-MD vs. 8.7% Primary MD, $p = 0.016$).

Table 1. Sociodemographic and family history data.

Sample Characteristics	Primary MD N = 47 (%)	AI-MD N = 33 (%)	p [a]
Age (Mean ± SD)	49.87 ± 11.32	50.39 ± 8.89	0.140 [b]
Gender			0.678
Men	22 (46.8)	17 (51.5)	
Women	25 (53.2)	16 (48.5)	
Household structure			0.736
Alone	14 (29.8)	11 (33.3)	
With others	33 (70.2)	22 (66.7)	
Education level			0.041
Primary or Secondary education	20 (42.6)	21 (65.6)	
Upper secondary education	27 (57.4)	11 (34.4)	
Employment situation			0.271
Employed	16 (34)	6 (18.8)	
Unemployed	1 (2.1)	0	
Disability	27 (57.4)	25 (78.1)	
Retired	3 (6.4)	1 (3.1)	
Medical comorbidities			
Serious illness (SI)	14 (29.8)	18 (54.5)	0.026 *
Hospitalization due to SI [c]	14 (100)	17 (94.4)	0.370
Current medication [d]	46 (100)	29 (96.7)	0.213
Family History			
Depression [e]	35 (79.5)	17 (56.7)	0.042 *
Alcohol use disorder [f]	13 (28.3)	16 (53.3)	0.033 *
Substance use disorder [g]	4 (8.7)	10 (31.3)	0.016 *

Notes: [a] Chi-Square; [b] Student's T-Test; [c] n = 32; [d] n = 76; [e] n = 74; [f] n = 76; [g] n = 78; * Significance ($p < 0.05$). MD: Major Depression; AI-MD: Alcohol Induced Major Depression.

3.1.2. Clinical Assessment

Characteristics of AUD in the AI-MD group were collected with a PRISM interview: The mean age of onset of alcohol abuse was 33.42 years (12.26 SD) and 37.34 years (12.49 DS) for alcohol dependence. According to the DSM-IV TR diagnosis criteria, 100% of subjects fulfilled a lifetime criteria for alcohol dependence and 94% for the last 12 months. The mean age for first alcohol disorder treatment in the AI-MD patients was 37.55 years (15.96 SD).

The main results in clinical severity for depression are described in Table 2. There were no differences in the age of onset of depression between the two groups. Moreover, there were no differences between groups for any of the instruments assessing the severity of depression (HAM-D, BDI and SSI) or anxiety (HAM-A and STAI). Furthermore, the severity of depression was not associated with the age of onset of alcohol addiction in the AI-MD group. A trauma and life events instrument

(LSC-R) showed a higher mean score in patients with AI-MD diagnosis compared to Primary MD patients, ((14.21 ± 11.35 SD) vs. 9.30 ± 7.38 SD; $p = 0.021$)). There were no differences for the temperament and character (dimensions between groups). There were differences between groups regarding the following subscales: "disorderliness" trait from "novelty seeking" dimension ($p = 0.035$), showing AI-MD patients with higher scores in comparison to Primary MD patients (51.81 ± 10.05 and 46.29 ± 11.44, respectively). In addition, differences ($p = 0.034$) were found between groups regarding "conformity" trait from "reward dependence" dimension; patients in the Primary MD group showed a higher mean score (50.79 ± 9.41) than patients with an AI-MD diagnosis (44.87 ± 13.92).

Table 2. Results of Clinical Assessment on depression, anxiety, personality and stressful events.

Variables	Primary MD N = 47 (Mean ± SD/Mean (%))	AI-MD N = 33 (Mean ± SD/Mean (%))	p [a]
Age onset depression (years)	37.64 (13.53)	39.18 (11.26)	0.593
HAM-D	15.64 ± 10.34	11.88 ± 7.54	0.79
BDI	22.37 ± 14.65	23.41 ± 11.59	0.739
SSI	11.68 ± 8.12	12.36 ± 8.48	0.156
HAM-A	25.22 ± 14.32	25.67 ± 12	0.884
STAI			
STAI- State	28.17 ± 13.82	27.44 ± 13.78	0.817
STAI- Trait	30.00 ± 13.16	32.28 ± 11.17	0.425
LSC-R	9.30 (7.38)	14.21 (11.35)	0.021 *
Personality Dimensions			
Temperament			
Novelty seeking (NS)	47.38 ± 11.07	50.84 ± 9.89	0.172
Harm avoidance (HA)	54.60 ± 11.82	60.87 ± 11.61	0.415
Reward dependence (RD)	43.57 ± 9.65	45.68 ± 10.66	0.381
Persistence (PS)	44.45 ± 9.92	47.55 ± 11.62	0.224
Character			
Self-directedness (SD)	42.33 ± 11.92	39.61 ± 11.12	0.325
Cooperativeness (CO)	45.14 ± 11.42	45 ± 12.22	0.959
Self-transcendence (ST)	48.74 ± 10.57	50.35 ± 11.53	0.536
Depression Criteria			
Criteria 1: depressed mood	46 (97.9)	32 (94.1)	0.377
Criteria 2: diminished interest or pleasure	46 (97.9)	28 (82.4)	0.014 *
Criteria 3: significant unintentional weight loss or gain	34 (72.3)	31 (91.2)	0.036 *
Criteria 4: insomnia or sleeping too much	43 (91.5)	27 (79.4)	0.117
Criteria 5: agitation or psychomotor retardation	34 (72.3)	22 (64.7)	0.463
Criteria 6: fatigue	44 (93.6)	27 (79.4)	0.055
Criteria 7 feelings of worthlessness or excessive guilt	43 (91.5)	28 (82.4)	0.217
Criteria 8: diminished ability to think or concentrate	46 (97.9)	27 (79.4)	0.006 *
Criteria 9: recurrent thoughts of death	30 (63.8)	10 (29.4)	0.002 *

Notes: [a] Student's T-Test * Significance ($p < 0.05$). HAM-D: Hamilton Depression Rating Scale, BDI: Beck Depression Inventory, SSI: Suicidal Ideation Scale, HAM-A: Hamilton Anxiety Rating Scale, STAI: State-Trait Anxiety Inventory, LSC-R: Life Stressor Checklist-Revised.

Taking into account the DSM-IV-TR depression criteria for the diagnosis of depression, five (or more) criteria should be present during the same 2-week period and should represent a change from previous functioning; at least one of the symptoms is either: depressed mood or loss of interest or pleasure. The nine criteria are described in Table 2. First, there were no differences between groups for the first criteria (depressed mood), showing both groups with a similar prevalence of these criteria (97.9% in Primary MD vs. 94.1% in AI-MD). However, differences were found for the second criteria (anhedonia). The majority of Primary MD participants (97.9%) reported this symptom while a lower number in AI-MD participants reported it (82.4%) ($p = 0.014$). There were differences in relation to the third criterion, changes in weight and/or appetite; AI-MD patients showed a higher prevalence (91.2%) than patients with primary episodes (72.3%) ($p = 0.036$). There were also differences in the eight criteria (diminished ability to concentrate), more frequent among PMD patients (97.9%) than AI-MD group of patients (79.4%) ($p = 0.006$). Finally, differences were found in recurrent thoughts of death (criteria 9), where 63.8% of PMD patients showed these criteria and 29.4% of AI-MD patients ($p = 0.002$). There were no differences in other depression criteria.

3.2. Blood Test Results

Regarding the blood test results, AI-MD participants had more significant abnormal results in comparison with Primary MD in the following: TSH ($p = 0.016$), AST ($p < 0.001$), ALT ($p < 0.001$), ALP ($p = 0.043$) and GGT ($p < 0.001$). There were no significant differences in the results of CRP levels, bilirubin, cholesterol and triglycerides between groups. Table 3 shows the total number of participants (or percentage) with pathological results in both groups.

Table 3. Results of pathological blood test in Primary MD and AI-MD groups.

Biochemical Paramaters	Subjects with Abnormal Values *		p
(Normal Values)	Primary MD N (%)	AI-MD N (%)	
TSH [a] (10–38 mcUI/mL)	0	4 (12.5)	0.016 **
Bilirubin [b] (0.2–1.2 mg/dL)	2 (5)	4 (12.1)	0.270
AST [c] (UI/L) 10–38 UI/L	4 (9.3)	17 (51.5)	<0.001 **
ALT [d] (UI/L) 7–41 UI/L	14 (32.6)	26 (76.5)	<0.001 **
ALP [e] (40–129 UI/L)	3 (8.6)	9 (27.3)	0.043 **
GGT [f] (8–61 UI/L)	11 (32.4)	26 (78.8)	<0.001 **
Cholesterol [g] (50–129 mg/dL)	25 (59.5)	16 (48.5)	0.340
Triglycerides [h] (40–150 mg/dL)	14 (33.3)	7 (21.9)	0.279
CRP [i] (0–0.8 mg/dL)	13 (31.7)	15 (57.7)	0.378

Notes: [a] Chi-Square. * There were no patients with values below the lower range in all the parameters analysed. The parameters were considered abnormal when the value was above the highest range; ** Significance ($p < 0.05$), Thyroid-stimulating hormone (TSH), alanine transaminase (ALT), aspartate transaminase (AST), alkaline phosphatase (ALP), and gamma-glutamyl transpeptidase (GGT), C Reactive Protein (CRP). [a] n = 76, [b] n = 73, [c] n = 76, [d] n = 77, [e] n = 68, [f] n = 67, [g] n = 74, [h] n = 74, [i] n = 67.

3.3. GWAS Results

Variants with a missing rate higher than 5% or having a minor allele frequency lower than 1% or deviating significantly from Hardy–Weinberg equilibrium were filtered out. From the original 814,923 variants, 508,097 were considered for further analysis. A total of 24 samples were removed after quality control. For 16 individuals, unusual Identity By Descent (IBD) values were observed when compared to the rest of patients and were discarded due to possible contamination. An additional individual showed an heterozygosity rate deviating from the heterozygosity observed in the rest of patients. Principal component analysis (PCA) was performed to assess ancestry and seven patients with non-European ancestry were discarded for further analysis. As association analyses are generally performed considering only variants with a high frequency in the population, variants with a frequency lower than 5% in the sequenced samples were filtered out. For each single variant, among the 341,946 common variants for genotyping data, three different tests were performed separately: (i) basic allelic chi-square, (ii) Fisher's exact test and (iii) logistic regression. A Manhattan plot resulted from each test (Figure 1). For each test, we created a table that contains the odd-ratios obtained (effect of the variants) and *p*-values, for more information about this tables see Tables A1–A3.

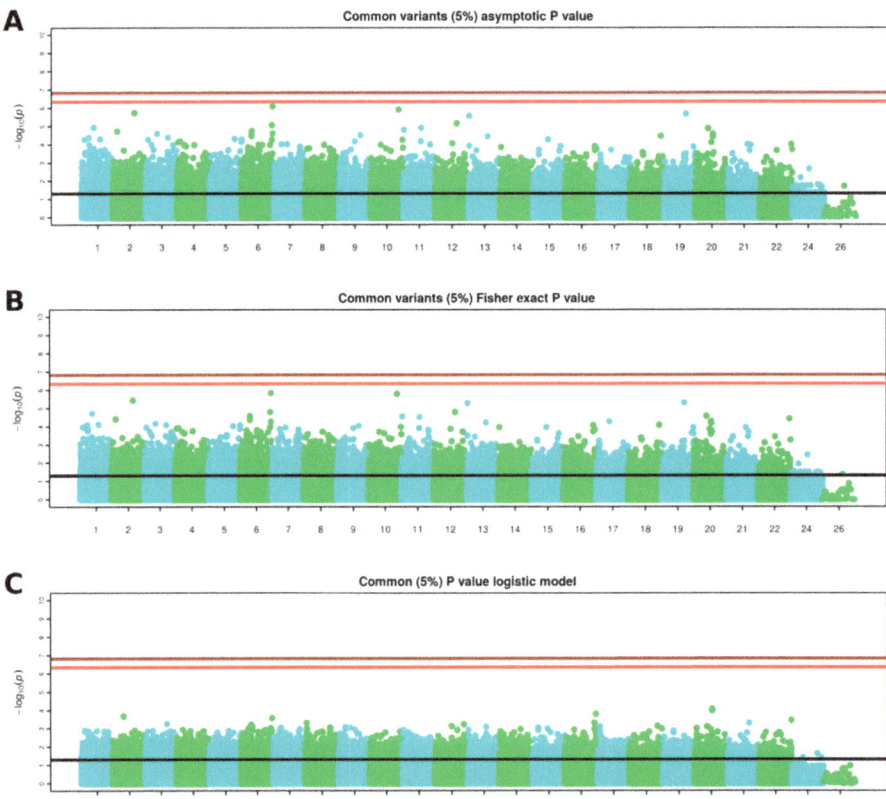

Figure 1. Manhattan plots indicating the negative base 10 logarithm of the *p*-values obtained performing: basic allele chi-square test (**A**) and Fisher's exact test (**B**) and logistic regression model (**C**) on 341,946 common variants obtained from whole genome genotyping data. The black horizontal line represents a significance level of 0.05. The light red horizontal line represents the multiple testing obtained considering the number of independent loci; the dark red horizontal line represents the multiple testing threshold obtained considering the total number of considered common variants. Chromosomes over 22 represent sexual and mitochondrial chromosomes.

Apart from testing each single variant, covariates were also included into the logistic model. When including all the provided covariates into the logistic model even the most minimal differences between two groups of samples disappeared, suggesting that correcting for all these covariates jointly is not useful to identify the genetic differences between the two groups of individuals in our study. On the other hand, covariates were also analysed separately in Figure 2 and none of the variants reached statistical significance.

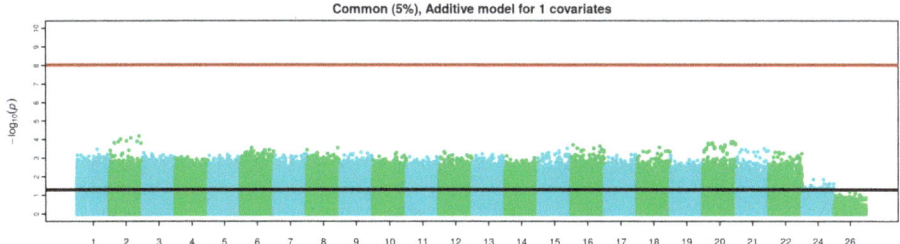

Figure 2. Manhattan plot indicating the negative base 10 logarithm of the *p*-values obtained when including each single covariate into the logistic regression model for 341,946 common variants from whole genome genotyping data. For each individual variant, a single test for each covariate was performed, so for each variant, 16 different tests were performed and each test is represented by a point in the Manhattan plot. The black horizontal line represents a significance level of 0.05. The dark red horizontal line represents the multiple testing threshold obtained considering the total number of performed tests (Number of variants × Number of covariates). Chromosomes over 22 represent sexual and mitochondrial chromosomes.

Overall, none of the variants reached significance beyond multiple testing thresholds, although, some suggestive variants were observed in chromosomes 2, 6, 10, 13 and 19 in the basic allele chi-square test and Fisher's exact test (Figure 2).

Interestingly, variants rs3130531, rs7772901, rs73115241, rs386580033 and rs529060937 were among the top 20 variants for all the three different applied association tests; moreover 17 over the 20 SNPs listed in Table 4 were also represented in Table 4 meaning that a basic allele chi-square test and Fisher's exact test produced very similar results. Covariates analyses in a regression model did not provided any significant result. Table 4 shows further information of the five relevant variants.

Table 4. Genetic information of the five relevant variants.

SNP	Gene	Function	Probeset ID	Genotype Category
rs3130531		intergenic	AX-11435435	PolyHighResolution
rs7772901	PDE10A	intron variant	AX-11644567	PolyHighResolution
rs73115241		intergenic	AX-13511810	PolyHighResolution
rs386580033	PSORS1C1	intron variant	AX-35729741	PolyHighResolution
rs529060937	PSORS1C1	intron variant	AX-35729743	PolyHighResolution

4. Discussion

AI-MD is a common and clinically relevant condition that should be better characterized to improve its diagnosis and adequate treatment. This study has found clinical and biological features that may help physicians in differentiating AI-MD from primary MD and improve the knowledge about their etiopathology and also, its therapeutic approach. Clinical differences were found mainly in family history of diseases; criteria used for depression diagnosis, lifetime traumatic stressors and medical comorbidities. However, non-genetic differences were found.

AI-MD patients showed greater alcohol use and a family history of other substances use disorders, whilst in contrast, MD patients showed greater family history of depression. Interestingly, AI-MD patients showed greater lifetime stressors events such as physical abuse, childhood abuse, intimate partner violence, etc. These findings are consistent with other animal and human studies reporting an association between traumatic events and SUDs [63–67]. Furthermore, as expected, AI-MD showed more medical comorbidity possibly by the effects related to the alcohol use, and its toxicity [68]. Finally, overall, personality dimensions and traits did not show large differences between groups.

We identified some further differences in the criteria used to diagnose MD according to DSM-IV-TR [69]. We only found differences in four of the nine criterions used to diagnose depression. AI-MD patients met with more frequency the criteria related to changes in weight. The high medical comorbidity found among AI-MD patients may explain this significant difference related to weight criteria [70,71] although we have not detected this association in our sample. Other authors have found different criteria between Primary and Induced depression associated with cocaine use disorder [72]; however, these authors found more "weight changes" in the primary depression group compared to induced depression group. In contrast, Primary MD patients met more criteria related to anhedonia, loss of concentration and recurrent thoughts of death. Our results are not according to other studies and show that depressive co-morbidity in patients with AUD may thus be characterized by more pronounced levels of anhedonia, as compared to other symptom domains of depression [73]. Animal and human studies were the focus in the paper of anhedonia as a transdiagnostic symptom. Anhedonia is a core symptom in depression and it is also involved in addictive disorders [74]. In this sense, dysregulation of the reward system and alterations in ventral extrapyramidal circuits were described in both disorders [75,76]. These findings imply acute dysfunction within mesolimbic dopamine pathways, although the cause of such alterations is unclear [77].

The differences in the blood test in terms of liver enzymes having a greater prevalence of abnormal results in the AI-MD group, in the same line as the severe medical condition, were expected due to the well recognized association between alcohol use and liver disease (for review Fuster and Samet, 2018) [78], ranging from steatosis to cirrhosis and liver cancer. A relationship between liver disease, AUD and depressive symptoms has also been described [79]; the underlying mechanism could be associated with inflammatory processes that are worsened by alcohol consumption [80]. Finally, animal and human studies have described an association between changes in the hypothalamus–pituitary–thyroid (HPT) axis and AUD [81]; these changes seems to normalize after detoxification [82,83]. The mechanism that has been related with changes in TSH levels is that alcohol could affect the feedback inhibition of the thyroid hormones by having a direct toxic effect on the thyroid gland and a compensatory increase in the thyroid release hormone secretion.

Regarding GWAS findings, single variant association analysis did not produce any significant result nor when including clinical covariates (jointly, separately or combinations of them). Nevertheless, some suggestive variants were identified: 5 SNPs having the lowest P-values for the 3 types of statistical analysis were: rs3130531, rs7772901, rs73115241, rs386580033 and rs529060937. As far as we know, none of those SNPs have been previously associated to depression, nor alcohol use disorder. For the rs3130531, the T allele was more prevalent in the AI-MD group compared to Primary MD group of patients. This SNP has been implicated in somatic illness as rheumatoid arthritis [84] and diabetes [85], but at this moment, no association has been described previously with depression nor AUD. The rs73115241 is an intergenic variant, located in Chromosome 20 with no currently known function. The T allele was more prevalent in the AI-MD group compared to the Primary MD group. The rs7772901, is an intronic variant; in our sample, the C allele was more prevalent in the AI-MD group than in the Primary MD group of patients. Finally, rs386580033 and rs529060937 correspond both to intronic variants, probably with a regulatory function. In our sample, the A and the G allele, respectively, were more prevalent in the Primary MD group than in the AI-MD diagnosed patients.

Our findings have some limitations that should be considered. The main limitation is related to the small sample size and not having control groups to compare (healthy controls and AUD non-depressed controls). The analysis performed did not show differences in women, but this could be related with the sample size, which has made it not possible to study the effect of gender. Depressive disorders are more common in women than men, moreover, depression associated with addictive disorders (either primary or induced) is more prevalent in women with SUD than in men, and more frequent than expected in women without any SUD [86]. Differences have also been found in clinical presentation and some neurobiological markers [87]. A bigger sample size could help to detect gender differences. Furthermore, replication is required in an independent set of samples and/or using alternative and more complex genomic risk score methods. In addition, MD and AUD has a modest heritability, both are polygenic disorders meaning that many genetic variants have an individual small effect size. Finally, due to the effects of alcohol consumption in inflammatory pathways which also have been related with depression, it would be important to replicate these findings, comparing them with a group of AUD without any depression.

In spite of these limitations, the accurate process of phenotype and genotype of the samples is a strong point of the study. AI-MD has crucial implications for both prognosis and therapeutic approaches. In two previous meta-analyses of antidepressant treatments in comorbid depression with substance use, the lack of response to selective serotonin reuptake inhibitors (SSRIs) was explained by the possible confounding factor of the presence of substance-induced depression in the samples [17,18]. In this context, the distinction between Primary MD and AI-MD might be crucial to improve treatment strategies and outcomes. To date, the diagnosis is based on clinical criteria (using DSM-5 (American Psychiatric Association 2013) or ICD-10 (Organización Mundial de la Salud 2000)) but there is still a need for specific biomarkers to facilitate the identification of AI-MD to improve diagnosis and clinical management. In this sense, genetic studies including expression studies, pharmacogenomics and epigenetics can improve the diagnosis, therapeutic approach and prognosis of these prevalent diseases.

5. Conclusions

This preliminary study has found clinical and biological features that may help physicians in differentiating AI-MD from primary MD. These results will facilitate future studies to increase the knowledge about their etiopathology and its therapeutic approach.

Author Contributions: Conceptualization, M.T., F.F. and J.T.; methodology M.T., F.F. and J.T.; software, A.F., J.T., N.S. and M.A.-F.; validation, A.F., J.T., N.S. and M.A.-F.; formal analysis, A.F., J.T., N.S. and M.A.-F.; investigation A.F., J.T. and M.A.-F.; resources A.F., J.T. and M.A.-F.; data curation, A.F., J.T., N.S. and M.A.-F.; writing—original draft preparation, A.F.; writing—review and editing, M.T., F.F., N.S. and A.F.; visualization, A.F.; supervision, M.T. and F.F.; project administration, M.T., F.F. and J.T.; funding acquisition, M.T., F.F. and J.T. All authors have read and agreed to the published version of the manuscript.

Funding: This project has received funding from the European Union's Horizon 2020 research and innovation programme 2014–2020 under Grant Agreement No. 634143 (MedBioinformatics) and ISCIII-Red de Trastornos Adictivos-RTA-FEDER (RD12/0028/0009 and RD16/0017/0010). Acció instrumental d'Intensificació de Professionals de la Salut—Facultatius especialistes (PERIS: SLT006/17/00014).

Acknowledgments: We would like to thank E.M., M.P., C.G. and the CAS Barceloneta nursing for their valuable assistance throughout the clinical part of the study. The authors thank the participants and the psychiatry research support staff for their generosity and interest, which made this study possible.

Conflicts of Interest: The authors have no conflicts of interest.

Appendix A

For the purpose of this report, a table reporting those relevant differences (not achieving statistically significance) in allele frequency between the two groups were created for each test. The tables only contain those variants showing higher differences between groups. For each table we report different fields (columns) according to the specific test conducted. The psychical position (Pos) reported in the tables refers to GRCH 38 version from the Genome Reference Consortium. In Tables A1–A3 are listed the 20 SNPs showing the lowest p-values for basic allele chi-square test, Fisher's exact test, and logistic regression, respectively.

Table A1. Basic allele chi-square test.

SNP	Chr	Pos	Effect Allele	Alternative Allele	F_AI-MD	F_Primary MD	OR	p Value
rs73250026	6	165960669	G	A	0.35	0.01429	37.15	7.991×10^{-7}
rs12355672	10	123921288	A	G	0.3	0	NA	0.000001204
rs2602186	2	159271306	A	G	0.3421	0.01471	34.84	0.000001802
rs2245046	19	47858424	A	G	0.3684	0.02857	19.83	0.000002057
rs61955462	13	21009654	A	G	0.45	0.07143	10.64	0.000002643
rs76785029	12	94882905	T	C	0.3421	0.02857	17.68	0.000006816
rs77332950	6	162137147	T	C	0.375	0.04412	13	0.000008363
rs11163044	1	81002495	T	C	0.25	0	NA	0.00001147
rs61893521	11	76392642	A	G	0.425	0.07353	9.313	0.0000119
rs73124405	20	20515790	T	G	0.3421	0.0303	16.64	0.00001311
rs10839772	11	1850324	A	G	0.55	0.1571	6.556	0.00001524
rs3130531	6	31206616	A	G	0.7105	0.2794	6.33	0.00001749
rs116179105	2	19494199	A	G	0.2895	0.01471	27.3	0.00001855
rs7772901	6	165959846	C	A	0.475	0.1143	7.012	0.00002349
rs28504201	3	58573163	A	G	0.4	0.07143	8.667	0.00002465
rs73115241	20	38797004	T	C	0.425	0.08571	7.884	0.00002561
rs386580033	6	31091163	A	G	0.2	0.6176	0.1548	0.00002629
rs2771040	9	108152199	G	A	0.4737	0.1143	6.975	0.00003021
rs529060937	6	31091197	G	A	0.2105	0.6286	0.1576	0.00003293
rs73485007	18	74495070	T	C	0.2778	0.01471	25.77	0.00003323

Notes: Chr: Chromosome, SNP: SNP ID, Pos: Physical position (base-pair), F_AI_MD: Frequency of this allele in AI-MD, F_Primary MD: Frequency of this allele in Primary MD, OR: Estimated odds ratio, P: Asymptotic p-value for this test.

Table A2. Fisher's exact test.

SNP	Chr	Pos	Effect Allele	Alternative Allele	F_AI-MD	F_Primary MD	OR	p Value
rs73250026	6	165960669	G	A	0.35	0.01429	37.15	0.000001416
rs12355672	10	123921288	A	G	0.3	0	NA	0.000001588
rs2602186	2	159271306	A	G	0.3421	0.01471	34.84	0.000003575
rs2245046	19	47858424	A	G	0.3684	0.02857	19.83	0.000004805
rs61955462	13	21009654	A	G	0.45	0.07143	10.64	0.000005148
rs77332950	6	162137147	T	C	0.375	0.04412	13	0.00001555
rs76785029	12	94882905	T	C	0.3421	0.02857	17.68	0.00001572
rs11163044	1	81002495	T	C	0.25	0	NA	0.00001807
rs386580033	6	31091163	A	G	0.2	0.6176	0.1548	0.00002548
rs73124405	20	20515790	T	G	0.3421	0.0303	16.64	0.00002572
rs10839772	11	1850324	A	G	0.55	0.1571	6.556	0.00002733
rs61893521	11	76392642	A	G	0.425	0.07353	9.313	0.0000293
rs3130531	6	31206616	A	G	0.7105	0.2794	6.33	0.00003134
rs137916	22	50491713	A	G	0.025	0.3529	0.04701	0.00003637
rs116179105	2	19494199	A	G	0.2895	0.01471	27.3	0.00003841
rs529060937	6	31091197	G	A	0.2105	0.6286	0.1576	0.00004234
rs7772901	6	165959846	C	A	0.475	0.1143	7.012	0.00005108
rs915476	17	32288009	C	T	0	0.2857	0	0.00005113
rs73115241	20	38797004	T	C	0.425	0.08571	7.884	0.00005121
rs17780066	13	78448090	T	C	0.2368	0	NA	0.00005933

Notes: Chr: Chromosome, SNP: SNP ID, Pos: Physical position (base-pair), F_AI_MD: Frequency of this allele in AI-MD, F_Primary MD: Frequency of this allele in Primary MD, OR: Estimated odds ratio, P: Asymptotic p-value for this test.

Table A3. Logistic regression.

SNP	Chr	Pos	Effect Allele	OR	p Value
rs73115241	20	38797004	T	14.1	0.00008067
rs6028915	20	38786218	C	13.63	0.0001002
rs9933149	16	87226206	T	0.06377	0.0001541
rs2162380	2	64556555	A	12	0.0002039
rs7772901	6	165959846	C	9.49	0.0002534
rs2301584	22	51171497	A	11.89	0.0003368
rs4876226	8	2059004	T	9.259	0.0004704
rs4876226	8	2059004	T	9.259	0.0004704
rs4876226	8	2059004	T	9.259	0.0004704

Table A3. *Cont.*

SNP	Chr	Pos	Effect Allele	OR	p Value
rs16843122	3	135278749	C	0.08456	0.0005255
rs4765145	12	124843104	C	0.05933	0.0005727
rs3130531	6	31206616	A	5.473	0.0005918
rs386580033	6	31091163	A	0.1706	0.0006138
rs7407243	18	70010868	G	9.425	0.000684
rs529060937	6	31091197	G	0.1759	0.0007074
rs4913427	12	68631620	T	0.1561	0.0007113
rs499691	6	32194339	T	7.06	0.0007266
rs1048677	17	3564716	G	7.575	0.0007284
rs6046396	20	19852503	G	6.717	0.0007339
rs34058147	13	75567543	G	0.1383	0.0007866

Notes: Chr: Chromosome, SNP: SNP ID, Pos: Physical position (base-pair), F_AI_MD: Frequency of this allele in AI-MD, F_Primary MD: Frequency of this allele in Primary MD, OR: Estimated odds ratio, P: Asymptotic *p*-value for this test.

References

1. World Health Organization. *Global Status Report on Alcohol and Health 2018*; Poznyak, V., Rekve, D., Eds.; Licence: CC BY-NC-SA 3.0 IGO; World Health Organization: Geneva, Switzerland, 2018; ISBN 978-92-4-156563-9.
2. WHO. *Depression and Other Common Mental Disorders*; WHO: Geneva, Switzerland, 2017.
3. Davis, L.; Uezato, A.; Newell, J.M.; Frazier, E. Major depression and comorbid substance use disorders. *Curr. Opin. Psychiatry* 2008, *21*, 14–18. [CrossRef] [PubMed]
4. Zimmerman, M. What should the standard of care for psychiatric diagnostic evaluations be? *J. Nerv. Ment. Dis.* 2003, *191*, 281–286. [CrossRef] [PubMed]
5. Boschloo, L.; Vogelzangs, N.; Smit, J.H.; Van Den Brink, W.; Veltman, D.J.; Beekman, A.T.F.; Penninx, B.W.J.H. Comorbidity and risk indicators for alcohol use disorders among persons with anxiety and/or depressive disorders Findings from the Netherlands Study of Depression and Anxiety (NESDA). *J. Affect. Disord.* 2011, *131*, 233–242. [CrossRef] [PubMed]
6. Melartin, T.K.; Rytsala, H.J.; Leskela, U.S.; Lestela-Mielonen, P.S.; Sokero, T.P.; Isometsa, E.T. Current Comorbidity of Psychiatric Disorders Among DSM-IV Major Depressive Disorder Patients in Psychiatric Care in the Vantaa Depression Study. *J. Clin. Psychiatry* 2002, *63*, 126–134. [CrossRef] [PubMed]
7. Karpyak, V.M.; Geske, J.R.; Hall-Flavin, D.K.; Loukianova, L.L.; Schneekloth, T.D.; Skime, M.K.; Seppala, M.; Dawson, G.; Frye, M.A.; Choi, D.S.; et al. Sex-specific association of depressive disorder and transient emotional states with alcohol consumption in male and female alcoholics. *Drug Alcohol Depend.* 2019, *196*, 31–39. [CrossRef]
8. Hasin, D.S.; Goodwin, R.D.; Stinson, F.S.; Grant, B.F. Epidemiology of Major Depressive Disorder. *Arch. Gen. Psychiatry* 2005, *62*, 1097. [CrossRef]
9. Hasin, D.S.; Stinson, F.S.; Ogburn, E.; Grant, B.F. Prevalence, Correlates, Disability, and Comorbidity of DSM-IV Alcohol Abuse and Dependence in the United States. *Arch. Gen. Psychiatry* 2007, *64*, 830. [CrossRef]
10. Kessler, R.C. The epidemiology of dual diagnosis. *Biol. Psychiatry* 2004, *56*, 730–737. [CrossRef]
11. Conner, K.R.; Pinquart, M.; Gamble, S.A. Meta-analysis of depression and substance use among individuals with alcohol use disorders. *J. Subst. Abuse Treat.* 2009, *37*, 127–137. [CrossRef]
12. Ehlers, C.L.; Gilder, D.A.; Gizer, I.R.; Wilhelmsen, K.C. Indexing the 'dark side of addiction': Substance-induced affective symptoms and alcohol use disorders. *Addiction* 2019, *114*, 139–149. [CrossRef]
13. Boden, J.M.; Fergusson, D.M. Alcohol and depression. *Addiction* 2011, *106*, 906–914. [CrossRef] [PubMed]
14. Lai, H.M.X.; Cleary, M.; Sitharthan, T.; Hunt, G.E. Prevalence of comorbid substance use, anxiety and mood disorders in epidemiological surveys, 1990–2014: A systematic review and meta-analysis. *Drug Alcohol Depend.* 2015, *154*, 1–13. [CrossRef] [PubMed]
15. McHugh, R.K.; Weiss, R.D. Alcohol Use Disorder and Depressive Disorders. *Alcohol Res.* 2019, *40*. [CrossRef] [PubMed]
16. Schuckit, M.A. Comorbidity between substance use disorders and psychiatric conditions. *Addiction* 2006, *101*, 76–88. [CrossRef]

17. Nunes, E.V.; Levin, F.R. Treatment of depression in patients with alcohol or other drug dependence: A meta-analysis. *JAMA* **2004**, *291*, 1887–1896. [CrossRef]
18. Torrens, M.; Fonseca, F.; Mateu, G.; Farré, M. Efficacy of antidepressants in substance use disorders with and without comorbid depression A systematic review and meta-analysis. *Drug Alcohol Depend.* **2005**, *78*, 1–22. [CrossRef]
19. Niciu, M.J.; Chan, G.; Gelernter, J.; Arias, A.J.; Douglas, K.; Weiss, R.; Anton, R.F.; Farrer, L.; Cubells, J.F.; Kranzler, H.R. Subtypes of major depression in substance dependence. *Addiction* **2009**, *104*, 1700–1709. [CrossRef]
20. Samet, S.; Fenton, M.C.; Nunes, E.; Greenstein, E.; Aharonovich, E.; Hasin, D. Effects of independent and substance-induced major depressive disorder on remission and relapse of alcohol, cocaine and heroin dependence. *Addiction* **2013**. [CrossRef]
21. Magidson, J.F.; Wang, S.; Lejuez, C.W.; Iza, M.; Blanco, C. Prospective study of substance-induced and independent major depressive disorder among individuals with substance use disorders in a nationally representative sample. *Depress. Anxiety* **2013**, *30*, 538–545. [CrossRef]
22. Conner, K.R.; Gamble, S.A.; Bagge, C.L.; He, H.; Swogger, M.T.; Watts, A.; Houston, R.J. Substance-Induced Depression and Independent Depression in Proximal Risk for Suicidal Behavior. *J. Stud. Alcohol Drugs* **2014**, *75*, 567–572. [CrossRef]
23. Foulds, J.A.; Adamson, S.J.; Boden, J.M.; Williman, J.A.; Mulder, R.T. Depression in patients with alcohol use disorders: Systematic review and meta-analysis of outcomes for independent and substance-induced disorders. *J. Affect. Disord.* **2015**, *185*, 47–59. [CrossRef] [PubMed]
24. Preuss, U.W.; Schuckit, M.A.; Smith, T.L.; Danko, G.P.; Dasher, A.C.; Hesselbrock, M.N.; Hesselbrock, V.M.; Nurnberger, J.I. A comparison of alcohol-induced and independent depression in alcoholics with histories of suicide attempts. *J. Stud. Alcohol* **2002**, *63*, 498–502. [CrossRef] [PubMed]
25. Schuckit, M.A.; Tipp, J.E.; Bergman, M.; Reich, W.; Hesselbrock, V.M.; Smith, T.L. Comparison of induced and independent major depressive disorders in 2945 alcoholics. *Am. J. Psychiatry* **1997**, *154*, 948–957. [CrossRef]
26. Schuckit, M.A.; Smith, T.L.; Danko, G.P.; Pierson, J.; Trim, R.; Nurnberger, J.I.; Kramer, J.; Kuperman, S.; Bierut, L.J.; Hesselbrock, V. A comparison of factors associated with substance-induced versus independent depressions. *J. Stud. Alcohol Drugs* **2007**, *68*, 805–812. [CrossRef] [PubMed]
27. Cohn, A.M.; Epstein, E.E.; McCrady, B.S.; Jensen, N.; Hunter-Reel, D.; Green, K.E.; Drapkin, M.L. Pretreatment clinical and risk correlates of substance use disorder patients with primary depression. *J. Stud. Alcohol Drugs* **2011**, *72*, 151–157. [CrossRef] [PubMed]
28. Tirado Muñoz, J.; Farré, A.; Mestre-Pintó, J.; Szerman, N.; Torrens, M. Dual diagnosis in Depression: Treatment recommendations. *Adicciones* **2018**, *30*, 66–76. [CrossRef]
29. Raimo, E.B.; Schuckit, M.A. Alcohol dependence and mood disorders. *Addict. Behav.* **1998**, *23*, 933–946. [CrossRef]
30. Muench, C.; Schwandt, M.; Jung, J.; Cortes, C.R.; Momenan, R.; Lohoff, F.W. The major depressive disorder GWAS-supported variant rs10514299 in TMEM161B-MEF2C predicts putamen activation during reward processing in alcohol dependence. *Transl. Psychiatry* **2018**, *8*, 131. [CrossRef]
31. Tawa, E.A.; Hall, S.D.; Lohoff, F.W. Overview of the Genetics of Alcohol Use Disorder. *Alcohol Alcohol.* **2016**, *51*, 507–514. [CrossRef]
32. Lohoff, F.W. Overview of the Genetics of Major Depressive Disorder. *Curr. Psychiatry Rep.* **2010**, *12*, 539–546. [CrossRef]
33. Bland, R.C.; Newman, S.C.; Orn, H. Recurrent and Nonrecurrent Depression. *Arch. Gen. Psychiatry* **1986**, *43*, 1085. [CrossRef] [PubMed]
34. Kendler, K.S.; Kuhn, J.W.; Vittum, J.; Prescott, C.A.; Riley, B. The Interaction of Stressful Life Events and a Serotonin Transporter Polymorphism in the Prediction of Episodes of Major Depression. *Arch. Gen. Psychiatry* **2005**, *62*, 529. [CrossRef] [PubMed]
35. Weissman, M.M. Onset of Major Depression in Early Adulthood. *Arch. Gen. Psychiatry* **1984**, *41*, 1136. [CrossRef] [PubMed]
36. Klein, D.N.; Lewinsohn, P.M.; Rohde, P.; Seeley, J.R.; Durbin, C.E. Clinical features of major depressive disorder in adolescents and their relatives: Impact on familial aggregation, implications for phenotype definition, and specificity of transmission. *J. Abnorm. Psychol.* **2002**, *111*, 98–106. [CrossRef] [PubMed]

37. Lyons, M.J.; Eisen, S.A.; Goldberg, J.; True, W.; Lin, N.; Meyer, J.M.; Toomey, R.; Faraone, S.V.; Merla-Ramos, M.; Tsuang, M.T. A Registry-Based Twin Study of Depression in Men. *Arch. Gen. Psychiatry May* **1998**, *55*, 468–472. [CrossRef]
38. Luo, X.; Kranzler, H.R.; Zuo, L.; Wang, S.; Blumberg, H.P.; Gelernter, J. CHRM2 gene predisposes to alcohol dependence, drug dependence and affective disorders: Results from an extended case–control structured association study. *Hum. Mol. Genet.* **2005**, *14*, 2421–2434. [CrossRef]
39. Wang, J.C.; Hinrichs, A.L.; Stock, H.; Budde, J.; Allen, R.; Bertelsen, S.; Kwon, J.M.; Wu, W.; Dick, D.M.; Rice, J.; et al. Evidence of common and specific genetic effects: Association of the muscarinic acetylcholine receptor M2 (CHRM2) gene with alcohol dependence and major depressive syndrome. *Hum. Mol. Genet.* **2004**, *13*, 1903–1911. [CrossRef]
40. Sjöholm, L.K.; Kovanen, L.; Saarikoski, S.T.; Schalling, M.; Lavebratt, C.; Partonen, T. CLOCK is suggested to associate with comorbid alcohol use and depressive disorders. *J. Circadian Rhythm.* **2010**. [CrossRef]
41. Tambs, K.; Harris, J.R.; Magnus, P. Genetic and Environmental Contributions to the Correlation Between Alcohol Consumption and Symptoms of Anxiety and Depression. Results from a Bivariate Analysis of Norwegian Twin Data. *Behav. Genet.* **1997**, *27*, 241–250. [CrossRef]
42. Nurnberger, J.I.; Foroud, T.; Flury, L.; Su, J.; Meyer, E.T.; Hu, K.; Crowe, R.; Edenberg, H.; Goate, A.; Bierut, L.; et al. Evidence for a locus on chromosome 1 that influences vulnerability to alcoholism and affective disorder. *Am. J. Psychiatry* **2001**, *158*, 718–724. [CrossRef]
43. Andersen, A.M.; Pietrzak, R.H.; Kranzler, H.R.; Ma, L.; Zhou, H.; Liu, X.; Kramer, J.; Kuperman, S.; Edenberg, H.J.; Nurnberger, J.I.; et al. Polygenic Scores for Major Depressive Disorder and Risk of Alcohol Dependence. *JAMA Psychiatry* **2017**, *74*, 1153–1160. [CrossRef] [PubMed]
44. Gelernter, J.; Kranzler, H.; Sherva, R.; Almasy, L.; Koesterer, R.; Smith, A.; Anton, R.; Preuss, U.; Ridinger, M.; Rujescu, D.; et al. Genome-wide association study of alcohol dependence: Significant findings in African-and European-Americans including novel risk loci. *Mol. Psychiatry* **2014**, *19145*, 41–49. [CrossRef] [PubMed]
45. Treutlein, J.; Cichon, S.; Ridinger, M.; Wodarz, N.; Soyka, M.; Zill, P.; Maier, W.; Moessner, R.; Gaebel, W.; Dahmen, N.; et al. Genome-wide association study of alcohol dependence. *Arch. Gen. Psychiatry* **2009**, *66*, 773–784. [CrossRef] [PubMed]
46. CONVERGE. Consortium Sparse whole genome sequencing identifies two loci for major depressive disorder. *Nature* **2015**, *523*, 588–591. [CrossRef] [PubMed]
47. Okbay, A.; Baselmans, B.M.; De Neve, J.-E.; Turley, P.; Nivard, M.G.; Fontana, M.A.; Meddens, S.F.W.; Linnér, R.K.; Rietveld, C.A.; Derringer, J.; et al. Genetic variants associated with subjective well-being, depressive symptoms and neuroticism identified through genome-wide analyses. *Nat. Genet.* **2016**, *48*, 624–633. [CrossRef]
48. Hyde, C.L.; Nagle, M.W.; Tian, C.; Chen, X.; Paciga, S.; Wendland, J.; Tung, J.; Hinds, D.; Perlis, R.; Winslow, A. Identification of 15 genetic loci associated with risk of major depression in individuals of European descent. *Nat. Genet.* **2017**, *48*, 1031–1036. [CrossRef]
49. Balliet, W.E.; Edwards-Hampton, S.; Borckardt, J.J.; Morgan, K.; Adams, D.; Owczarski, S.; Madan, A.; Galloway, S.K.; Serber, E.R.; Malcolm, R. Depressive symptoms, pain, and quality of life among patients with nonalcohol-related chronic pancreatitis. *Pain Res. Treat.* **2012**. [CrossRef]
50. Edwards, A.C.; Aliev, F.; Bierut, L.J.; Bucholz, K.K.; Edenberg, H.; Hesselbrock, V.; Kramer, J.; Kuperman, S.; Nurnberger, J.I.; Schuckit, M.A.; et al. Genome-wide association study of comorbid depressive syndrome and alcohol dependence. *Psychiatr. Genet.* **2012**, *22*, 31–41. [CrossRef]
51. Edwards, A.C. Challenges in the Study of Genetic Variants of Comorbid Alcohol Use Disorder and Major Depression. *JAMA Psychiatry* **2017**, *74*, 1193–1194. [CrossRef]
52. Zhou, H.; Polimanti, R.; Yang, B.-Z.; Wang, Q.; Han, S.; Sherva, R.; Nuñez, Y.Z.; Zhao, H.; Farrer, L.A.; Kranzler, H.R.; et al. Genetic Risk Variants Associated With Comorbid Alcohol Dependence and Major Depression. *JAMA Psychiatry* **2017**, *74*, 1234–1241. [CrossRef]
53. American Psychiatric Association. *DSM-IV TR. Manual Diagnóstico y Estadístico de los Trastornos Mentales*; Masson: Barcelona, Spain, 2002.
54. Hasin, D.S.; Samet, W.E.; Nunes, J.; Meydan, K.; Matseoane, B.A.R.; Waxman, B.A. Diagnosis of Comorbid Psychiatric Disorders in Substance Users Assessed With the Psychiatric Research Interview for Substance and Mental Disorders for DSM-IV. *Am. J. Psychiatry* **2006**, *163*, 689–696. [CrossRef] [PubMed]

55. Torrens, M.; Serrano, D.; Astals, M.; Pérez-Domínguez, G.; Martín-Santos, R. Diagnosing comorbid psychiatric disorders in substance abusers: Validity of the Spanish versions of the psychiatric research interview for substance and mental disorders and the structured clinical interview for DSM-IV. *Am. J. Psychiatry* **2004**, *161*, 1231–1237. [CrossRef] [PubMed]
56. Lobo, A.; Chamorro, L.; Luque, A.; Dal-Ré, R.; Badia, X.; Baró, E.; Lacámara, C.; González-Castro, G.; Gurrea-Escajedo, A.; Elices-Urbano, N.; et al. Validation of the Spanish versions of the Montgomery-Asberg Depression and Hamilton Anxiety Rating Scales. *Med. Clin.* **2002**, *118*, 493–499. [CrossRef]
57. Bonicatto, S.; Dew, A.M.; Soria, J.J. Analysis of the psychometric properties of the Spanish version of the Beck Depression Inventory in Argentina. *Psychiatry Res.* **1998**, *79*, 277–285. [CrossRef]
58. Beck, A.T.; Kovacs, M.; Weissman, A. Assessment of suicidal intention: The Scale for Suicide Ideation. *J. Consult. Clin. Psychol.* **1979**, *47*, 343–352. [CrossRef] [PubMed]
59. Hamilton, M. The assessment of anxiety states by rating. *Br. J. Med. Psychol.* **1959**, *32*, 50–55. [CrossRef]
60. Spielberger, C.D. Manual for the State-Trait Anxiety Inventory (STAI Form Y). 1983. Available online: https://doi.org/10.1002/9780470479216.corpsy0943 (accessed on 29 April 2020).
61. Cloninger, R.C. *The Temperament and Character Inventory (TCI): A Guide to Its Development and Use*; Center for Psychobiology of Personality, Washington University: St. Louis, MO, USA, 1994; ISBN 978-0-9642917-1-3.
62. Wolf, J.P.; Kimerling, R. PsycNET Record Display—PsycNET. In *Assessing Psychological Trauma and PTSD*; Wilson, J.P., John, P., Keane, T.M., Eds.; The Guilford Press: New York, NY, USA, 1997; pp. 192–238.
63. Kok, T.; De Haan, H.; Van Der Meer, M.; Najavits, L.; De Jong, C. Assessing traumatic experiences in screening for PTSD in substance use disorder patients: What is the gain in addition to PTSD symptoms? *Psychiatry Res.* **2015**, *226*, 328–332. [CrossRef]
64. Enoch, M.-A. The Role of Early Life Stress as a Predictor for Alcohol and Drug Dependence. *Psychopharmacology* **2011**, *214*, 17–31. [CrossRef]
65. Noori, H.R.; Helinski, S.; Spanagel, R. Cluster and meta-analyses on factors influencing stress-induced alcohol drinking and relapse in rodents. *Addict. Biol.* **2014**, *19*, 225–232. [CrossRef]
66. Reilly, M.T.; Noronha, A.; Goldman, D.; Koob, G.F. Genetic studies of alcohol dependence in the context of the addiction cycle. *Neuropharmacology* **2017**, *122*, 3–21. [CrossRef]
67. Gilpin, N.W.; Weiner, J.L. Neurobiology of comorbid post-traumatic stress disorder and alcohol-use disorder. *Genes Brain Behav.* **2017**, *16*, 15–43. [CrossRef] [PubMed]
68. Mannelli, P.; Pae, C.U. Medical comorbidity and alcohol dependence. *Curr. Psychiatry Rep.* **2007**, *9*, 217–224. [CrossRef] [PubMed]
69. American Psychiatric Association. *DSM 5. Manual Diagnóstico y Estadístico de Los Trastornos Mentales*; Masson: Barcelona, Spain, 2013; ISBN 9788498358100.
70. Calder, P.C.; Albers, R.; Antoine, J.-M.; Blum, S.; Bourdet-Sicard, R.; Ferns, G.A.; Folkerts, G.; Friedmann, P.S.; Frost, G.S.; Guarner, F.; et al. Inflammatory Disease Processes and Interactions with Nutrition. *Br. J. Nutr.* **2009**, *101*, 1–45. [CrossRef] [PubMed]
71. Swanson, G.R.; Sedghi, S.; Farhadi, A.; Keshavarzian, A. Pattern of Alcohol Consumption and its Effect on Gastrointestinal Symptoms in Inflammatory Bowel Disease. *Alcohol* **2010**, *44*, 223–228. [CrossRef] [PubMed]
72. Alías-Ferri, M.; García-Marchena, N.; Mestre-Pintó, J.I.; Araos, P.; Vergara-Moragues, E.; Fonseca, F.; González-Saiz, F.; Rodríguez de Fonseca, F.; Torrens, M.; Group, N. Trastorno por uso de cocaína y depresión: Cuando el diagnóstico clínico no es suficiente. *Adicciones* **2020**. [CrossRef]
73. Levchuk, L.A.; Meeder, E.M.G.; Roschina, O.V.; Loonen, A.J.M.; Boiko, A.S.; Michalitskaya, E.V.; Epimakhova, E.V.; Losenkov, I.S.; Simutkin, G.G.; Bokhan, N.A.; et al. Exploring Brain Derived Neurotrophic Factor and Cell Adhesion Molecules as Biomarkers for the Transdiagnostic Symptom Anhedonia in Alcohol Use Disorder and Comorbid Depression. *Front. Psychiatry* **2020**, *11*. [CrossRef]
74. Destoop, M.; Morrens, M.; Coppens, V.; Dom, G. Addiction, Anhedonia, and Comorbid Mood Disorder. A Narrative Review. *Front. Psychiatry* **2019**, *10*, 311. [CrossRef]
75. Batalla, A.; Homberg, J.R.; Lipina, T.V.; Sescousse, G.; Luijten, M.; Ivanova, S.A.; Schellekens, A.F.A.; Loonen, A.J.M. The role of the habenula in the transition from reward to misery in substance use and mood disorders. *Neurosci. Biobehav. Rev.* **2017**, *80*, 276–285. [CrossRef]
76. Becker, A.; Ehret, A.M.; Kirsch, P. From the neurobiological basis of comorbid alcohol dependence and depression to psychological treatment strategies: Study protocol of a randomized controlled trial. *BMC Psychiatry* **2017**, *17*. [CrossRef]

77. Felger, J.C.; Treadway, M.T. Inflammation Effects on Motivation and Motor Activity: Role of Dopamine. *Neuropsychopharmacology* **2017**, *42*, 216–241. [CrossRef]
78. Fuster, D.; Samet, J.H. Alcohol use in patients with chronic liver disease. *N. Engl. J. Med.* **2018**, *379*, 1251–1261. [CrossRef] [PubMed]
79. Le Strat, Y.; Le Foll, B.; Dubertret, C. Major depression and suicide attempts in patients with liver disease in the United States. *Liver Int.* **2015**, *35*, 1910–1916. [CrossRef] [PubMed]
80. Huang, X.; Liu, X.; Yu, Y. Depression and chronic liver diseases: Are there shared underlying mechanisms? *Front. Mol. Neurosci.* **2017**, *10*, 134. [CrossRef] [PubMed]
81. Aoun, E.G.; Lee, M.R.; Haass-Koffler, C.L.; Swift, R.M.; Addolorato, G.; Kenna, G.A.; Leggio, L. Relationship between the thyroid axis and alcohol craving. *Alcohol Alcohol.* **2015**, *50*, 24–29. [CrossRef] [PubMed]
82. Liappas, I.; Piperi, C.; Malitas, P.N.; Tzavellas, E.O.; Zisaki, A.; Liappas, A.I.; Kalofoutis, C.A.; Boufidou, F.; Bagos, P.; Rabavilas, A.; et al. Interrelationship of hepatic function, thyroid activity and mood status in alcohol-dependent individuals. *In Vivo* **2006**, *20*, 293–300.
83. Hermann, D.; Heinz, A.; Mann, K. Dysregulation of the hypothalamic-pituitary-thyroid axis in alcoholism. *Addiction* **2002**, *97*, 1369–1381. [CrossRef]
84. Lee, H.-S.; Lee, A.T.; Criswell, L.A.; Seldin, M.F.; Amos, C.I.; Carulli, J.P.; Navarrete, C.; Remmers, E.F.; Kastner, D.L.; Plenge, R.M.; et al. Several regions in the major histocompatibility complex copnfer risk for anti-CCP-antibody positive rheumatoid arthritis, independent of the DRB1 locus. *Mol. Med.* **2008**, *14*, 293–300. [CrossRef]
85. Nejentsev, S.; Howson, J.M.M.; Walker, N.M.; Szeszko, J.; Field, S.F.; Stevens, H.E.; Reynolds, P.; Hardy, M.; King, E.; Masters, J.; et al. Localization of type 1 diabetes susceptibility to the MHC class I genes HLA-B and HLA-A. *Nature* **2007**, *450*, 887–892. [CrossRef]
86. Farré, A.; Tirado-Muñoz, J.; Torrens, M. Dual Depression: A Sex Perspective. *Addict. Disord. Their Treat.* **2017**, *16*, 180–186. [CrossRef]
87. Labaka, A.; Goñi-Balentziaga, O.; Lebeña, A.; Pérez-Tejada, J. Biological Sex Differences in Depression: A Systematic Review. *Biol. Res. Nurs.* **2018**, *20*, 383–392. [CrossRef]

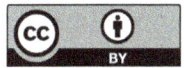

© 2020 by the authors. Licensee MDPI, Basel, Switzerland. This article is an open access article distributed under the terms and conditions of the Creative Commons Attribution (CC BY) license (http://creativecommons.org/licenses/by/4.0/).

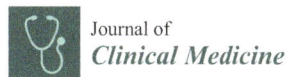

Article

The Tryptophan System in Cocaine-Induced Depression

Francina Fonseca [1,2,3,†], Joan-Ignasi Mestre-Pintó [1,4,*,†], Àlex Gómez-Gómez [4,5], Diana Martinez-Sanvisens [2], Rocío Rodríguez-Minguela [1], Esther Papaseit [3,6], Clara Pérez-Mañá [3,6], Klaus Langohr [5,7], Olga Valverde [8,9], Óscar J. Pozo [5], Magí Farré [3,6], Marta Torrens [1,2,3,*] and on behalf of NEURODEP GROUP [‡]

1. Addiction Research Group (GRAd), Neuroscience Research Program, Hospital del Mar Medical Research Institute (IMIM), 08003 Barcelona, Spain; MFFonseca@parcdesalutmar.cat (F.F.); roromin1@hotmail.com (R.R.-M.)
2. Institut de Neuropsiquiatria i Addiccions, Hospital del Mar, 08003 Barcelona, Spain; 98459@parcdesalutmar.cat
3. Department of Psychiatry and Department of Pharmacology, School of Medicine, Universitat Autònoma de Barcelona (UAB), 08290 Cerdanyola del Vallès, Spain; epapaseit.germanstrias@gencat.cat (E.P.); cperezm.mn.ics@gencat.cat (C.P.-M.); mfarre.germanstrias@gencat.cat (M.F.)
4. Department of Experimental and Health Sciences (CEXS), Universitat Pompeu Fabra, 08002 Barcelona, Spain; agomez@imim.es
5. Integrative Pharmacology and Systems Neuroscience Research Group, Neuroscience Research Programme, Hospital del Mar Medical Research Institute (IMIM), 08003 Barcelona, Spain; klangohr@imim.es (K.L.); opozo@imim.es (Ó.J.P.)
6. Clinical Pharmacology Department, Hospital Universitari Germans Trias i Pujol (IGTP), 08003 Badalona, Spain
7. Department of Statistics and Operations Research, Universitat Politècnica de Catalunya Barcelonatech, 08034 Barcelona, Spain
8. Neurobiology of Behaviour Research Group (GReNeC-NeuroBio), Department of Experimental and Health Sciences, Universitat Pompeu Fabra, 08002 Barcelona, Spain; olga.valverde@upf.edu
9. Neurobiology of Behaviour Research Group, Neuroscience Research Programme, IMIM-Hospital Del Mar Research Institute, 08003 Barcelona, Spain
* Correspondence: jmestre@imim.es (J.-I.M.-P.); mtorrens@parcdesalutmar.cat (M.T.); Tel.: +34-932483175 (M.T.)
† These authors contributed equally to this study.
‡ NEURODEP GROUP: Josep Martí Bonany (J.M.B.), Julián Mateus (J.M.), Paola Rossi (P.R.), Claudio Tamarit (C.T.), Gabriel Vallecillo (G.V.).

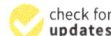

Received: 23 October 2020; Accepted: 17 December 2020; Published: 19 December 2020

Abstract: Major depression disorder (MDD) is the most prevalent psychiatric comorbid condition in cocaine use disorder (CUD). The comorbid MDD might be primary-MDD (CUD-primary-MDD) or cocaine-induced MDD (CUD-induced-MDD), and their accurate diagnoses and treatment is a challenge for improving prognoses. This study aimed to assess the tryptophan/serotonin (Trp/5-HT) system with the acute tryptophan depletion test (ATD), and the kynurenine pathway in subjects with CUD-primary-MDD, CUD-induced-MDD, MDD and healthy controls. The ATD was performed with a randomized, double-blind, crossover, and placebo-controlled design. Markers of enzymatic activity of indoleamine 2,3-dioxygenase/tryptophan 2,3-dioxygenase, kynurenine aminotransferase (KAT) and kynureninase were also established. Following ATD, we observed a decrease in Trp levels in all groups. Comparison between CUD-induced-MDD and MDD revealed significant differences in 5-HT plasma concentrations (512 + 332 ng/mL vs. 107 + 127 ng/mL, $p = 0.039$) and the Kyn/5-HT ratio (11 + 15 vs. 112 + 136; $p = 0.012$), whereas there were no differences between CUD-primary-MDD and MDD. Effect size coefficients show a gradient for all targeted markers (d range 0.72–1.67). Results suggest different pathogenesis for CUD-induced-MDD, with lower participation of the tryptophan system, probably more related to other neurotransmitter pathways and accordingly suggesting the need for a different pharmacological treatment approach.

Keywords: primary/substance-induced depression; cocaine use disorder; tryptophan; serotonin; kynurenine

1. Introduction

Major depression disorder (MDD) is the most prevalent psychiatric comorbid condition in subjects with cocaine use disorder (CUD), and its treatment constitutes a challenge [1]. In clinical practice, the co-occurrence of substance use hinders both the diagnosis of depressive symptoms and the differentiation between primary depressive and cocaine-induced episodes. Indeed, such a distinction could prove crucial in improving diagnostics and treatment, and therefore the prognoses [2,3]. Accordingly, there is a growing interest in putative biomarker research that enhances a better approach to this comorbid pathology.

Depression and substance use disorder (SUD) share some common neurobiological pathways [4] such as the monoaminergic, endocannabinoid and, inflammatory ones. Traditionally, the serotoninergic (5-HT) pathway has been the most studied in major depression, and there is clear evidence of its implication in the neurobiology of primary-MDD [5]. There are various models to investigate 5-HT pathways, including modulation of the tryptophan (Trp) system, which has been reported as playing a critical role in both the pathogenesis of depression [6] and SUD [5]. Trp undergoes two main metabolic pathways (Figure 1). On the one hand, by the subsequent action of tryptophan hydroxylase and aromatic L-aminoacid decarboxylase, Trp is converted into 5-HT. Reduced 5-HT synthesis and bioavailability due to the depletion of Trp (5-HT precursor) has been postulated as a tool to study MDD mechanisms and potential biomarkers. The acute tryptophan depletion test (ATD) is a standardized method of reducing brain 5-HT through the administration of large neutral amino acids (LNAAs). This limits the transport of endogenous Trp across the blood–brain barrier by competition with other LNAAs and subsequently decreases serotonergic neurotransmission. It has shown to be useful in studying the effect of 5-HT on mood [7–9]. After a depletion of Trp, and the consequent temporary reduction in 5-HT levels, a lowering in mood has been observed in patients with previous MDD history, but not in those without a personal or familial diagnosis of depression [10]. On the other hand, through the kynurenine pathway, Trp is transformed into kynurenine (Kyn) by the action of indoleamine 2,3-dioxygenase (IDO) and tryptophan 2,3-dioxygenase (TDO). The dysregulation of metabolites in both pathways has been associated with MDD. In this regard, a decrease in the synthesis of 5-HT has been linked to depressive symptoms, and a stimulation of IDO followed by an increase in Kyns can trigger depression [11–13]. Raised IDO activity has been associated with MDD [11,14–16]. Kyn has also been involved in several neuropsychiatric disorders, including depression and schizophrenia-like cognitive deficits (for a revision see Savitz et al., 2020) [17]. Many Kyns are neuroactive, modulating neuroplasticity and/or exerting neurotoxic effects in part through their effects on N-methyl-D-aspartate (NMDA) receptor signaling and glutamatergic neurotransmission. Their involvement in neuropsychiatric disorders is related to inflammation; this system has been described as being a regulator of the immune system. In addition, depression has been associated with inflammatory factors [18,19], for instance, increased levels of pro-inflammatory cytokines including interleukin (IL)-6, tumor necrosis factor (TNF) α, and IL-1β. Moreover, elevated concentrations of acute phase proteins have been reported in patients with MDD [20] and there are studies describing the response to immunotherapy in depression [21]. On the other hand, the Kyn system and SUD have not been researched as extensively as depression, although it has been observed that MDD could be involved in SUD mediated by the glutamatergic system. Kyn acid is an antagonist of the NMDA receptor, therefore increasing its concentrations has been proposed as a possible treatment strategy for the craving and relapse in alcohol addiction in animal models [22]. Although some authors have reported no significant differences in Kyn levels between MDD and healthy controls [23], it is generally agreed that higher Kyn levels are found in MDD subjects [24–26]. Methodological variations, as the type of sample or statistical analyses, could explain the differences found in the studies and reviews. The majority of studies are based on analyses that look for statistically significant differences in concentrations and ratios rather than effect sizes. Remarkably, Kyn levels have been observed to correlate with the addition of celecoxib, a cyclooxygenase-2 inhibitor, nonsteroidal anti-inflammatory drug indicated for the treatment of osteoarthritis and rheumatoid arthritis [27,28] in managing MDD [29]. They have also been described as predictors of acute responses to ketamine treatment for severe depression [30]. Despite the increasing evidence regarding the role of Kyn in MDD, no findings with respect to CUD and CUD-induced-MDD have been reported.

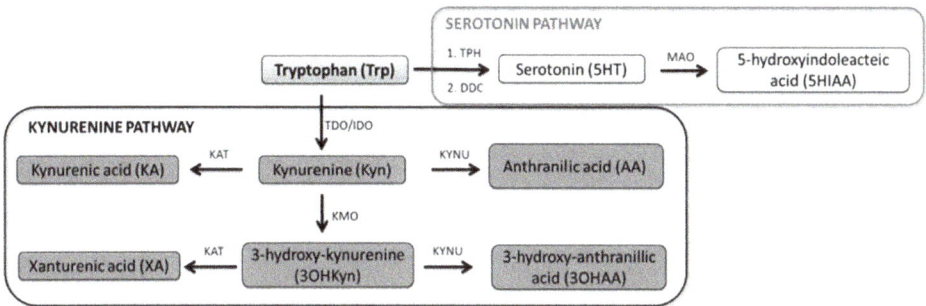

Figure 1. Tryptophan metabolic pathways. Metabolites involved in the tryptophan system including serotonin and kynurenine pathways. TPH, tryptophan hydroxylase; DDC, aromatic L-aminoacid decarboxylase; MAO, monoamine oxidase; IDO, indoleamine 2,3-dioxygenase; TDO, tryptophan 2,3-dioxygenase; KAT, kynurenine aminotransferase; KYNU, L-kynurenine hydrolase; and KMO, kynurenine 3-monooxygenase.

Furthermore, the 5-HT hypothesis in depression has been empirically confirmed through the use of selective serotonin reuptake inhibitors (SSRI), antidepressants that block the presynaptic 5-HT transporter and thus increase 5-HT concentrations in the synapses. When considering substance-induced MDD, however, this theoretical basis is less clear due to the lack of response to SSRI in comorbid MDD [31], suggesting the involvement of other neurotransmitter systems in the neurobiology of induced depression. Comorbid depression is one of the most relevant indicators of a poor prognosis in CUD patients, therefore providing effective treatment is crucial.

We have hypothesized that differences on markers of tryptophan pathways between cocaine-induced depression (CUD-induced-MDD), CUD-primary depression (CUD-primary-MDD) and MDD, are significant and of medium–large magnitude. To test this hypothesis, we have designed a study aimed at assessing the Trp system in both the 5-HT pathway, through ATD, and the Kyn pathway, in subjects diagnosed CUD-primary-MDD, CUD-induced-MDD, MDD, and matched healthy controls (HC).

2. Experimental Section

2.1. Subjects

A total of 35 subjects participated in the study. All diagnoses were performed according to DSM-IV-TR criteria [32]. Patients were recruited at the addiction treatment facilities of the Institute of Neuropsychiatry and Addiction at Parc Salut Mar in Barcelona (Spain).

HC were included from a database of healthy subjects willing to participate in medical research projects at the Pharmacology Unit of the IMIM-Hospital del Mar Medical Research Institute, Barcelona (Spain).

Inclusion criteria were: both genders, age > 18 years, Caucasian origin, and body mass index 19–29 kg/m^2. In the MDD groups (primary and induced), the most recent episode had to be in remission, and 17-item Hamilton Depression Rating Scale (HDRS) [33] score ≤ 6. In the CUD groups, subjects had to have maintained at least 4 weeks of substance abstinence prior to the trial as confirmed by detection in random urine controls.

Exclusion criteria included: cognitive or language limitations that precluded evaluations (based on the clinical criteria of the evaluators), pregnant or breastfeeding women, use of anti-inflammatory drugs or monoamine oxidase inhibitors (MAOIs), and any medical problem that could interfere in the study procedures. In the comorbid CUD and MDD groups: any psychiatric disorder in Axis I other than MDD, and/or any substance use disorders other than cocaine or nicotine. In the HC group: any psychiatric disorder in Axis I, family history of depressive disorder, and any substance use disorder (except nicotine).

The clinical protocol was approved by the local Research Ethical Committee CEIC-Parc de Salut Mar, Barcelona, Spain (2009/3494/I and 2012/4751/I) and the study was conducted in accordance with the Declaration of Helsinki and Spanish laws concerning clinical research. Volunteers were financially compensated. All subjects gave written informed consent prior to their participation in the study.

2.2. Clinical Assessments

A close-ended questionnaire was used to record patients' sociodemographic characteristics, family history, medical assessment, history of substance use, and previous psychiatric treatment. Depression severity was evaluated with the 17-item Spanish version of the HDRS [34].

2.3. Psychiatric Assessment

SUD and non-SUD were diagnosed according to DSM-IV-TR criteria [32] using the Spanish version of the Psychiatric Research Interview for Substance and Mental Disorders IV (PRISM-IV) [35]. The PRISM is a semi-structured interview designed to differentiate primary disorders, SUD, and the expected effects of intoxication and withdrawal when evaluating current and life-time DSM-IV-TR disorders. Diagnoses obtained through the PRISM interview have shown good to excellent validity and test–retest reliability for primary-MDD and substance-induced MDD [35,36].

2.4. Acute Tryptophan Depletion Test (ATD)

In one of the sessions, subjects were given an amino acid mixture lacking Trp. ATD-session: L-alanine 5.5 g, L-arginine 4.9 g, L-cysteine 2.7 g, glycine 3.2 g, L-histidine 3.2 g, L-isoleucine 8.0 g, L-leucine 13.5 g, L-lysine 11 g, L-methionine 3.0 g, L-proline 12.2 g, L-phenylalanine 5.7 g, L-serine 6.9 g, L-threonine 6.9 g, L-tyrosine 6.9 g, and L-valine 8.9 g. Non-ATD: L-Trp: 2.3 g was administered. The order of ATD and non-ATD sessions was randomly determined, and investigators and subjects were blinded to the amino acid content of the mixture.

Subjects were admitted to the IMIM Clinical Research Unit facilities at 08.00 after an overnight fast (from 21.00 h). The day before the experimental sessions they were required to follow a low-Trp diet [7,9] (see Supplementary Material). Subjects presenting nicotine addiction were treated during the experimental session with patches according to their nicotine daily dose. A urine sample was collected for drug testing (Instant-View®, Multipanel 10 Test Drug Screen, Alfa Scientific Designs Inc., Poway, CA, USA). Participants were required to be drug-free before inclusion in each experimental session. The capsules and amino acid drink with/without tryptophan were administered between 08:15 and 08:30. The subjects remained sitting/lying in a calm laboratory environment during the session, with restricted social interactions. Blood for platelet-poor plasma was obtained at different time points: basal and 5 h. It was collected by venipuncture in a 4 mL plastic tube containing EDTA and immediately centrifuged at $12,000 \times g$ for 10 min. The remaining platelet-poor plasma was divided into aliquots and stored at $-20\,°C$ until analysis.

After 5 h of the mixture intake, all subjects were given an enriched Trp diet (containing pasta, chicken, and banana). To control for undesired Trp depletion side effects (such as sustained depressed mood or suicidal ideation) patients remained on the laboratory premises until 17:00 and were requested to return 24 h after session commencement.

2.5. Selection of the Serotonin–Kynurenine Pathway Biomarkers

Markers belonging to the serotonin–kynurenine pathway were quantified by a previously validated method based on liquid chromatography tandem mass spectrometry (LC-MS/MS) [37]. Six markers of the serotonergic pathway were included in the present study. Plasmatic levels of 5-HT and

5-hydroxyindoleacteix acid (5HIAA) were measured and some amino acid ratios were calculated. Values of 5-HT/Trp and 5HIAA/5-HT were used to assess the enzymatic activity of tryptophan hydroxylase (TPH) and MAO, respectively (Figure 1). Kyn/5-HT provided information about the preferential pathway in Trp metabolism and 5HIAA/Trp was calculated as an indicator of the whole serotoninergic pathway. Additionally, seven markers belonging to the kynurenine pathway were evaluated. The plasmatic concentrations of Kyn, kynurenic acid (KA), and anthranilic acid (AA) were measured. The enzymatic activity of IDO/TDO, kynurenine aminotransferase) KAT, and kynureninase was established by the calculation of Kyn/Trp, KA/Kyn, and AA/Kyn ratios, respectively (Figure 1).

2.6. Statistical Analysis

A descriptive analysis of all variables of interest was carried out separately in each of the four study groups. For this purpose, the mean, median, standard deviation, and range were calculated. Repeated measures ANOVA models were used to analyze the changes after 5 h of both the tryptophan and the Hamilton Depression Rating Scale scores. The models included ATD and group condition as main factors as well as all two-way and three-way interactions and the computation of simultaneous confidence intervals and adjusted p-values to guarantee that a family-wise error rate of 0.05 was based on the multivariate t distribution of the vector of test statistics.

Concerning the targeted markers, given the skewed distribution of most them, these data were log-transformed prior to the inferential analyses. Next, 1-way ANOVA models were fitted to compare the study groups with respect to the mean of the log-transformed variables. The model assumptions (homoscedasticity and normally distributed residuals) were checked with residual plots as well as with the Levene test (homoscedasticity) and the Kolmogorov–Smirnov test, respectively. If assumptions held and group differences were statistically significant, the Tukey test was applied for the post-hoc pairwise comparisons. Otherwise, nonparametric analyses were carried out. For this purpose, the Kruskal–Wallis test was used to compare the study groups with respect to the median, and the post-hoc comparisons (if applied) were performed with Dunn's Test [38]. Cohen's d was used to quantify the effect size of the pairwise differences among study groups (small: $d \leq 0.20$; medium: $d \geq 0.50$; large: $d \geq 0.80$; very large: $d \geq 1.30$). Cohen's d is a standardized score, analogous to a z score. Following Cohen's effect-size conventions, only differences higher than a medium effect size ($d \geq 0.50$) were considered of relevance [39,40].

All data were analyzed using the statistical software R, version 3.4.3. (Vienna, Austria; http://www.rproject.org). In the case of the group comparisons, statistical significance was set at 0.05 (to protect against Type-I errors), and for model assumption tests at 0.1 (to protect against Type-II errors).

3. Results

3.1. Demographic and Clinical Characteristics

A total of 35 subjects were included in the study. The main sociodemographic and clinical characteristics of the sample are described in Table 1. The final groups were: 8 HC, 8 CUD-Induced-MDD, 14 CUD-Primary-MDD, and 5 MDD.

The groups diagnosed with primary depression had a similar age at the onset of depressive disorders, and the incidence of previous depressive episodes did not differ substantially among all groups. The CUD-primary-MDD group showed a highly prevalent history of family depression. The number of subjects under antidepressant treatment was lower in the CUD-induced-MDD group (37.5%) than the CUD-primary-MDD group (57.1%).

Regarding substance use data, there were no differences in the age of cocaine use onset. More than 70% of the sample of the CUD groups presented a nicotine use disorder, whereas the MDD and HC groups were non-smokers (Table 1).

Table 1. Sociodemographic and clinical characteristics of the sample at baseline ($n = 35$).

	HC $n = 8$	CUD-Induced-MDD $n = 8$	CUD-Primary-MDD $n = 14$	MDD $n = 5$
Sex (Male n)	5 (50)	6 (75)	12 (85.7)	5 (100)
Age (Mean ± SD)	32.13 ± 3.94	38 ± 12.17	44.21 ± 8.26	43.80 ± 13.9
Civil status (% Single)	62.5	62.5	35.7	40
Work status (% Employed)	25	37.5	50	40
Depression (MDD)				
Age of onset first primary-MDD (Mean ± SD)	NA	NA	34.29 ± 10.56	36.4 ± 11.97
Age of onset first induced-MDD (Mean ± SD)	NA	34.01 ± 12.47	NA	NA
Number of episodes (Mean ± SD)	NA	6.63 ± 8.23	2.08 ± 1.04	1.6 ± 0.89
Months since last episode (Mean ± SD)	NA	22.75 ± 31.23	36.29 ± 55	34.4 ± 40.9
Family history of depression (%)	NA	37.5	71.4	80
Current antidepressant treatment (%)	NA	37.5	57.1	100
Age of onset CUD	NA	26.75 ± 10.29	31.43 ± 7.39	NA
Age of cocaine problematic use	NA	26.38 ± 9.61	31.21 ± 7.43	NA
Maximum cocaine abstinence period (Months)	NA	19.50 ± 18.42	37.77 ± 54.17	NA
No. 1st and 2nd degree relatives with CUD	0	0	0.64 ± 0.93	0
Nicotine use disorder (%)	0	75	78.6	0

HC, healthy controls; MDD, major depression disorder; CUD, cocaine use disorder; NA, not applicable.

3.2. Acute Tryptophan Depletion Test (ATD)

Based on the repeated measures ANOVA model, except for the HC, the levels of Trp in all the ATD groups were significantly decreased in a similar way (Figure 2a). In the non-ATD test, there was a significant increase in Trp levels only in CUD-Primary-MDD between baseline and 5 h (Figure 2b). In the non-ATD session there was only a significant increase in Trp levels in CUD-primary-MDD group between baseline and 5 h (Figure 2d). Regarding HDRS scores, there were no significant changes between basal and 5 h in either session (Figure 2c,d). See Table S1 of Supplementary Material.

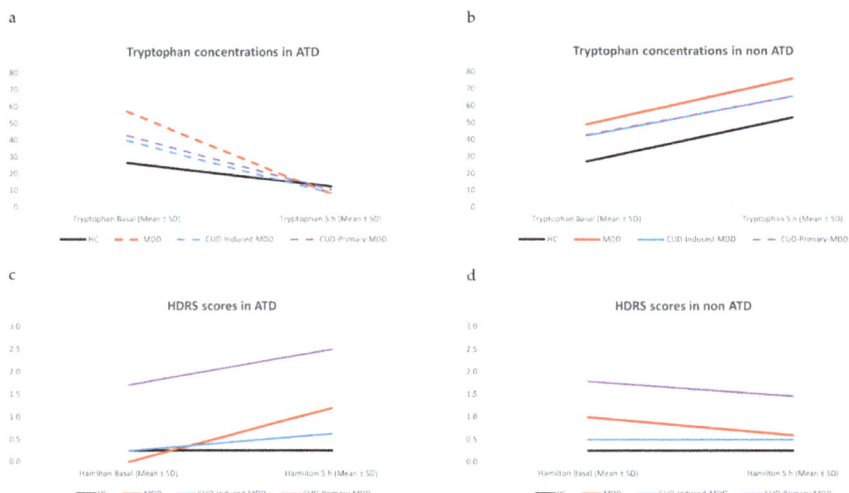

Figure 2. Variations in tryptophan concentrations and Hamilton Depression Rating Scale (HDRS) scores in both acute tryptophan depletion (ATD) and non-ATD tests. Dotted lines indicate significant changes (according to repeated measures ANOVA) between basal and 5 h follow up. 2a $p < 0.020$, 2b $p = 0.030$. (**a**) Tryptophan concentrations in ATD. (**b**) Tryptophan concentrations in non ATD. (**c**) HDRS scores in ATD. (**d**) HDRS scores in non ATD.

3.3. Kynurenine Pathway

As a first step, the basal values obtained for the 13 targeted markers (serotonin and Kyn pathways) in the HC group were compared with those in the MDD to select the most appropriate markers for MDD. Results for the values for each of the selected markers are summarized in Table 2.

Table 2. Basal values for the serotonin–kynurenine pathways (ng/mL for concentrations and adimensional for ratio values).

	HC	CUD-Induced-MDD	CUD-Primary-MDD	MDD
	n = 8	n = 8	n = 14	n = 5
Kyn	2716 ± 847	2971 ± 1171	3358 ± 894	4293 ± 1424
KA	247 ± 95	272 ± 135	304 ± 128	370 ± 205
AA	64 ± 23	79 ± 61	54 ± 32	32 ± 12
5-HT	729 ± 456	512 ± 332	521 ± 584	107 ± 127
5-HIAA	52 ± 14	87 ± 76	68 ± 21	75 ± 15
Kyn/Trp	0.016 ± 0.004	0.019 ± 0.006	0.021 ± 0.006	0.027 ± 0.015
KA/Kyn	0.093 ± 0.028	0.091 ± 0.026	0.094 ± 0.037	0.084 ± 0.021
AA/Kyn	0.026 ± 0.014	0.031 ± 0.023	0.016 ± 0.009	0.008 ± 0.004
KA/AA	4.2 ± 1.6	6.8 ± 7.3	9.4 ± 10.2	13.8 ± 9.4
Kyn/5-HIAA	56 ± 22	43 ± 17	58 ± 37	60 ± 16
5-HT/Trp	0.0042 ± 0.0022	0.0032 ± 0.0018	0.0031 ± 0.0033	0.0008 ± 0.0003
5-HIAA /5-HT	0.088 ± 0.038	0.26 ± 0.29	0.91 ± 1.12	2.08 ± 2.67
5-HT/Kyn	0.286 ± 0.188	0.183 ± 0.114	0.164 ± 0.184	0.027 ± 0.032
5-HIAA/Trp	0.00031 ± 0.00009	0.00053 ± 0.00038	0.00044 ± 0.00015	0.00043 ± 0.00014
Kyn/5-HT	4.8 ± 2.5	11 ± 15	44 ± 55	112 ± 136

Note: Descriptive data are presented as mean ± standard deviation (SD). HC, healthy controls; MDD, major depression disorder; CUD, cocaine use disorder; Kyn, kynurenine; KA, kynurenic acid; AA, anthranilic acid; 5-HT, serotonin; 5-HIAA, 5-hydroxyindoleacetic acid; Trp, tryptophan.

3.3.1. Controls vs. MDD

The main differences were observed in the plasmatic concentration of the two principal tryptophan metabolites, 5-HT and Kyn: the former was significantly decreased in MDD ($p = 0.006$) whilst the latter was found to be increased ($p = 0.042$) (Figure 3A,B). Differences were observed in 5HIAA/5-HT (marker of MAO enzymatic activity) and Kyn/5-HT (marker of the balance between both pathways) (Figure 3C,D). Both ratios were significantly raised ($p = 0.002$ and $p = 0.001$, respectively) for the MDD volunteers. No significant differences were reported for the rest of the tryptophan metabolites in either the 5-HT or Kyn pathways. Based on these results, 5HIAA/5-HT and Kyn/5-HT were selected as potential depression markers. The effect size coefficients of all these comparisons were large ($d \geq 1.24$) (Table 3).

Table 3. Effect size coefficient (Cohen's d) comparisons between groups in the four targeted markers.

		CUD-Induced-MDD (n = 8)	CUD-Primary-MDD (n = 14)	MDD (n = 5)
5-HT	HC (n = 8)	0.54	0.38	1.67 **
	CUD-Induced-MDD	—	0.02	1.47 *
	CUD-Primary-MDD	—	—	0.80
Kyn	HC	0.25	0.73	1.44 *
	CUD-Induced-MDD	—	0.39	1.04
	CUD-Primary-MDD	—	—	0.90
5-HIAA/5-HT	HC	0.83	0.91	1.24 **
	CUD-Induced-MDD	—	0.71	1.12
	CUD-Primary-MDD	—	—	0.72
Kyn/5-HT	HC	0.58	0.88	1.31 **
	CUD-Induced-MDD	—	0.73	1.22 **
	CUD-Primary-MDD	—	—	0.83

Cohen's effect size: small ($d > 0.20$), medium ($d > 0.50$), large ($d > 0.80$), and very large ($d > 1.30$). HC, healthy controls; MDD, major depression disorder; CUD, cocaine use disorder; Kyn, Kynurenine; 5-HT, Serotonin; 5-HIAA, 5-hydroxyindoleacetic acid. * $p < 0.05$ ** $p < 0.01$.

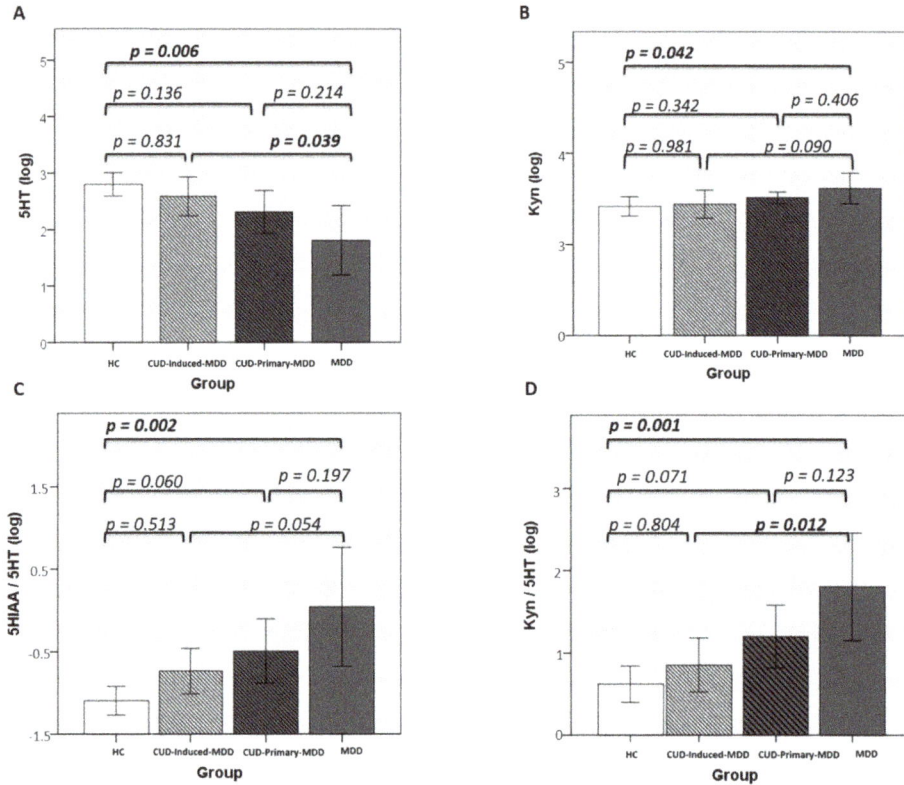

Figure 3. Variations observed in the four selected markers for the CUD-induced/primary depression groups compared with HC and MDD. (**A**) 5-HT, (**B**) Kyn, (**C**) 5HIAA/5-HT, and (**D**) Kyn/5-HT. Post-hoc comparisons were performed with Dunn's Test.

3.3.2. Cocaine Use Disorder Groups

CUD-induced-MDD showed a significantly higher concentration of 5-HT ($p = 0.039$) when compared with MDD levels, and a lower, but not significant, Kyn concentration was found ($p = 0.090$) (Figure 3A,B). The values of the ratios presented significant differences for Kyn/5-HT (increased in MDD, $p = 0.012$) but only a trend for 5HIAA/5-HT ($p = 0.054$) (Figure 3C,D). Remarkably, no significant differences were observed in any marker for the comparison between HC and CUD-induced-MDD.

CUD-induced-MDD showed large or very large differences ($d > 1$) when comparing all targeted markers with MDD (Table 3) in terms of magnitude of the effect. Additionally, CUD-primary-MDD presented medium to large differences from MDD ($d \geq 0.72 \leq 0.90$) when performing the same comparisons.

3.3.3. Overall Perspective

When looking at the results as a whole, with MDD group as reference, effect size coefficient shows a gradient where for all targeted markers the biggest magnitude of the effect is HC (d ranging from 1.24 to 1.67), followed by CUD-Induced-MDD (d ranging from 1.04 to 1.47), and ending with CUD-Primary-MDD (d ranging from 0.72 to 0.90).

Taking HC group as reference, the same gradients appear where largest magnitude of the effect is MDD (d ranging from 1.24 to 1.67), followed by CUD-primary-MDD (d ranging from 0.73 to 0.91), and ending with CUD-induced-MDD (d ranging from 0.25 to 0.83), except for 5-HT where CUD groups flip their positions (CUD-induced-MDD d= 0.54 and CUD-primary-MDD $d = 0.38$).

4. Discussion

The present study suggests a preservation of the Trp system in CUD-induced-MDD because its results are similar to the HC and significantly different from MDD in 5-HT and Kyn/5-HT. Furthermore, the results also show the already known differences between HC and MDD in 5-HT and Kyn values (and ratios). All this points to the existence of similar patterns in MDD and CUD-primary-MDD groups on the one hand, and between HC and CUD-induced-MDD groups on the other.

To the best of our knowledge, this is the first study to evaluate ATD in the CUD-primary/induced-MDD. In 1995, Satel et al. studied the implications of a reduction in Trp levels in the addiction symptoms of CUD patients, mainly referring to drug craving. They observed that following depletion there was a decrease in craving scores [41]. Cocaine craving, and the subsequent loss of control, is a key factor associated with relapse, and research has been carried out regarding the neurobiological mechanisms involved [42]. With respect to comorbid MDD, one study assessed the effect of ATD on depression scores depending on smoker status [43]. The authors proposed that, apart from 5-HT, other neurotransmitters could be involved, probably the acetylcholine pathway and receptors; however, they did not discriminate between primary and substance-induced MDD. Findings from the functional test follow similar trends when studying the biological markers.

Our results pose that subjects with CUD-induced-MDD present differences at the biochemical level when compared with MDD. Gradients showed by the effect size coefficients for all targeted markers suggest that biochemical alterations in both the 5-HT and Kyn pathways in CUD-primary-MDD resemble those observed in MDD. Moreover, the changes suffered in these pathways by patients with CUD-induced-MDD are less prominent and closer to HC values.

According to these results and previously published research [44] it can be presumed that the biochemical basis of induced-MDD differs from primary-MDD. The neurobiological basis for induced depression in CUD does not seem to be primarily mediated by 5-HT dysfunction and other neurotransmitter pathways may be involved. In this regard, research has presented promising results showing alterations in dopamine pathways [45], the cocaine and amphetamine-regulated transcript (CART) peptide [46], and neurotrophins [47]. Cocaine reinforcing effects are directly related to the dopamine concentration in the mesocortical system. As a result, the pathogenesis of CUD-induced-MDD could be associated with changes in the dopaminergic system, also associated with motivation and anhedonia [48] and with changes in Brain-derived Neurotrophic Factor (BDNF) signaling [47,49].

There are several limitations to this study. Firstly, the sample size was small for all groups; the strict inclusion criteria made it difficult to find pure cocaine/depressed only patients. For this reason, although our results suggest biochemical differences between MDD and CUD-induced-MDD, such findings should be confirmed by the analysis of a larger set of samples. A second limitation is that the MDD patients were under remission. Although this helped in the depletion test, it could have contributed to the moderate differences observed in some comparisons. It is expected that greater differences could be obtained in the analysis of some of these markers in patients suffering from moderate–severe depressive symptoms. Additionally, we cannot discard the fact that significant differences can be found for some additional biomarkers when analyzing samples from patients with depressive symptoms. Such could be the case of the ratio Kyn/Trp (targeting TDO and IDO activities) that has been reported to be increased in SUD patients with depressive symptoms [50], although no significant differences were found in our study. An added limitation which should be resolved in further investigation is the lack of an experimental group made up of subjects diagnosed with CUD without major depression disorder. Finally, the small sample size also hampered a proper evaluation of the effect of gender on the results. Although performing such studies based on the tryptophan depletion test would be difficult, the basal bioanalytical changes would allow detailed assessment of several aspects including gender effect. Depressive disorders are more common in women than men, moreover, depression associated with addictive disorders (primary or induced) is more prevalent in women with SUD than men, and more frequent than expected in women without any SUD [51]. Differences have also been found in clinical presentation and some neurobiological markers [52] including the Kyn pathway. For example, in a study in a Finnish population, IDO levels associated with depressive symptoms differed between the genders [15]. In this regard, we tried to minimize the impact of gender differences by performing the tests in all the women during their follicular phase.

Despite such limitations, results of this study indicate a different pathogenesis for CUD-induced depression. The participation of the Trp system varies and is probably more related to other neurotransmitter pathways. The lack of efficacy of SSRI in the treatment of dual depression, at least in CUD patients, and the efficacy of tricyclic antidepressants, is probably due to a greater range of neurotransmitters system effects through their mechanism of action [3,31]. Further studies are needed to confirm the role of the Kyn pathway and to explore other neurobiological systems in CUD patients with comorbid depression to improve treatment approach and prognosis.

The results of this study are a first step to the better knowledge of the differential mechanisms in primary and induced MDD. As previously mentioned, depression and substance use disorders represent 7% of the disease burden measured in disability-adjusted life years worldwide, they also contribute to general mortality with no contemporary decrease [53]. The joint presence of an MDD and SUD increases the severity of both disorders due to their high prevalence and poor prognosis [3,54]. Although induced MDD has been traditionally appraised as a minor condition that could improve spontaneously with substance abstinence, research has demonstrated that it could imply a worse prognosis for both affective and SUD [55]. Samet et al. (2013) [55] reported that patients with substance induced MDD showed a higher risk of relapse than those with primary-MDD. Moreover, longitudinal studies have reported that primary-MDD has been detected in patients initially diagnosed with induced-MDD [56]. Finally, there are treatment implications that could benefit from a thorough diagnosis of primary and induced-MDD as differential responses to antidepressants in both type of depression [57] have been described, with poor response to SSRI in the latter. Our results concur; CUD-primary-MDD showed a similar pattern of Trp system to MDD, and CUD-induced-MDD 5-HT and Kyn/5-HT were significantly different from MDD groups. Our hypothesis is that tryptophan metabolic pathways could be less involved in the pathogenesis of induced depression. Additionally, the kynurenine pathway can be useful as a biomarker in patients with any kind of depression; nevertheless, other neurobiological systems (dopamine, glutamate, endogenous opioid, and endocannabinoid systems) should be explored to define the pathophysiology of induced depressions.

5. Conclusions

The tryptophan system, including the serotonin and kynurenine pathways, might help in differentiating among primary-depressive episodes and those which are cocaine-induced in subjects with CUD. This differentiation could be crucial in improving treatment approach and prognosis.

Supplementary Materials: The following are available online at http://www.mdpi.com/2077-0383/9/12/4103/s1, Table S1. ADT tryptophan and Hamilton Depression Rating Scale scores, Appendix 1. NEURO-DEP Study diet.

Author Contributions: M.T. was the principal investigator of the grants supporting the research. M.T. and M.F. were responsible for the study concept and design. M.T., M.F., J.-I.M.-P. and F.F. designed the protocol. F.F., on behalf of NEURODEP GROUP, D.M.-S., C.P.-M. and E.P. selected the participants. J.-I.M.-P., R.R.-M., C.P.-M., E.P., on behalf of NEURODEP GROUP and M.F. conducted the ATD test sessions. À.G.-G. and Ó.J.P. performed the quantification of kynurenines analyses in human plasma. J.-I.M.-P. and K.L. performed the statistical analysis and F.F., Ó.J.P., M.F. and M.T. interpreted findings. F.F., J.-I.M.-P. and Ó.J.P. wrote the initial draft of the manuscript. M.T., M.F. and O.V. provided critical revision of the manuscript for key intellectual content. All authors have read and agreed to the published version of the manuscript.

Funding: This work was supported by grants from the Instituto de Salud Carlos III–ISCIII Red de Trastornos Adictivos 2016 (RD16/0017/0010, RD16/0017/0003; Fondo de Investigación Sanitaria (FIS) (PI09/02121, PI12/01838, PI14/00178, PI16/00603); National R + D+I and funded by the Instituto de Salud Carlos III (ISCIII) and the European Regional Development Fund (FEDER) grant Juan Rodes (JR 16/00020); Ministerio de Sanidad, Política Social e Igualdad, Plan Nacional Sobre Drogas (PNSD) (2012I054); Suport Grups de Recerca AGAUR-Gencat (2017 SGR 316, 2017 SGR 530); Acció instrumental d'Intensificació de Professionals de la Salut - Facultatius especialistes (PERIS) (SLT006/17/00014); and Ministerio de Economía y Competitividad (MTM2015-64465-C2-1-R). The funding agencies had no role in study design, data collection, interpretation, or had influence on the writing.

Acknowledgments: We would like to thank E. Menoyo, M. Pérez, S. Martin, C. Gibert and the CAS Barceloneta nursing for their valuable assistance throughout the clinical part of the study. The authors thank the participants and the psychiatry research support staff for their generosity and interest which made this study possible.

Conflicts of Interest: F.F. has received travel grants during the last 3 years from Lundbeck, Otsuka, Indivior, Pfizer, Gilead and Servier; she has also received grant/research support from Indivior and Servier. M.T. has been consultant/advisor and/or speaker for Gilead Sciences, Merck Sharp & Dohme Corp, Indivior, Mundipharma Pharmaceutics, Servier and Adamed. The authors declare no conflict of interest, and the funders had no role in the design of the study, data collection, analyses, and interpretation, in the writing of the manuscript, or in the decision to publish the results.

References

1. Pettinati, H.M.; O'Brien, C.P.; Dundon, W.D. Current Status of Co-Occurring Mood and Substance Use Disorders: A New Therapeutic Target. *Am. J. Psychiatry* **2013**, *170*, 23–30. [CrossRef]
2. Alías-Ferri, M.; García-Marchena, N.; Mestre-Pintó, J.I.; Araos, P.; Vergara-Moragues, E.; Fonseca, F.; González-Saiz, F.; De Fonseca, F.R.; Torrens, M.; Neurodep Group. Cocaine and depressive disorders: When standard clinical diagnosis is insufficient. *Adicciones* **2020**, *6*, 1321. [CrossRef]
3. Muñoz, J.T.; Farré, A.; Mestre-Pintó, J.; Szerman, N.; Torrens, M. Dual diagnosis in Depression: Treatment recommendations. *Adicciones* **2017**, *30*, 66–76. [CrossRef]
4. Gómez-Coronado, N.; Sethi, R.; Bortolasci, C.C.; Arancini, L.; Berk, M.; Dodd, S. A review of the neurobiological underpinning of comorbid substance use and mood disorders. *J. Affect. Disord.* **2018**, *241*, 388–401. [CrossRef]
5. Müller, C.P.; Homberg, J.R. The role of serotonin in drug use and addiction. *Behav. Brain Res.* **2015**, *277*, 146–192. [CrossRef]
6. Dell'Osso, L.; Carmassi, C.; Mucci, F.; Marazziti, D. Depression, Serotonin and Tryptophan. *Curr. Pharm. Des.* **2016**, *22*, 949–954. [CrossRef]
7. Delgado, P.L.; Charney, D.S.; Price, L.H.; Aghajanian, G.K.; Landis, H.; Heninger, G.R. Serotonin Function and the Mechanism of Antidepressant Action. Reversal of antidepressant-induced remission by rapid depletion of plasma tryptophan. *Arch. Gen. Psychiatry* **1990**, *47*, 411–418. [CrossRef]
8. Toker, L.; Amar, S.; Bersudsky, Y.; Benjamin, J.; Klein, E. The biology of tryptophan depletion and mood disorders. *Isr. J. Psychiatry Relat. Sci.* **2010**, *47*, 46–55.
9. Young, S.N. Acute tryptophan depletion in humans: A review of theoretical, practical and ethical aspects. *J. Psychiatry Neurosci.* **2013**, *38*, 294–305. [CrossRef]
10. Ruhé, H.G.; Mason, N.S.; Schene, A.H. Mood is indirectly related to serotonin, norepinephrine and dopamine levels in humans: A meta-analysis of monoamine depletion studies. *Mol. Psychiatry* **2007**, *12*, 331–359. [CrossRef]
11. Oxenkrug, G.F. Tryptophan kynurenine metabolism as a common mediator of genetic and environmental impacts in major depressive disorder: The serotonin hypothesis revisited 40 years later. *Isr. J. Psychiatry Relat. Sci.* **2010**, *47*, 56–63. [CrossRef] [PubMed]
12. Ogyu, K.; Kubo, K.; Noda, Y.; Iwata, Y.; Tsugawa, S.; Omura, Y.; Wada, M.; Tarumi, R.; Plitman, E.; Moriguchi, S.; et al. Kynurenine pathway in depression: A systematic review and meta-analysis. *Neurosci. Biobehav. Rev.* **2018**, *90*, 16–25. [CrossRef] [PubMed]
13. Savitz, J. Role of Kynurenine Metabolism Pathway Activation in Major Depressive Disorders. *Curr. Top. Behav. Neurosci.* **2017**, *31*, 249–267. [CrossRef]
14. Dantzer, R.; O'Connor, J.C.; Freund, G.G.; Johnson, R.W.; Kelley, K.W. From inflammation to sickness and depression: When the immune system subjugates the brain. *Nat. Rev. Neurosci.* **2008**, *9*, 46–56. [CrossRef]

15. Elovainio, M.; Hurme, M.; Jokela, M.; Pulkki-Råback, L.; Kivimäki, M.; Hintsanen, M.; Hintsa, T.; Lehtimäki, T.; Viikari, J.; Raitakari, O.T.; et al. Indoleamine 2,3-Dioxygenase Activation and Depressive Symptoms: Results from the Young Finns Study. *Psychosom. Med.* **2012**, *74*, 675–681. [CrossRef]
16. Barreto, F.S.; Filho, A.J.C.; De Araújo, M.C.; De Moraes, M.O.; De Moraes, M.E.; Maes, M.; De Lucena, D.F.; Macedo, D.S. Tryptophan catabolites along the indoleamine 2,3-dioxygenase pathway as a biological link between depression and cancer. *Behav. Pharmacol.* **2018**, *29*, 165–180. [CrossRef]
17. Savitz, J. The kynurenine pathway: A finger in every pie. *Mol. Psychiatry* **2020**, *25*, 131–147. [CrossRef]
18. Miller, A.H.; Raison, C.L. The role of inflammation in depression: From evolutionary imperative to modern treatment target. *Nat. Rev. Immunol.* **2016**, *16*, 22–34. [CrossRef]
19. Kowalczyk, M.; Szemraj, J.; Bliźniewska, K.; Maes, M.; Berk, M.; Su, K.-P.; Gałecki, P. An immune gate of depression – Early neuroimmune development in the formation of the underlying depressive disorder. *Pharmacol. Rep.* **2019**, *71*, 1299–1307. [CrossRef]
20. Maes, M. Depression is an inflammatory disease, but cell-mediated immune activation is the key component of depression. *Prog. Neuro-Psychopharmacol. Biol. Psychiatry* **2011**, *35*, 664–675. [CrossRef]
21. Roman, M.; Irwin, M.R. Novel neuroimmunologic therapeutics in depression: A clinical perspective on what we know so far. *Brain Behav. Immun.* **2020**, *83*, 7–21. [CrossRef] [PubMed]
22. Vengeliene, V.; Cannella, N.; Takahashi, T.T.; Spanagel, R. Metabolic shift of the kynurenine pathway impairs alcohol and cocaine seeking and relapse. *Psychopharmacology* **2016**, *233*, 3449–3459. [CrossRef] [PubMed]
23. Quak, J.; Doornbos, B.; Roest, A.M.; Duivis, H.E.; Vogelzangs, N.; Nolen, W.A.; Penninx, B.W.; Kema, I.P.; De Jonge, P. Does tryptophan degradation along the kynurenine pathway mediate the association between pro-inflammatory immune activity and depressive symptoms? *Psychoneuroendocrinology* **2014**, *45*, 202–210. [CrossRef] [PubMed]
24. Sublette, M.E.; Galfalvy, H.C.; Fuchs, D.; Lapidus, M.; Grunebaum, M.F.; Oquendo, M.A.; Mann, J.J.; Postolache, T.T. Plasma kynurenine levels are elevated in suicide attempters with major depressive disorder. *Brain Behav. Immun.* **2011**, *25*, 1272–1278. [CrossRef] [PubMed]
25. Oxenkrug, G.F. Serotonin-Kynurenine Hypothesis of Depression: Historical Overview and Recent Developments. *Curr. Drug Targets* **2013**, *14*, 514–521. [CrossRef] [PubMed]
26. Réus, G.Z.; Jansen, K.; Titus, S.; Carvalho, A.F.; Gabbay, V.; Quevedo, J. Kynurenine pathway dysfunction in the pathophysiology and treatment of depression: Evidences from animal and human studies. *J. Psychiatr. Res.* **2015**, *68*, 316–328. [CrossRef] [PubMed]
27. Fidahic, M.; Kadic, A.J.; Radic, M.; Puljak, L. Celecoxib for rheumatoid arthritis. *Cochrane Database Syst. Rev.* **2017**, *6*, CD012095. [CrossRef]
28. Puljak, L.; Marin, A.; Vrdoljak, D.; Markotic, F.; Utrobicic, A.; Tugwell, P. Celecoxib for osteoarthritis. *Cochrane Database Syst. Rev.* **2017**, *5*, CD009865. [CrossRef]
29. Krause, D.; Myint, A.-M.; Schuett, C.; Musil, R.; Dehning, S.; Cerovecki, A.; Riedel, M.; Arolt, V.; Schwarz, M.J.; Müller, N. High Kynurenine (a Tryptophan Metabolite) Predicts Remission in Patients with Major Depression to Add-on Treatment with Celecoxib. *Front. Psychiatry* **2017**, *8*, 16. [CrossRef]
30. Zhou, Y.-L.; Liu, W.; Zheng, W.; Wang, C.; Zhan, Y.; Lan, X.; Zhang, B.; Zhang, C.; Xiang, Y.-T. Predictors of response to repeated ketamine infusions in depression with suicidal ideation: An ROC curve analysis. *J. Affect. Disord.* **2020**, *264*, 263–271. [CrossRef]
31. Torrens, M.; Fonseca, F.; Mateu, G.; Farré, M. Efficacy of antidepressants in substance use disorders with and without comorbid depression: A systematic review and meta-analysis. *Drug Alcohol Depend.* **2005**, *78*, 1–22. [CrossRef] [PubMed]
32. American Psychiatric Association. *Diagnostic and Statistical Manual of Mental Disorders*, 4th ed.; Text Revision (DSM-IV-TR); American Psychiatric Association: Washington, DC, USA, 2000; ISBN 0890423342.
33. Hamilton, M. A rating scale for depression. *J. Neurol. Neurosurg. Psychiatry* **1960**, *23*, 56–62. [CrossRef] [PubMed]
34. Bobes, J.; Bulbena, A.; Luque, A.; Dal-Ré, R.; Ballesteros, J.; Ibarra, N.; Grupo de Validacion en Espanol de Escalas Psicometricas. A comparative psychometric study of the Spanish versions with 6, 17, and 21 items of the Hamilton Depression Rating Scale. *Med. Clin.* **2003**, *120*, 693–700. [CrossRef]
35. Torrens, M.; Serrano, D.; Astals, M.; Pérez-Domínguez, G.; Martín-Santos, R. Diagnosing Comorbid Psychiatric Disorders in Substance Abusers: Validity of the Spanish Versions of the Psychiatric Research Interview for Substance and Mental Disorders and the Structured Clinical Interview for DSM-IV. *Am. J. Psychiatry* **2004**, *161*, 1231–1237. [CrossRef] [PubMed]

36. Hasin, D.S.; Samet, S.; Nunes, E.; Meydan, J.; Matseoane, K.; Waxman, R. Diagnosis of Comorbid Psychiatric Disorders in Substance Users Assessed With the Psychiatric Research Interview for Substance and Mental Disorders for DSM-IV. *Am. J. Psychiatry* **2006**, *163*, 689–696. [CrossRef] [PubMed]
37. Marcos, J.; Renau, N.; Valverde, O.; Aznar-Laín, G.; Gracia-Rubio, I.; Gonzalez-Sepulveda, M.; Pérez-Jurado, L.A.; Ventura, R.; Segura, J.; Pozo, Ó.J. Targeting tryptophan and tyrosine metabolism by liquid chromatography tandem mass spectrometry. *J. Chromatogr. A* **2016**, *1434*, 91–101. [CrossRef]
38. Dunn, O.J. Multiple Comparisons Using Rank Sums. *Technometrics* **2012**, *6*, 241–252. [CrossRef]
39. Cohen, J. *Statistical Power Analysis for the Behavioral Sciences*; Revised Edition; Academic Press: New York, NY, USA, 1977.
40. Sullivan, G.M.; Feinn, R. Using Effect Size—Or Why the P Value Is Not Enough. *J. Grad. Med Educ.* **2012**, *4*, 279–282. [CrossRef]
41. Satel, S.L.; Krystal, J.; Delgado, P.L.; Kosten, T.R.; Charney, D.S. Tryptophan depletion and attenuation of cue-induced craving for cocaine. *Am. J. Psychiatry* **1995**, *152*, 778–783. [CrossRef]
42. Volkow, N.D.; Fowler, J.S.; Wang, G.-J.; Telang, F.; Logan, J.; Jayne, M.; Ma, Y.; Pradhan, K.; Wong, C.; Swanson, J.M. Cognitive control of drug craving inhibits brain reward regions in cocaine abusers. *NeuroImage* **2010**, *49*, 2536–2543. [CrossRef]
43. Knott, V.; Bisserbe, J.-C.; Eshah, D.; Thompson, A.; Bowers, H.; Blais, C.; Eilivitsky, V. The moderating influence of nicotine and smoking on resting-state mood and EEG changes in remitted depressed patients during tryptophan depletion. *Biol. Psychol.* **2013**, *94*, 545–555. [CrossRef] [PubMed]
44. Keller, B.; Mestre-Pintó, J.-I.; Álvaro-Bartolomé, M.; Martínez-Sanvisens, D.; Farré, M.; García-Fuster, M.J.; García-Sevilla, J.A.; Torrens, M.; Fonseca, F.; Mateus, J.; et al. A Biomarker to Differentiate between Primary and Cocaine-Induced Major Depression in Cocaine Use Disorder: The Role of Platelet IRAS/Nischarin (I1-Imidazoline Receptor). *Front. Psychiatry* **2017**, *8*, 258. [CrossRef] [PubMed]
45. Gryz, M.; Lehner, M.; Wisłowska-Stanek, A.; Płaźnik, A. Dopaminergic system activity under stress condition—seeking individual differences, preclinical studies. *Psychiatr. Pol.* **2018**, *52*, 459–470. [CrossRef] [PubMed]
46. Meng, Q.; Kim, H.-C.; Oh, S.; Lee, Y.-M.; Hu, Z.; Oh, K.-W. Cocaine- and Amphetamine-Regulated Transcript (CART) Peptide Plays Critical Role in Psychostimulant-Induced Depression. *Biomol. Ther.* **2018**, *26*, 425–431. [CrossRef] [PubMed]
47. Pedraz, M.; Martin, A.I.; García-Marchena, N.; Araos, P.; Serrano, A.; Romero-Sanchiz, P.; Suárez, J.; Castilla-Ortega, E.; Barrios, V.; Campos-Cloute, R.; et al. Plasma Concentrations of BDNF and IGF-1 in Abstinent Cocaine Users with High Prevalence of Substance Use Disorders: Relationship to Psychiatric Comorbidity. *PLoS ONE* **2015**, *10*, e0118610. [CrossRef] [PubMed]
48. Cléry-Melin, M.-L.; Jollant, F.; Gorwood, P. Reward systems and cognitions in Major Depressive Disorder. *CNS Spectr.* **2019**, *24*, 64–77. [CrossRef]
49. Thomas, M.J.; Kalivas, P.W.; Shaham, Y. Neuroplasticity in the mesolimbic dopamine system and cocaine addiction. *Br. J. Pharmacol.* **2008**, *154*, 327–342. [CrossRef]
50. Neupane, S.P.; Lien, L.; Martinez, P.; Hestad, K.; Bramness, J.G. The Relationship of Alcohol Use Disorders and Depressive Symptoms to Tryptophan Metabolism: Cross-Sectional Data from a Nepalese Alcohol Treatment Sample. *Alcohol. Clin. Exp. Res.* **2015**, *39*, 514–521. [CrossRef]
51. Farré, A.; Tirado-Muñoz, J.; Torrens, M. Dual Depression: A Sex Perspective. *Addict. Disord. Treat.* **2017**, *16*, 180–186. [CrossRef]
52. Labaka, A.; Goñi-Balentziaga, O.; Lebeña, A.; Pérez-Tejada, J. Biological Sex Differences in Depression: A Systematic Review. *Biol. Res. Nurs.* **2018**, *20*, 383–392. [CrossRef]
53. Rehm, J.; Shield, K.D. Global Burden of Disease and the Impact of Mental and Addictive Disorders. *Curr. Psychiatry Rep.* **2019**, *21*, 10. [CrossRef] [PubMed]
54. Davis, L.L.; Uezato, A.; Newell, J.M.; Frazier, E. Major depression and comorbid substance use disorders. *Curr. Opin. Psychiatry* **2008**, *21*, 14–18. [CrossRef] [PubMed]
55. Samet, S.; Fenton, M.C.; Nunes, E.; Greenstein, E.; Aharonovich, E.; Hasin, D.S. Effects of independent and substance-induced major depressive disorder on remission and relapse of alcohol, cocaine and heroin dependence. *Addiction* **2013**, *108*, 115–123. [CrossRef] [PubMed]

56. Magidson, J.; Wang, S.; Lejuez, C.W.; Iza, M.; Blanco, C. Prospective study of substance-induced and independent major depressive disorder among individuals with substance use disorders in a nationally representative sample. *Depress. Anxiety* **2013**, *30*, 538–545. [CrossRef]
57. Foulds, J.A.; Adamson, S.J.; Boden, J.M.; Williman, J.A.; Mulder, R.T. Depression in patients with alcohol use disorders: Systematic review and meta-analysis of outcomes for independent and substance-induced disorders. *J. Affect. Disord.* **2015**, *185*, 47–59. [CrossRef]

Publisher's Note: MDPI stays neutral with regard to jurisdictional claims in published maps and institutional affiliations.

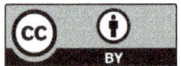 © 2020 by the authors. Licensee MDPI, Basel, Switzerland. This article is an open access article distributed under the terms and conditions of the Creative Commons Attribution (CC BY) license (http://creativecommons.org/licenses/by/4.0/).

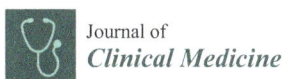

Article

Temperament and Character Profile and Its Clinical Correlates in Male Patients with Dual Schizophrenia

Laura Río-Martínez [1,2], Julia E. Marquez-Arrico [1], Gemma Prat [1] and Ana Adan [1,2,*]

[1] Department of Clinical Psychology and Psychobiology, School of Psychology, University of Barcelona, Passeig de la Vall d'Hebrón 171, 08035 Barcelona, Spain; laurario@ub.edu (L.R.-M.); jmarquez@ub.edu (J.E.M.-A.); gprat@ub.edu (G.P.)
[2] Institute of Neurosciences, University of Barcelona, 08035 Barcelona, Spain
* Correspondence: aadan@ub.edu; Tel.: +34-9331-25060

Received: 8 May 2020; Accepted: 12 June 2020; Published: 16 June 2020

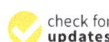

Abstract: Personality traits are relevant in understanding substance use disorders (SUD) and schizophrenia (SZ), but few works have also included patients with dual schizophrenia (SZ+) and personality traits. We explored personality profile in a sample of 165 male patients under treatment, using the Temperament and Character Inventory-Revised. The participants were assigned to three groups of 55 patients each, according to previous diagnosis: SUD, SZ- and SZ+ (without/with SUD). We analyzed their clinical characteristics, relating them to personality dimensions. The SUD and SZ+ groups scored higher than SZ- in Novelty/Sensation Seeking. SZ- and SZ+ presented higher Harm Avoidance and lower Persistence than the SUD group. SZ+ patients showed the lowest levels of Self-directedness, while SZ- and SZ+ had higher scores in Self-transcendence than the SUD group. Several clinical characteristics were associated with personality dimensions depending on diagnosis, and remarkably so for psychiatric symptoms in the SZ- and SZ+ groups. The three groups had a maladaptive personality profile compared to general population. Our results point to different profiles for SUD versus SZ, while both profiles appear combined in the SZ+ group, with extreme scores in some traits. Thus, considering personality endophenotypes in SZ+ could help in designing individualized interventions for this group.

Keywords: temperament; character; personality; substance use disorder; schizophrenia; dual schizophrenia; psychiatric symptoms; global functioning

1. Introduction

Personality can be broadly defined as the pattern of a person's thoughts, behaviors, and feelings in different contexts throughout their life. From a dimensional perspective, some research supports the existence of a series of features that follow a normal distribution along a continuum, whose extremes would imply some vulnerability for the development of psychopathology [1]. Studying the relationships between mental disorders and personality traits, as well as between the latter and the clinical characteristics of some disorders, can contribute to generating new approaches and tools aimed at the prevention and treatment of psychopathology from an individualized perspective [2].

On the other hand, substance use disorders (SUD) constitute a public health problem given their high prevalence and consequences on individuals, their environment, and society as a whole [3]. Schizophrenia (SZ) is one of the mental disorders causing the greatest deterioration and stigma [4]. Furthermore, there is a high comorbidity between SUD and SZ [5], with prevalence rates of SUD of around 50% among patients diagnosed with SZ or other psychotic disorders [4,6]. This condition, called dual schizophrenia (SZ+), is more prevalent in men, as is the case with other profiles of dual diagnosis (DD) [7,8]. SZ+ has aroused great interest due to its severity, since these patients present a worse clinical and sociodemographic profile [9–11], less adherence to treatment, worse therapeutic results [5,12], an earlier onset of SZ and of the SUD [13–15], more suicide attempts [16] and more violent behavior [17], when compared to patients with a single diagnosis. Furthermore, treatment of SZ+ patients involves significant difficulties associated with their own characteristics, but also with those of the healthcare system [18].

Although much of the research on personality in DD has followed a categorical perspective in the analysis of relationships between personality disorders and SUD [19,20], studying personality from a dimensional perspective has become relevant in understanding entities such as SUD [21,22], SZ [23,24], and DD [25,26]. However, there are few available papers addressing personality traits in patients with SZ+. Collecting scientific evidence regarding SZ+ patients is a complex process, and sometimes the data have been obtained by extrapolation from works analyzing either SUD or SZ- patients separately [27]. Among the available personality trait models, Cloninger's [28] stands out as a theoretically robust model based on a psychobiological perspective, and has been used in several studies with these diagnostic groups [29–31]. This model defines personality through individual differences in the adaptive systems that receive, process and store information. It is structured around two basic concepts: temperament and character. Temperament is characterized by those biological traits of personality with a larger genetic load, developing in earlier life phases, and remaining relatively stable through the life cycle. Character, on the other hand, is formed by those traits learned through experience, more related to social interactions and thus being less stable in comparison. In Cloninger's model, personality is understood as the result of the interaction between temperament and character.

Furthermore, the evidence points to some personality traits acting as endophenotypes or risk factors for SUD development, the most relevant being Impulsivity [32,33] and Neuroticism [22,34], although some works point to an interaction between Impulsivity and anxious personality [35,36]. Furthermore, Novelty/Sensation Seeking has also been consistently associated with substance use [37,38], and high scores in Impulsivity and Novelty/Sensation Seeking have been found to be associated with a higher number of relapses [39,40], more craving and greater severity of addiction [41,42], more risk of suicide [43], higher rates of abandonment of treatment [44] and worse therapeutic results [42,45]. Using Cloninger's model, SUD patients have scored lower in Self-directedness, Persistence, and Cooperativeness [38,44,46], low scores in the latter two being also associated with a greater probability of abandonment of treatment [47].

Research on personality has also highlighted the existence of possible endophenotypes for SZ, with Harm Avoidance, measured using Cloninger's model, receiving the most attention [29,48]. Some studies have found an association between high Harm Avoidance and an increased risk of suicide in stabilized and under-treatment SZ patients [49,50]. Thus, studies focusing on personality assessment following Cloninger's model point to a specific character and temperament profile made up of two components: the asocial component, characterized by high Harm Avoidance and low Reward Dependence; and the schizotypal component, characterized by high Self-transcendence, and low Self-directedness and Cooperativeness. This schizotypal profile has been proposed as a possible vulnerability marker for the development of SZ [29,31,51].

The scarce data published on SZ+ patients suggest that they have a character and temperament profile different from that observed in other groups with DD [25,30]. In some studies, the SZ+ group presented a profile similar to that of the SZ- group, but with higher scores in Novelty/Sensation Seeking [30,52], this trait also being associated with greater severity of addiction [9]. Moreover, increased Harm Avoidance was associated with the presence of more psychiatric symptoms in SZ+ patients [30]. Finally, the data point to the existence of a more marked profile in SZ+ patients when compared to those with SZ- or SUD, which worsens with age or time of consumption [52,53].

We consider that research on personality traits and possible behavioral endophenotypes is of special interest, since such knowledge can improve the design of strategies aimed at prevention as well as personalized interventions. For this reason, we decided to investigate the possible differences in temperament and character profiles among groups of SUD, SZ+, and SZ- patients under treatment, following Cloninger's psychobiological model, and then compared them with the corresponding normative data. In addition, we analyzed whether personality traits are associated with some clinical characteristics of these disorders. To our knowledge, this is the first work focused on studying the temperament and character profile in these three diagnostic groups, and one of the few that also analyzes their personality profile.

2. Experimental Section

2.1. Participants

The total sample of our study consisted of 165 patients, all of them males, assigned to three groups of 55 patients each, according to their previous diagnosis. All the participants were under treatment in different public or private centers in the province of Barcelona (Catalonia). In the SUD and SZ+ groups, abstinence was verified by urinalysis in the referral centers.

The inclusion criteria were: (1) male sex (given the higher prevalence rates of the diagnoses studied for this sex); (2) aged 18 to 55; (3) under treatment and stabilized; (4) with a SUD diagnosis in initial remission for the SUD and SZ+ groups, according to Diagnostic and Statistical Manual of Mental Disorders (DSM-5) criteria [54]; (5) with a diagnosis of schizophrenia for the SZ- and SZ+ groups, according to DSM-5 criteria [54]. The exclusion criteria were: (1) presenting a disorder induced by substance use or medical illness, according to DSM-5 criteria [54]; (2) not yet stabilized; (3) presenting any physical and/or mental condition that could affect either understanding or taking the tests.

2.2. Procedure

First, the reference professionals from the collaborating centers screened those patients who met our inclusion criteria. Then, we contacted each participant, provided more detailed information, and obtained their informed and signed consent. Participation in the study was voluntary, and the only compensation the participants received was an individualized return of their results. The Research Committee of the University of Barcelona approved our study (IRB00003099), which complied with the ethical principles of the Declaration of Helsinki [55]. A psychologist from our research team administered the assessment protocol in a variable number of sessions, depending on the state of each patient. The sessions included the assessment of other areas as part of a larger research project, with a total average of 4–5 sessions per patient. The research project, named "Psychobiology of dual diagnosis", aims to assess the genetic polymorphisms, neuropsychological functioning, circadian rhythmicity, and personality traits in patients with SUD, DD, and severe mental illness. As a comorbid condition, the DD and severe mental illness groups include SZ, bipolar disorder, and major depressive disorder.

2.3. Measures

2.3.1. Sociodemographic and Clinical Variables

For our study, we designed an *ad hoc* structured interview, in order to collect data regarding age, marital status, cohabitation, educational level, and employment situation, among others. In addition, through contact with the reference professionals in each center, we obtained information on the diagnoses, age of onset, family psychiatric history, suicide attempts, medical comorbidities, and relevant prescribed medication (the doses of antipsychotic drugs were converted to milligrams of chlorpromazine). Regarding substance use, we recorded the quantity and type of substances consumed, period of abstinence, and number of previous relapses. In addition, we administered the Structured Clinical Interview (SCID-I) for the DSM-IV [56] to confirm the diagnoses and complete the data collected. We applied the DSM-IV version of the SCID-I because, at the time of assessment, the Spanish version for the DSM-5 was not yet available. Additionally, we administered the Global Assessment of Functioning (GAF) scale [57] to assess each patient's general functioning.

We used the Spanish version of the Positive and Negative Syndrome Scale (PANSS) [58] to assess psychotic symptoms in the SZ+ and SZ- participants. This instrument provides scores on a positive symptom scale, a negative symptom scale, and a general psychopathology scale. Severity of addiction in the SUD and SZ+ groups was assessed with the Spanish version of the Drug Abuse Screening Test (DAST-20) [59]. This instrument provides a total score ranging from 0 to 20, with five cut-off points (0 no addiction; 1–5 mild addiction; 6–10 intermediate addiction; 11–15 high addiction; 16–20 severe addiction).

2.3.2. Temperament and Character Assessment

We administered the Temperament and Character Inventory-Revised (TCI-R) [60], based on Cloninger's personality model [28], to obtain the temperament and character profile of the participants in our study. This inventory consists of 240 items (5 of which are validity items) with a Likert-type response format ranging from 1 (false) to 5 (true), and offers direct scores and percentiles in seven dimensions. The four Temperament dimensions are Novelty Seeking (tendency to avoid routine and monotony, and to present a marked exploratory activity in the face of novelty); Harm Avoidance (tendency to experience negative affect, pessimism and behavioral inhibition); Reward Dependence (intense responses to rewards, including social rewards); and Persistence (persisting despite frustration or fatigue). The three Character dimensions are Self-directedness (ability to self-regulate and take responsibility for one's behavior according to interests and values, as well as to set goals for oneself); Cooperativeness (adapting to the social environment, being able to put oneself in the place of others); and Self-transcendence (tendency to spirituality and magical thinking). This inventory has previously shown good psychometric properties, and in our total sample the internal consistency was adequate for all the scales, with the following Cronbach's alpha coefficients: Novelty Seeking 0.745, Harm Avoidance 0.872, Reward Dependence 0.866, Persistence 0.893, Self-directedness 0.850, Cooperativeness 0.835, and Self-transcendence 0.825.

2.4. Data Analysis

Main descriptive data (mean, standard deviation or standard errors and percentages) were obtained for all the measured variables. For the clinical and sociodemographic data, we explored possible differences among the three groups with univariate analyses of variance (ANOVA) for continuous data, and with Kruskal-Wallis tests for non-continuous or categorical data. When the variables affected only two groups (data relating to SZ or SUD diagnoses), we applied the Student's t-test (t) if the quantitative data fulfilled the necessary conditions; otherwise, we used the Mann-Whitney U test. Chi-Square contrast was applied for categorical variables. Regarding internal consistency, we calculated Cronbach's alpha coefficient for the seven TCI-R dimensions.

We also performed multivariate analyses of covariance (MANCOVA), introducing the TCI-R dimensions as dependent variables, the group as independent variable, and age as a covariate, since it could act a confounding factor [61]. Post hoc comparisons were Bonferroni corrected to adjust the level of significance to the multiple comparisons made, and the partial squared Eta (η_p^2) statistic was used to measure the effect size, with the cut-off points being 0.01 (small), 0.06 (moderate), and 0.14 (large) [62]. Finally, we conducted stepwise linear regressions considering only the significant variables ($p \leq 0.05$) found in the previous bivariate correlation analysis performed between each TCI-R dimension and the clinical data.

All the data were analyzed using the SPSS software (IBM Corp, Armonk, NY, USA) for Windows, version 25, and tests were two-tailed with the type I error set at 5%.

3. Results

3.1. Sociodemographic and Clinical Characteristics

Table 1 presents the sociodemographic data for the three groups. Mean age for the total sample was 36.95 ± 8.09 years old. Most of the participants were single, lived in company, and were inactive from work; the average years of schooling for the total sample was 9.90 ± 2.23. We found differences in civil status between the SUD and SZ- groups ($p = 0.013$). In the SUD group, a higher proportion of patients were married or had a stable partner. Furthermore, this group presented a higher proportion of working patients than the other two groups ($p \leq 0.010$ in both cases).

Table 1. Sociodemographic data for the three groups. Mean, standard deviation or percentages, and statistical contrasts.

Sociodemographic Variables	SUD (N = 55)	SZ+ (N = 55)	SZ- (N = 55)	Statistical Contrasts
Age	35.78 ± 6.98	36.00 ± 8.19	39.07 ± 8.72	$F_{(2,162)} = 2.91$
Civil status				$\chi^2_{(2)} = 9.75$ *
Single	58.2%	76.4%	83.6%	
Married/Stable partner	25.5%	12.7%	9.1%	
Separated/Divorced	16.4%	10.9%	7.3%	
Living arrangements				$\chi^2_{(1)} = 2.16$
Alone	10.9%	7.3%	3.6%	
Accompanied	89.1%	92.7%	96.4%	
Employment situation				$\chi^2_{(4)} = 62.19$ ***
Working	30.9%	10.9%	9.1%	
Unemployment compensation	25.5%	5.5%	3.6%	
On sick leave	16.4%	7.3%	0%	
Disability pension	12.7%	61.8%	81.8%	
No income	14.5%	14.5%	5.5%	
Years of schooling	10.38 ± 2.20	9.62 ± 2.31	9.71 ± 2.15	$F_{(2,162)} = 1.94$

SUD: Substance use disorder; SZ+: Dual schizophrenia; SZ-: Schizophrenia; * $p < 0.05$; *** $p < 0.001$.

Regarding the clinical data in Table 2, we did not find differences among the groups in the presence of a family history of mental disorders, but there were differences in the family history of SUD, which were higher in the SZ+ and SUD groups compared to the SZ group ($p \leq 0.031$ in both cases). No differences were observed in the number of comorbid organic pathologies.

The SZ+ group presented a higher number of suicide attempts than the SUD group ($p = 0.011$), with no differences among the rest of the contrasts, although the SUD group had the lowest rate of previous suicide attempts. Furthermore, the SUD group presented a higher GAF than the two groups with SZ ($p < 0.001$ in both cases). Regarding medication, the SUD group had fewer prescribed drugs compared to the other two groups ($p < 0.001$ in both cases), with no differences between the groups with SZ. When we analyzed the prescription of antipsychotic drugs, no patient in the SUD group had received typical antipsychotics, and only 3.6% of these patients had received atypical antipsychotics. Thus, we found differences in the type of antipsychotic drug prescribed between the SUD group and the two groups with SZ ($p < 0.001$, in all cases), while there were no differences between the SZ+ and SZ- groups. However, when we looked at the doses of antipsychotics converted to milligrams of chlorpromazine (of which the SUD group presented a residual amount), the SZ- group had been prescribed almost twice as many milligrams than the SZ+ group ($p < 0.001$). In the SZ+ group, there were more participants who had been prescribed an interdictory drug compared to the SUD group ($p = 0.049$).

Considering the clinical characteristics of SZ, we found no differences between groups in age of onset or duration of the disorder. We also found no differences in positive or negative symptoms measured with the PANSS, but the SZ+ group had a higher score than the SZ- group on the general psychopathology scale ($p = 0.004$).

With respect to the clinical characteristics of SUD, we observed that the SZ+ group presented an earlier onset of the disorder with respect to the SUD group ($p = 0.019$), as well as a longer duration of the disorder ($p = 0.049$). Furthermore, the SZ+ group had consumed a greater number of substances on average ($p = 0.033$), but we found no differences in the main type of substance, with a majority of polyconsumers in both groups. Most of the participants had been cocaine and alcohol users, with no differences found between the SUD and SZ+ groups. Neither did we find differences in the consumption of hallucinogens or opioids, although in both cases the rates were higher in the SZ+ group. In contrast, use of cannabis ($p = 0.010$), and of hypnotics and anxiolytics ($p = 0.008$), were higher in the SZ+ group compared to the SUD group. We also found no difference in abstinence time or severity of addiction. Finally, the SZ+ group presented a greater number of previous relapses than the SUD group ($p = 0.002$).

Table 2. Clinical data for the three groups. Mean, standard deviation or percentages, and statistical contrasts.

Clinical Characteristics	SUD (N = 55)	SZ+ (N = 55)	SZ− (N = 55)	Statistical Contrasts
Family history of psychiatric disorders	21.8%	29.1%	34.5%	$\chi^2_{(1)} = 2.20$
Family history of SUD	29.1%	21.8%	7.3%	$\chi^2_{(1)} = 8.68$ *
Suicide attempts	0.42 ± 0.90	1.25 ± 1.82	0.69 ± 1.57	$F_{(2,162)} = 4.56$ *
GAF	74.50 ± 10.06	63.13 ± 11.22	59.75 ± 10.15	$F_{(2,162)} = 29.52$ ***
Number of psychiatric medications	0.93 ± 1.14	3.30 ± 1.68	3.22 ± 1.46	$F_{(2,162)} = 47.81$ ***
Typical antipsychotics	0%	22.2%	25.5%	$\chi^2_{(1)} = 15.80$ ***
Atypical antipsychotics	3.6%	96.3%	94.5%	$\chi^2_{(1)} = 134.74$ ***
CPZ equivalent dosage (mg)	6.06 ± 32.13	350.55 ± 281.35	617.07 ± 522.12	$F_{(2,162)} = 43.56$ ***
Interdictor	20%	37%		$\chi^2_{(1)} = 3.89$ *
Medical disease comorbidity	0.47 ± 0.69	0.53 ± 0.77	0.64 ± 0.80	$F_{(2,162)} = 0.67$
Onset age of SZ		23.35 ± 6.96	23.65 ± 6.71	$t_{(1,108)} = 0.237$
Duration of SZ (years)		12.65 ± 8.01	15.42 ± 9.30	$t_{(1,108)} = 1.67$
PANSS scores				
Positive symptoms		11.83 ± 5.70	10.30 ± 4.19	$t_{(1,108)} = 1.46$
Negative symptoms		15.58 ± 7.39	14.18 ± 7.40	$t_{(1,108)} = 0.89$
General psychopathology		31.10 ± 10.91	24.70 ± 9.01	$t_{(1,108)} = 2.99$ **
Onset age of SUD	20.55 ± 7.24	17.60 ± 5.65		$t_{(1,108)} = 2.38$ *
Duration of SUD (years)	14.61 ± 8.94	17.85 ± 8.03		$t_{(1,108)} = 2.00$ *
Number of substances used	2.93 ± 1.61	3.62 ± 1.75		$t_{(1,108)} = 2.16$ *
Main substance of dependence				$\chi^2_{(4)} = 6.66$
Cocaine	12.7%	10.9%		
Alcohol	9.1%	12.7%		
Alcohol + Cocaine	27.3%	9.1%		
Polydrug use	50.9%	67.3%		
Type of substances used [a]				
Cocaine	89.10%	92.70%		$\chi^2_{(1)} = 0.44$
Alcohol	80.00%	76.0%		$\chi^2_{(1)} = 0.21$
Cannabis	52.70%	76.40%		$\chi^2_{(1)} = 6.71$ **
Psychodysleptics	27.30%	40.00%		$\chi^2_{(1)} = 1.99$
Opioids	14.50%	25.50%		$\chi^2_{(1)} = 2.05$
Sedatives	1.80%	16.40%		$\chi^2_{(1)} = 7.04$ **
Abstinence period (months)	7.55 ± 2.61	6.57 ± 3.64		$t_{(1,108)} = 1.62$
Number of relapses	0.82 ± 1.48	2.25 ± 2.97		$t_{(1,108)} = 3.21$ **
DAST-20 (severity of addiction)	13.05 ± 3.47	13.44 ± 2.86		$t_{(1,108)} = 0.54$

SUD: Substance use disorder; SZ+: Dual schizophrenia; SZ−: Schizophrenia; GAF: Global Assessment of Functioning; CPZ: Chlorpromazine; SZ: Schizophrenia; PANSS: Positive and Negative Syndrome Scale; DAST-20: Drug Abuse Screening Test; * $p < 0.05$; ** $p < 0.01$; *** $p < 0.001$; [a] Percentages will not equal 100 as each patient may have taken more than one substance.

3.2. Personality Dimensions

Table 3 shows the results obtained in the TCI-R for the three groups. Regarding the Temperament dimensions, the MANCOVA showed differences among the groups in Novelty Seeking, Harm Avoidance, and Persistence. Thus, the groups with consumption (SZ+ and SUD) presented higher scores in Novelty Seeking, compared to the SZ- group ($p \leq 0.001$ in both cases). In contrast, the two groups with SZ (SZ+ and SZ-) obtained higher scores in Harm Avoidance ($p < 0.001$ in both cases) and lower Persistence scores ($p \leq 0.024$ in both cases) with respect to the SUD group.

For the Character dimensions, the MANCOVA contributed differences in Self-directedness and Self-transcendence. Post hoc contrasts showed a lower score for Self-directedness in the SZ+ group compared to the other two groups ($p < 0.001$ in both cases). Finally, the two groups with SZ presented higher scores in Self-transcendence compared to the SUD group ($p \leq 0.002$ in both cases).

Table 3. Results for the Temperament and Character Inventory-Revised (TCI-R) dimensions for the three groups. Mean, standard error, and MANCOVA results.

TCI-R Dimensions	SUD (N = 55)	SZ+ (N = 55)	SZ- (N = 55)	$F_{(2,161)}$	η_p^2	Bonferroni *Post-Hoc* Analyses
Temperament						
Novelty Seeking	106.88 ± 1.86	106.06 ± 1.86	96.23 ± 1.88	9.86 ***	0.11	SUD,SZ+ > SZ-
Harm Avoidance	95.27 ± 2.60	112.12 ± 2.60	111.18 ± 2.62	13.22 ***	0.14	SZ+,SZ- > SUD
Reward Dependence	97.88 ± 2.14	91.50 ± 2.14	95.70 ± 2.16	2.31	0.03	
Persistence	113.48 ± 2.66	103.45 ± 2.65	99.38 ± 2.68	7.38 ***	0.08	SZ+,SZ -< SUD
Character						
Self-directedness	137.82 ± 3.08	116.54 ± 3.08	134.64 ± 3.11	13.90 ***	0.15	SZ+ < SZ-,SUD
Cooperativeness	130.75 ± 2.44	123.24 ± 2.43	131.40 ± 2.46	3.46	0.04	
Self-transcendence	58.66 ± 2.20	77.26 ± 2.20	69.77 ± 2.22	18.19 ***	0.18	SZ+,SZ- > SUD

SUD: Substance use disorder; SZ+: Dual schizophrenia; SZ-: Schizophrenia; *** $p < 0.001$.

Analysis of the percentiles (Figure 1) showed that the two groups with consumption (SZ+ and SUD) presented high scores in Novelty Seeking, while those of the SZ- group were slightly low in this dimension. On the other hand, the two groups with SZ presented a very high score in Harm Avoidance, while all three groups presented low scores in Reward Dependence, more so in the SZ+ group. Regarding the Persistence scale, the scores for the two groups with SZ were low in this dimension. Regarding the character dimensions, the three groups showed low scores in Self-directedness and Cooperativeness, especially the SZ+ group. Finally, the two groups with SZ presented high scores in Self-transcendence, although more markedly so in the SZ+ group.

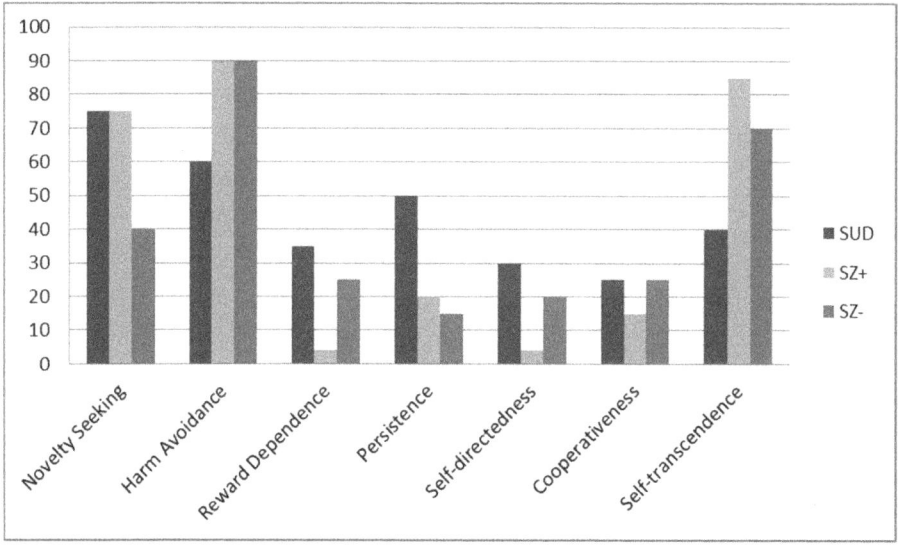

Figure 1. Percentile scores for the three groups for the Temperament and Character Inventory-Revised according to population norms. SUD: Substance use disorder; SZ+: Dual schizophrenia; SZ-: Schizophrenia.

3.3. Clinical Variates Associated with Personality Dimensions

Table 4 shows the stepwise regression analyses for the TCI-R dimensions. We observed that, for the SUD group, onset age of SUD was negatively related to Novelty Seeking, explaining 13.3% of the variance ($F_{(1,53)} = 9.227$; $p = 0.004$), while the GAF was positively linked to Reward Dependence, and explained 24.9% of the variance ($F_{(81,53)} = 18.885$; $p < 0.001$). Regarding the SZ+ group, general psychopathology (PANSS) was positively associated to Harm Avoidance, accounting for 11.7% of the variance ($F_{(1,53)} = 6.156$; $p = 0.018$). Abstinence period measured in months ($p = 0.015$) was positively related to Self-directedness, whereas general psychopathology (PANSS) ($p = 0.028$) was negatively linked to this dimension, and both of them accounted for 31.3% for the variance ($F_{(1,53)} = 9.867$; $p < 0.001$) in Self-directedness. Likewise, 28.2% of the variance ($F_{(1,53)} = 8.058$; $p < 0.001$) in Cooperativeness was explained by number of relapses ($p = 0.001$), which were negatively related, duration of SZ (measured in years) ($p = 0.005$) and onset age of SUD ($p = 0.036$), which were positively related to Cooperativeness in this group. In addition, positive symptoms (PANSS) were positively associated to Self-transcendence and accounted for 8.4% of the variance ($F_{(1,53)} = 4.554$; $p = 0.039$). Finally, for the SZ- group, positive symptoms (PANSS) were positively related to Harm Avoidance and explained 9.1% of the variance ($F_{(1,53)} = 5.096$; $p = 0.019$). Similarly, 18.7% of the variance ($F_{(1,53)} = 6.627$; $p = 0.003$) in Reward Dependence was explained by the GAF ($p = 0.008$) and the PANSS negative symptoms ($p = 0.032$). The former was positively associated to Reward dependence, whereas the latter was negatively associated. General psychopathology was negatively linked both to Self-directedness, and explained 16.1% of the variance ($F_{(1,53)} = 10.37$; $p = 0.002$), and to Cooperativeness, accounting for 22.8% of the variance in this dimension ($F_{(1,53)} = 15.473$; $p < 0.001$). General psychopathology was also positively related to Self-transcendence, explaining 11.7% of the variance ($F_{(1,53)} = 11.569$; $p = 0.001$).

Table 4. Multiple linear regression models for the Temperament and Character Inventory-Revised (TCI-R) for the three groups.

TCI-R Dimensions	SUD (N = 55)			SZ+ (N = 55)			SZ- (N = 55)		
	R² Adjusted	IV	β Standardized	R² Adjusted	IV	β Standardized	R² Adjusted	IV	β Standardized
Temperament									
Novelty Seeking	0.133	Onset age of SUD	−0.386 **						
Harm Avoidance				0.117	PANSS_GP	0.373 *	0.091	PANSS_P	0.331 *
Reward Dependence	0.249	GAF	0.513 ***				0.187	GAF PANSS_N	0.360 ** −0.285 *
Character									
Self-directedness				0.313	Abstinence period (months) PANSS_GP	0.370 * −0.332 *	0.161	PANSS_GP	−0.421 **
Cooperativeness				0.282	Number of relapses Duration of SZ (years) Age of SUD onset	−0.412 *** 0.343 ** 0.249 *	0.228	PANSS_GP	−0.494 ***
Self-transcendence				0.084	PANSS_P	0.327 *	0.117	PANSS_GP	0.441 ***

SUD: Substance use disorder; SZ+: Dual schizophrenia; SZ-: Schizophrenia; GAF: Global Assessment of Functioning; SZ: Schizophrenia; PANSS_GP: Positive and Negative Syndrome Scale_General Psychopathology; PANSS_P: Positive and Negative Syndrome Scale_Positive Scale; PANSS_N: Positive and Negative Syndrome Scale_Negative Scale; * $p < 0.05$; ** $p < 0.01$; *** $p < 0.001$.

4. Discussion

Our work focused on studying the temperament and character profile of patients with SZ+, SZ- and SUD, comparing them among themselves as well as with respect to the normative reference data, in order to elucidate the existence of a possible endophenotype of SZ+. Furthermore, we tried to study the possible associations among personality traits and the clinical characteristics of each diagnosis.

Regarding the clinical and sociodemographic characteristics, our results are in line with the data provided by previous works analyzing similar groups of patients [14,63,64]. Thus, presenting a SUD, SZ- or SZ+ was associated with being single or without a stable partner, living with the family of origin, having a low educational level, and with being unemployed. Furthermore, the SUD group presented a better sociodemographic and clinical profile compared to the other two groups, thus confirming a greater deterioration associated with SZ compared to SUD [15,25].

The two groups with consumption presented more family history of SUD, which is consistent with the idea that such history is a risk factor for developing an addiction [65]. This reflects the importance of considering this factor in the prevention of addictions. On the other hand, the SZ+ group presented an earlier onset of the disorder, a longer duration of the SUD, and a greater quantity of substances consumed. All of these characteristics have been previously related to a worse clinical state, a greater number of relapses, and more suicide attempts [9,10,15]. In line with previous works [15,27], we observed a higher consumption of cannabis in the SZ+ group, which is of special interest since the evidence points to the consumption of this substance as a risk factor for the development of a SZ [66,67]. Moreover, it becomes even more relevant when we consider that, in our study, the onset of SUD happened earlier than that of SZ in the SZ+ group, in line with that found in previous studies [15,30]. Thus, it is important to pay attention to the consumption of cannabis (especially among people with a higher risk of developing a psychotic disorder), given the high prevalence of its consumption among the youth population [11]. However, in our sample, we have a majority of polyconsumers in both groups, and this does not allow us to analyze these data in greater depth at this time.

Regarding personality results, patients in the groups with consumption (SUD and SZ+) showed a greater tendency to present intense responses to novel stimuli, as well as to respond impulsively and to try to avoid monotony and routine (higher Novelty Seeking), compared with the SZ- group and with population data. This is consistent with the data pointing at Novelty/Sensation Seeking as a possible risk factor for addiction [37,68], regardless of whether or not there is an additional diagnosis of SZ [52]. Furthermore, in the SUD group, a higher Novelty Seeking score was associated with a lower onset age of SUD. This points to the importance of detecting extreme scores for this trait in the population at risk, since an earlier start of consumption has been related to a worse clinical course and higher rates of abandonment of treatment [9,27,44], worse strategies of coping during the therapeutic approach [64], and worse cognitive functioning [69]. Therefore, in interventions with these groups of patients it may be very useful to implement strategies aimed at improving decision making, managing routine or boredom, and directing the search for new sensations towards behaviors different from consumption.

Group members diagnosed with SZ tended to experience negative affect frequently, be pessimistic, have multiple concerns, and some behavioral inhibition (high Harm Avoidance). In line with that observed in other studies, which point to Harm Avoidance as a possible endophenotype for SZ [29,48], patients in our sample with a diagnosis of SZ had higher scores in this dimension than the SUD group or the general population. Furthermore, consistent with previous data [30], higher Harm Avoidance was associated in these groups with the presence of more psychiatric symptoms. This reflects the importance of using treatment interventions aimed at improving the management of negative affect in these patients.

In addition, the three groups were characterized as being less sentimental and more solitary and resistant to social pressure, compared to population data (lower Reward Dependence). This trend was especially marked in the SZ+ group, while the SUD group was more similar to the general population, although there were no differences among the groups in direct scores. These data are consistent with those provided by previous studies, especially regarding the groups with SZ [30,70]. In the SUD and

SZ- groups, a closer approach to social stimuli (high Reward Dependence) was associated with better general functioning and, additionally, in the SZ- group it was associated with a lower presence of negative symptoms. This reveals the importance of considering social behavior in order to design therapeutic interventions as well as in studying this dimension further. The two SZ groups showed more difficulties in persisting in a behavior or a task in the face of frustration or fatigue, thus showing a lack of constancy and activity (lower Persistence) compared to the SUD group and the normative data. These results agree with those obtained in previous works regarding groups with SZ [30,70]. This trait (lower Persistence) should also be taken into account, since it may impair treatment involvement and be associated with a higher dropout rate. Thus, at the clinical level, it could be useful to implement motivation and coping strategies to improve therapeutic alliance and adherence to treatment, since the treatment of SZ requires a high degree of compliance for it to be effective, and such treatments are long-lasting given the chronicity of the disorder.

Regarding the Character dimensions, and in line with previous studies [30,44,70], the three groups presented feelings of ineffectiveness as well as difficulties in taking responsibility for their own behavior, for directing it towards their goals and for adapting it to the demands of the situation (low Self-directedness). This trend was especially marked in the groups with SZ where, in addition, low Self-directedness was associated with the presence of more psychiatric symptoms. This reflects the importance of working on self-esteem and coping strategies in these patients, in order to improve not only their adaptive capacity, but also their own psychiatric symptoms.

Moreover, the three groups showed difficulties in adapting to society, a tendency to ignore other people's needs, and to show little or no interest in social relations (low Cooperativeness) [30,46,48]. This was associated with a greater number of psychiatric symptoms in the SZ group. In addition, in the SZ+ group the duration of the SZ and of the SUD was related to the scores in Cooperativeness, while a greater ease of adapting to social requirements was associated with fewer relapses in this group. Since in the SZ+ group a later SUD onset is associated with more Cooperativeness (feeling comfortable in a group and coping well), future studies may further investigate this trait as a potential protection factor for the onset of a SUD in patients with SZ. Thus, our result emphasizes the importance of paying attention to this personality trait, and of implementing interventions aimed at improving social skills and empathy in the diagnoses considered, in order to prevent relapses and to improve psychiatric symptoms.

Finally, according to previous data [29–31], the two SZ groups showed a tendency to spirituality and magical thinking, to have abstract beliefs, and to be carried away by their emotions (higher Self-transcendence), compared to the SUD group and to population data. This trend, which was especially marked in the SZ+ group, was associated in both SZ groups with the presence of more psychiatric symptoms. Thus, a diagnosis of SZ would imply the presence of ideas with a lower reality base, which is consistent with the type of mental disorder in these patients, and which may hinder their treatment. The trait of higher Self-transcendence may thus suppose a certain risk for SZ+ patients in not being realistic in establishing their recovery goals, as well as not being able to detect risk situations during the relapse prevention phase.

Taken as a whole, our results support the idea that there is a character and temperament profile more associated with SUD, and a different one more associated with SZ, and that both differ from the profile reflected by the population data. Thus, patients with SZ would present a specific profile [29,31] characterized by a tendency to negative affect, behavioral inhibition, spirituality and magical thinking, being lonely, with feelings of ineffectiveness and low control of their own behavior, and difficulties in adapting to the social environment. On the other hand, in line with the available data, our results suggest that the SZ+ group presents a personality profile similar to that of the SZ- group, together with the characteristics associated to SUD of low tolerance to routine and monotony, and a tendency to abandon tasks in the face of frustration or fatigue [30,52]. Finally, the SZ+ group presented more marked personality traits than those in the SUD and SZ- groups, in line with what has been observed in previous works [52,53]. This confirms the severity of this diagnostic condition and points to the possible existence of a shared endophenotype for SZ+, made up of traits characteristic of SZ and SUD, and with more extreme values than those observed in these diagnostic entities separately. Furthermore, given that the personality traits are modifiable, the consideration of these behavioral endophenotypes may be of help in designing specific intervention strategies, both for treatment and for relapse prevention.

This study has some strengths and limitations. One of the strengths is having studied these three groups of patients, thus allowing us to overcome the limitation of extrapolating data on patients with SZ+ from patients with SUD, on the one hand, and with SZ- on the other. Furthermore, we consider that the sample is representative of consuming patients, since the main pattern was that of poly-consumption, both with SZ and without psychiatric comorbidity. However, this point may also be a limitation, as it does not allow us to study the differential effects of each substance, nor study if certain personality profiles are associated with the consumption of a specific substance. In this sense, we consider it of special interest to explore further the possible implications of cannabis consumption, which was the largest in the SZ+ group. Moreover, our results are only generalizable to persons with a SUD diagnosis in initial remission, and we have not controlled for the possible effect of time of abstinence. Additionally, the fact that it is a multicenter study confers some external validity to our results. The fact that the sample is made up only of men means that the differences found are not due to sex but, in turn, does not allow us to generalize the results to the female population. This may be a future line of research, despite the greater difficulty of obtaining women undergoing treatment for SUD (around 20%). Furthermore, the study of personality traits has the specific limitations of self-reported measurements. Finally, the cross-sectional and retrospective design does not allow us to establish causal relationships or determine to what extent the results observed in personality traits reflect the effects of treatment. This aspect is of special relevance in the study of personality traits, since, as it has been already commented, several works point to the possibility that these traits may be endophenotypes for SUD and/or SZ. In this sense, we think that it is necessary to carry out longitudinal studies in order to study these aspects in greater depth.

5. Conclusions

To the best of our knowledge, this is the first work to study the temperament and character profiles of these three groups of patients, and to relate these dimensions to clinical characteristics of interest. In addition, it allows exploring the specific weight of the characteristics of each of the disorders (SUD and SZ) in SZ+.

The three diagnostic groups presented a different profile from that observed in the general population, with more maladaptive personality characteristics. Our results support the idea of the existence of a personality profile associated with SUD, a different one associated with SZ, and both emerging in combination in the SZ+ group. Thus, the groups with consumption issues presented higher scores in Novelty Seeking, while the groups with SZ presented higher scores in Harm Avoidance and Self-transcendence. In addition, the SZ+ group presented a character and temperament profile with more extreme scores. Regarding the therapeutic approach for these patients, it could be useful to work on their self-esteem, providing specific resources so that they feel capable of taking responsibility for their behavior, implementing strategies to improve their social skills, empathy and collaboration, and working on the interpretation of psychotic symptoms and the content of thoughts. On the other hand, the association of certain personality traits with clinical characteristics (GAF, psychiatric symptoms, onset age of SUD, abstinence period, relapses and duration of SZ) seems to us of special relevance based on the diagnosis, and we consider it a promising line of research, given its clinical applicability. Thus, future studies that overcome the limitations of this work could provide data of great interest in order to design personalized prevention and treatment strategies.

Author Contributions: Conceptualization, A.A.; methodology, A.A.; formal analysis, L.R.-M.; investigation, L.R.-M., J.E.M.-A. and A.A.; funding acquisition, A.A.; writing—original draft preparation, L.-R.-M. and A.A.; writing—review and editing, all authors. All authors have read and agreed to the published version of the manuscript.

Funding: This research was funded by Spanish Ministry of Economy, Industry, and Competitiveness (PSI2015-65026-MINECO/FEDER/UE); Generalitat de Catalunya (2017SGR-748) and the Spanish Ministry of Economy and Business (PSI2017-90806-REDT).

Acknowledgments: We thank the Mental Health division of Althaia Foundation, Gressol Man Project Foundation in Catalonia, ATRA group, Mental Health of Vall Hebron Hospital, and Addiction's Division of the Maresme Health Consortium, Ethos Association, Center for Attention and Follow-up on Drug Dependencies Les Corts, Els Tres Turons Foundation, Septimània and Sin Consumir for providing the sample of the study.

Conflicts of Interest: The authors declare no conflict of interest.

References

1. Andersen, A.M.; Bienvenu, O.J. Personality and psychopathology. *Int. Rev. Psychiatry* **2011**, *23*, 234–247. [CrossRef] [PubMed]
2. Szerman, N.; Peris, L. Precision Psychiatry and Dual Disorders. *J. Dual Diagn.* **2019**, *14*, 237–246. [CrossRef] [PubMed]
3. European Monitoring Centre for Drug and Addiction (EMCDDA). *Informe Europeo Sobre Drogas: Tendencias y Novedades*; Oficina de Publicaciones de la Unión Europea: Luxemburgo, 2018; ISBN 978-92-9497-318-4. [CrossRef]
4. Hunt, G.E.; Large, M.M.; Cleary, M.; Lai, H.M.X.; Saunders, J.B. Prevalence of comorbid substance use in schizophrenia spectrum disorders in community and clinical settings, 1990–2017: Systematic review and meta-analysis. *Drug Alcohol Depend.* **2018**, *191*, 234–258. [CrossRef] [PubMed]
5. European Monitoring Centre for Drug and Addiction (EMCDDA). *European Drug Report 2015: Comorbidity of Substance Use and Mental Disorders in Europe*; Publications Office of the European Union: Luxembourg, 2019; ISBN 978-92-9168-834-0. [CrossRef]
6. Green, A.I.; Khokhar, J.Y. Addiction and schizophrenia: A translational perspective. *Schizophr. Res.* **2018**, *194*, 1–3. [CrossRef]
7. Sánchez-Peña, J.F.; Alvarez-Cotoli, P.; Rodríguez-Solano, J.J. Psychiatric disorders associated with alcoholism: 2 year follow-up of treatment. *Actas Esp. Psiquiatr.* **2012**, *40*, 129–135.
8. Jiménez-Castro, L.; Raventós-Vorst, H.; Escamilla, M. Substance use disorder and schizophrenia: Prevalence and sociodemographic characteristics in the Latin American population. *Actas Esp. Psiquiatr.* **2010**, *39*, 123–130. [CrossRef]
9. Marquez-Arrico, J.E.; Adan, A. Personality in patients with substance use disorders according to the co-occurring severe mental illness: A study using the alternative five factor model. *Pers. Individ. Differ.* **2016**, *97*, 76–81. [CrossRef]
10. Schmidt, L.M.; Hesse, M.; Lykke, J. The impact of substance use disorders on the course of schizophrenia-A 15-year follow-up study. Dual diagnosis over 15 years. *Schizophr. Res.* **2011**, *130*, 228–233. [CrossRef]
11. Torrens, M.; Mestre-Pintó, J.I.; Montanari, L.; Vicente, J.; Domingo-Salvany, A. Patología dual: Una perspectiva europea. *Adicciones* **2017**, *29*, 3–5. [CrossRef]
12. Lynn Starr, H.; Bermak, J.; Mao, L.; Rodriguez, S.; Alphs, L. Comparison of long-acting and oral antipsychotic treatment effects in patients with schizophrenia, comorbid substance abuse, and a history of recent incarceration: An exploratory analysis of the PRIDE study. *Schizophr. Res.* **2018**, *194*, 39–46. [CrossRef]
13. Donoghue, K.; Doody, G.A.; Murray, R.M.; Jones, P.B.; Morgan, C.; Dazzan, P.; Hart, J.; Mazzoncini, R.; MacCabe, J.H. Cannabis use, gender and age of onset of schizophrenia: Data from the ÆSOP study. *Psychiatry Res.* **2014**, *215*, 528–532. [CrossRef] [PubMed]
14. Arias, F.; Szerman, N.; Vega, P.; Mesías, B.; Basurte, I. Psicosis y drogas. Estudio Madrid sobre prevalencia de patología dual. *Rev. Patol. Dual* **2015**, *2*, 4. [CrossRef]
15. Benaiges, I.; Serra-Grabulosa, J.M.; Prat, G.; Adan, A. Neuropsychological functioning and age-related changes in schizophrenia and/or cocaine dependence. *Psychopharmacol. Biol. Psychiatry* **2013**, *40*, 298–305. [CrossRef] [PubMed]

16. Togay, B.; Noyan, H.; Tasdelen, R.; Ucok, A. Clinical variables associated with suicide attempts in schizophrenia before and after the first episode. *Psychiatry Res.* **2015**, *229*, 252–256. [CrossRef] [PubMed]
17. Haddock, G.; Eisner, E.; Davies, G.; Coupe, N.; Barrowclough, C. Psychotic symptoms, self-harm and violence in individuals with schizophrenia and substance misuse problems. *Schizophr. Res.* **2013**, *151*, 215–220. [CrossRef]
18. Rubio, G.; Torrens, M.; Calatayud, M.; Haro, G. Modelos Asistenciales en Patología Dual. In *Tratado Sobre Patología Dual. Reintegrando la Salud Mental*; Haro, G., Bobes, J., Casas, M., Didia, J., Rubio, G., Eds.; MRA Editors: Barcelona, Spain, 2010; pp. 655–668.
19. Long, E.C.; Aggen, S.H.; Neale, M.C.; Knudsen, G.P.; Krueger, R.F.; South, S.C.; Czajkowski, N.; Nesvåg, R.; Ystrom, E.; Torvik, F.A.; et al. The association between personality disorders with alcohol use and misuse: A population-based twin study. *Drug Alcohol Depend.* **2017**, *174*, 171–180. [CrossRef]
20. Trull, T.J.; Freeman, L.K.; Vebares, T.J.; Choate, A.M.; Helle, A.C.; Wycoff, A.M. Borderline personality disorder and substance use disorders: An updated review. *Borderline Personal. Disord. Emot. Dysregulation* **2018**, *5*. [CrossRef]
21. Santens, E.; Claes, L.; Dierckx, E.; Luyckx, K.; Peuskens, H.; Dom, G. Personality profiles in substance use disorders: Do they differ in clinical symptomatology, personality disorders and coping? *Pers. Individ. Differ.* **2018**, *131*, 61–66. [CrossRef]
22. Zilberman, N.; Yadid, G.; Efrati, Y.; Neumark, Y.; Rassovsky, Y. Personality profiles of substance and behavioral addictions. *Addict. Behav.* **2018**, *82*, 174–181. [CrossRef]
23. Compton, M.T.; Bakeman, R.; Alolayan, Y.; Balducci, P.M.; Bernardini, F.; Broussard, B.; Crisafio, A.; Cristofaro, S.; Amar, P.; Johnson, S.; et al. Personality domains, duration of untreated psychosis, functioning, and symptom severity in first-episode psychosis. *Schizophr. Res.* **2015**, *168*, 113–119. [CrossRef] [PubMed]
24. Ridgewell, C.; Blackford, J.U.; McHugo, M.; Heckers, S. Personality traits predicting quality of life and overall functioning in schizophrenia. *Schizophr. Res.* **2017**, *182*, 19–23. [CrossRef] [PubMed]
25. Fernández-Mondragón, S.; Adan, A. Personality in male patients with substance use disorder and/or severe mental illness. *Psychiatry Res.* **2015**, *228*, 488–494. [CrossRef] [PubMed]
26. Marquez-Arrico, J.E.; Río-Martínez, L.; Navarro, J.F.; Prat, G.; Adan, A. Personality profile and clinical correlates of patients with substance use disorder with and without comorbid depression under treatment. *Front. Psychiatry* **2019**, *10*, 1–9. [CrossRef] [PubMed]
27. Roncero, C.; Barral, C.; Grau-López, L.; Bos-Cucuruli, E.; Casas, M. Patología dual en esquizofrenia. *Protoc. Interv. Patol. Dual* **2016**, 1–56.
28. Cloninger, C.R.; Svrakic, D.M.; Przybeck, T.R. A psychobiological model of temperament and character. *Arch. Gen. Psychiatry* **1993**, *50*, 975–990. [CrossRef] [PubMed]
29. Galindo, L.; Pastoriza, F.; Bergé, D.; Mané, A.; Picado, M.; Bulbena, A.; Robledo, P.; Pérez, V.; Vilarroya, O.; Cloninger, C.R. Association between neurological soft signs, temperament and character in patients with schizophrenia and non-psychotic relatives. *PeerJ* **2016**. [CrossRef]
30. Marquez-Arrico, J.E.; López-Vera, S.; Prat, G.; Adan, A. Temperament and character dimensions in male patients with substance use disorders: Differences relating to psychiatric comorbidity. *Psychiatry Res.* **2016**, *237*, 1–8. [CrossRef]
31. Miskovic, M.; Ravanic, D.; Bankovic, D.; Zivlak-Radulovic, N.; Banjac, V.; Dragisic, T. The risk model of developing schizophrenia based on temperament and character. *Psychiatr. Danub.* **2018**, *30*, 57–63. [CrossRef]
32. Khemiri, L.; Kuja-Halkola, R.; Larsson, H.; Jayaram-Lindström, N. Genetic overlap between impulsivity and alcohol dependence: A large-scale national twin study. *Psychol. Med.* **2016**, *46*, 1091–1102. [CrossRef]
33. Hamdan-Mansour, A.M.; Mahmoud, K.F.; Al Shibi, A.N.; Arabiat, D.H. Impulsivity and sensation-seeking personality traits as predictors of substance use among University students. *J. Psychosoc. Nurs. Ment. Health Serv.* **2018**, *56*, 57–63. [CrossRef]
34. Benotsch, E.G.; Jeffers, A.J.; Snipes, D.J.; Martin, A.M.; Koester, S. The five factor model of personality and the non-medical use of prescription drugs: Associations in a young adult sample. *Pers. Individ. Differ.* **2013**, *55*, 852–855. [CrossRef]
35. Ersche, K.D.; Turton, A.J.; Chamberlain, S.R.; Müller, U.; Bullmore, E.T.; Robbins, T.W. Cognitive dysfunction and anxious-impulsive personality traits are endophenotypes for drug dependence. *Am. J. Psychiatry* **2012**, *169*, 926–936. [CrossRef] [PubMed]

36. Valero, S.; Daigre, C.; Rodríguez-Cintas, L.; Barral, C.; Gomà-I-Freixanet, M.; Ferrer, M.; Casas, M.; Roncero, C. Neuroticism and impulsivity: Their hierarchical organization in the personality characterization of drug-dependent patients from a decision tree learning perspective. *Compr. Psychiatry* **2014**, *55*, 1227–1233. [CrossRef]
37. Arenas, M.C.; Aguilar, M.A.; Montagud-Romero, S.; Mateos-García, A.; Navarro-Francés, C.I.; Miñarro, J.; Rodríguez-Arias, M. Influence of the Novelty-Seeking Endophenotype on the Rewarding Effects of Psychostimulant Drugs in Animal Models. *Curr. Neuropharmacol.* **2015**, *14*, 87–100. [CrossRef] [PubMed]
38. Pedrero Pérez, E.J.; Rojo Mota, G. Diferencias de personalidad entre adictos a sustancias y población general. Estudio con el TCI-R de casos clínicos con controles emparejados. *Adicciones* **2008**, *20*, 251–261. [CrossRef]
39. Evren, C.; Durkaya, M.; Evren, B.; Dalbudak, E.; Cetin, R. Relationship of relapse with impulsivity, novelty seeking and craving in male alcohol-dependent inpatients. *Drug Alcohol Rev.* **2012**, *31*, 81–90. [CrossRef] [PubMed]
40. Stevens, L.; Goudriaan, A.E.; Verdejo-Garcia, A.; Dom, G.; Roeyers, H.; Vanderplasschen, W. Impulsive choice predicts short-term relapse in substance-dependent individuals attending an in-patient detoxification programme. *Psychol. Med.* **2015**, *45*, 2083–2093. [CrossRef] [PubMed]
41. Rodríguez-Cintas, L.; Daigre, C.; Grau-López, L.; Barral, C.; Pérez-Pazos, J.; Voltes, N.; Braquehais, M.D.; Casas, M.; Roncero, C. Impulsivity and addiction severity in cocaine and opioid dependent patients. *Addict. Behav.* **2016**, *58*, 104–109. [CrossRef]
42. Staiger, P.K.; Dawe, S.; Richardson, B.; Hall, K.; Kambouropoulos, N. Modifying the risk associated with an impulsive temperament: A prospective study of drug dependence treatment. *Addict. Behav.* **2014**, *39*, 1676–1681. [CrossRef]
43. Dvorak, R.D.; Lamis, D.A.; Malone, P.S. Alcohol use, depressive symptoms, and impulsivity as risk factors for suicide proneness among college students. *J. Affect. Disord.* **2013**, *149*, 326–334. [CrossRef]
44. Ávila-Escribano, J.J.; Sánchez-Barba, M.; Álvarez-Pedrero, A.; López-Villarreal, A.; Recio-Pérez, J.; Rodríguez-Rodilla, M.; Fraile-García, E. Capacidad de predicción del inventario de temperamento y carácter de cloninger (TCI-R) en la evolución de los trastornos por uso de alcohol. *Adicciones* **2016**, *28*, 136–143. [CrossRef]
45. Hershberger, A.R.; Um, M.; Cyders, M.A. The relationship between the UPPS-P impulsive personality traits and substance use psychotherapy outcomes: A meta-analysis. *Drug Alcohol Depend.* **2017**, *178*, 408–416. [CrossRef]
46. Andó, B.; Rózsa, S.; Kurgyis, E.; Szkaliczki, A.; Demeter, I.; Szikszay, P.; Demetrovics, Z.; Janka, Z.; Álmos, P.Z. Direct and indirect symptom severity indicators of alcohol dependence and the personality concept of the biosocial model. *Subst. Use Misuse* **2014**, *49*, 418–426. [CrossRef] [PubMed]
47. Zoccali, R.; Muscatello, M.R.A.; Bruno, A.; Bilardi, F.; De Stefano, C.; Felletti, E.; Isgrò, S.; Micalizzi, V.; Micò, U.; Romeo, A.; et al. Temperament and character dimensions in opiate addicts: Comparing subjects who completed inpatient treatment in therapeutic communities vs. incompleters. *Am. J. Drug Alcohol Abuse* **2007**, *33*, 707–715. [CrossRef] [PubMed]
48. Fresán, A.; León-Ortiz, P.; Robles-García, R.; Azcárraga, M.; Guizar, D.; Reyes-Madrigal, F.; Tovilla-Zárate, C.A.; de la Fuente-Sandoval, C. Personality features in ultra-high risk for psychosis: A comparative study with schizophrenia and control subjects using the Temperament and Character Inventory-Revised (TCI-R). *J. Psychiatr. Res.* **2015**, *61*, 168–173. [CrossRef]
49. Albayrak, Y.; Ekinci, O.; Çayköylü, A. Temperament and character personality profile in relation to suicide attempts in patients with schizophrenia. *Compr. Psychiatry* **2012**, *53*, 1130–1136. [CrossRef] [PubMed]
50. Vrbova, K.; Prasko, J.; Ociskova, M.; Holubova, M.; Kantor, K.; Kolek, A.; Grambal, A.; Slepecky, M. Suicidality, self-stigma, social anxiety and personality traits in stabilized schizophrenia patients—A cross-sectional study. *Neuropsychiatr. Dis. Treat.* **2018**, *14*, 1415–1424. [CrossRef] [PubMed]
51. Jetha, M.K.; Goldberg, J.O.; Schmidt, L.A. Temperament and its relation to social functioning in schizophrenia. *Int. J. Soc. Psychiatry* **2013**, *59*, 254–263. [CrossRef] [PubMed]
52. Zhornitsky, S.; Rizkallah, É.; Pampoulova, T.; Chiasson, J.P.; Lipp, O.; Stip, E.; Potvin, S. Sensation-seeking, social anhedonia, and impulsivity in substance use disorder patients with and without schizophrenia and in non-abusing schizophrenia patients. *Psychiatry Res.* **2012**, *200*, 237–241. [CrossRef]
53. Reno, R.M. Personality characterizations of outpatients with schizophrenia, schizophrenia with substance abuse, and primary substance abuse. *J. Nerv. Ment. Dis.* **2004**, *192*, 672–681. [CrossRef]

54. American Psychiatric Association. *Diagnostic and Statistical Manual of Mental Disorders*, 5th ed.; American Psychiatric Association: Washington, DC, USA, 2013.
55. WMA Declaration of Helsinki—Ethical Principles for Medical Research Involving Human Subjects—WMA—The World Medical Association. Available online: https://www.wma.net/policies-post/wma-declaration-of-helsinki-ethical-principles-for-medical-research-involving-human-subjects/ (accessed on 3 March 2020).
56. First, M.B.; Gibbon, M. The Structured Clinical Interview for DSM-IV Axis I Disorders (SCID-I) and the Structured Clinical Interview for DSM-IV Axis II Disorders (SCID-II). In *Comprehensive Handbook of Psychological Assessment, Vol. 2: Personality Assessment*; John Wiley & Sons: Hoboken, NJ, USA, 2004; pp. 134–143. ISBN 0-471-41612-6.
57. Hall, R.C.W. Global Assessment of Functioning: A Modified Scale. *Psychosomatics* **1995**, *36*, 267–275. [CrossRef]
58. Peralta Martín, V.; Cuesta Zorita, M.J. Validation of positive and negative symptom scale (PANSS) in a sample of Spanish schizophrenic patients. *Actas Luso. Esp. Neurol. Psiquiatr. Cienc. Afines* **1994**, *22*, 171–177. [PubMed]
59. Gálvez, B.P.; Fernández, L.G.; De Vicente Manzanaro, M.P.; Valenzuela, M.A.O.; Lafuente, M.L. Validación española del drug abuse screening test (DAST-20 y DAST-10). *Health Addict./Salud y Drog.* **2010**, *10*, 35–50. [CrossRef]
60. Gutiérrez-Zotes, J.A.; Bayón, C.; Montserrat, C.; Valero, J.; Labad, A.; Cloninger, C.R.; Fernández-Aranda, F. Inventario del Temperamento y el Carácter-Revisado (TCI-R). Baremación y datos normativos en una muestra de población general. *Actas Esp. Psiquiatr.* **2004**, *32*, 8–15. [PubMed]
61. Anusic, I.; Lucas, R.E.; Brent Donnellan, M. Cross-sectional age differences in personality: Evidence from nationally representative samples from Switzerland and the United States. *J. Res. Pers.* **2012**, *46*, 116–120. [CrossRef]
62. Richardson, J.T.E. Eta squared and partial eta squared as measures of effect size in educational research. *Educ. Res. Rev.* **2011**, *6*, 135–147. [CrossRef]
63. Adan, A.; Capella, M.D.M.; Prat, G.; Forero, D.A.; Lopez-Vera, S.; Navarro, J.F. Executive functioning in men with schizophrenia and substance use disorders. Influence of lifetime suicide attempts. *PLoS ONE* **2017**, *12*, 1–16. [CrossRef]
64. del Capella, M.M.; Adan, A. The age of onset of substance use is related to the coping strategies to deal with treatment in men with substance use disorder. *PeerJ* **2017**, 3660. [CrossRef]
65. Prom-Wormley, E.C.; Ebejer, J.; Dick, D.M.; Bowers, M.S. The genetic epidemiology of substance use disorder: A review. *Drug Alcohol Depend.* **2017**, *180*, 241–259. [CrossRef]
66. Belbasis, L.; Köhler, C.A.; Stefanis, N.; Stubbs, B.; van Os, J.; Vieta, E.; Seeman, M.V.; Arango, C.; Carvalho, A.F.; Evangelou, E. Risk factors and peripheral biomarkers for schizophrenia spectrum disorders: An umbrella review of meta-analyses. *Acta Psychiatr. Scand.* **2018**, *137*, 88–97. [CrossRef] [PubMed]
67. Ibarra-Lecue, I.; Mollinedo-Gajate, I.; Meana, J.J.; Callado, L.F.; Diez-Alarcia, R.; Urigüen, L. Chronic cannabis promotes pro-hallucinogenic signaling of 5-HT2A receptors through Akt/mTOR pathway. *Neuropsychopharmacology* **2018**, *43*, 2028–2035. [CrossRef] [PubMed]
68. Jupp, B.; Dalley, J.W. Behavioral endophenotypes of drug addiction: Etiological insights from neuroimaging studies. *Neuropharmacology* **2014**, *76*, 487–497. [CrossRef] [PubMed]
69. Capella, M.D.M.; Benaiges, I.; Adan, A. Neuropsychological performance in polyconsumer men under treatment. Influence of age of onset of substance use. *Sci. Rep.* **2015**, *5*, 1–10. [CrossRef] [PubMed]
70. Song, Y.Y.; Kang, J.I.; Kim, S.J.; Lee, M.K.; Lee, E.; An, S.K. Temperament and character in individuals at ultra-high risk for psychosis and with first-episode schizophrenia: Associations with psychopathology, psychosocial functioning, and aspects of psychological health. *Compr. Psychiatry* **2013**, *54*, 1161–1168. [CrossRef]

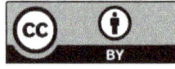

© 2020 by the authors. Licensee MDPI, Basel, Switzerland. This article is an open access article distributed under the terms and conditions of the Creative Commons Attribution (CC BY) license (http://creativecommons.org/licenses/by/4.0/).

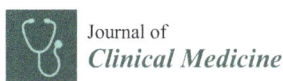

Article

Childhood Trauma Predicts Less Remission from PTSD among Patients with Co-Occurring Alcohol Use Disorder and PTSD

Paul Brunault [1,2,3,4,*], Kevin Lebigre [1,2], Fatima Idbrik [5], Damien Maugé [1,6], Philippe Adam [5], Servane Barrault [4,6], Grégoire Baudin [4,7], Robert Courtois [2,4], Hussein El Ayoubi [1,6], Marie Grall-Bronnec [8,9], Coraline Hingray [10], Nicolas Ballon [1,2,3] and Wissam El-Hage [2,3]

1. CHRU de Tours, Service d'Addictologie Universitaire, Équipe de Liaison et de Soins en Addictologie, 37044 Tours, France; k.lebigre@chu-tours.fr (K.L.); d.mauge@chu-tours.fr (D.M.); hussein.elayoubi@univ-tours.fr (H.E.A.); nicolas.ballon@univ-tours.fr (N.B.)
2. CHRU de Tours, Clinique Psychiatrique Universitaire, 37044 Tours, France; robert.courtois@univ-tours.fr (R.C.); wissam.elhage@univ-tours.fr (W.E.-H.)
3. UMR 1253, iBrain, Université de Tours, Inserm, 37020 Tours, France
4. Qualipsy EE 1901, Université de Tours, 37020 Tours, France; servane.barrault@univ-tours.fr (S.B.); gregoire.baudin@u-paris.fr (G.B.)
5. Soins de Suite et de Réadaptation en Addictologie "Le Courbat", 37460 Le Liège, France; medecin@lecourbat.fr (F.I.); padam@sante-escale41.fr (P.A.)
6. CHRU de Tours, Centre de Soins d'Accompagnement et de Prévention en Addictologie CSAPA-37, 37044 Tours, France
7. Laboratory of Psychopathology and Health Processes EA 4057, University Paris Descartes, Sorbonne Paris Cité, 92100 Boulogne-Billancourt, France
8. Addictology and Psychiatry Department, Hôpital Saint Jacques, University Hospital of Nantes, 85 rue Saint Jacques, Cedex 1, 44093 Nantes, France; marie.bronnec@chu-nantes.fr
9. Inserm, SPHERE U1246 methodS in Patients-Centered Outcomes and HEalth ResEarch, Université de Nantes, Université de Tours, 22 boulevard Benoni Goullin, 44200 Nantes, France
10. Pôle Universitaire du Grand Nancy, Centre Psychothérapique de Nancy, 54520 Laxou, France; c.hingray@chu-nancy.fr
* Correspondence: paul.brunault@univ-tours.fr; Tel.: +33-218-370-581

Received: 5 May 2020; Accepted: 27 June 2020; Published: 30 June 2020

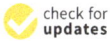

Abstract: Post-traumatic stress disorder (PTSD) is highly prevalent among patients hospitalized for an alcohol use disorder (AUD). Hospitalization can improve PTSD and AUD outcomes in some but not all patients, but we lack data on the baseline predictors of PTSD non-remission. This study aimed to determine the baseline risk factors for non-remitted PTSD in patients hospitalized for an AUD. Of 298 AUD inpatients recruited in a rehabilitation center (Le Courbat, France), we included 91 AUD inpatients with a co-occurring PTSD and a longitudinal assessment at baseline (T1) and before discharge (T2: 8 weeks later). Patients were assessed for PTSD diagnosis/severity (PCL-5=PTSD Checklist for DSM-5), different types of trauma including childhood trauma (LEC-5=Life Events Checklist for DSM-5/CTQ-SF=Childhood Trauma Questionnaire, Short-Form), and AUD diagnosis/severity (clinical interview/AUDIT=Alcohol Use Disorders Identification Test). Rate of PTSD remission between T1 and T2 was 74.1%. Non-remitted PTSD at T2 was associated with a history of childhood trauma (physical, emotional or sexual abuse, physical negligence), but not with other types of trauma experienced, nor baseline PTSD or AUD severity. Among patients hospitalized for an AUD with co-occurring PTSD, PTSD remission was more strongly related to the existence of childhood trauma than to AUD or PTSD severity at admission. These patients should be systematically screened for childhood trauma in order to tailor evidence-based interventions.

Keywords: Substance-use disorder; substance-related disorders; alcohol use disorder; post-traumatic stress disorder; dual disorders; childhood trauma; psychiatric disorders; rehabilitation centers; impulsive behavior; addictive disorders

1. Introduction

Alcohol use disorders (AUD), which are characterized by compulsive alcohol use and loss of control over alcohol intake [1], are a major public health problem worldwide [2]. AUD are among the most prevalent psychiatric disorders globally, affecting 8.6% (95% Confidence Interval=CI: 8.1–9.1) of men and 1.7% (95% CI: 1.6–1.9) of women (total point estimate: 5.1%, 95% CI: 4.9–5.4) [1], and they represent a significant health, social, and economic burden to Western societies [3]. AUD are often associated with other addictive and psychiatric disorders, and the co-occurrence of other addictive and psychiatric disorders (i.e., dual diagnosis) is a challenge for clinicians given their prevalence and poor outcome [4]. One of the most prevalent psychiatric disorders associated with AUD is post-traumatic stress disorder (PTSD); while the prevalence of PTSD ranges from 4.8% to 8% in the overall population [5,6], it is much higher in people with AUD and is estimated to be between 20% and 39% [7,8]. For these patients, a PTSD diagnosis is associated with a poorer AUD outcome, as well as a higher rate of hospitalization and a more severe social impairment [5,9,10].

Given the high prevalence of PTSD in patients with AUD and the major burden it represents, a better understanding of the variables associated with greater AUD or PTSD severity is of paramount importance to determine the most effective interventions for patients with this dual diagnosis. As the factors found to be associated with AUD or PTSD severity in cross-sectional studies may not necessarily be linked to poorer long-term outcomes, longitudinal studies are needed. One interesting research area is to identify the specific predictors of the course of PTSD and particularly of poorer remission rates. Based on the hypothesis that PTSD could be a causal risk or maintenance factor for AUD (i.e., improvement in PTSD associated with lower alcohol dependence) [11], identification of the factors associated with poor PTSD outcomes using a longitudinal approach could improve our ability to identify the patients who would benefit from tailor-made interventions, and ultimately improve AUD outcome [11].

In general, different predictors of poor PTSD outcomes have been identified, including being female, lower socio-economic status, childhood trauma, lifetime and childhood sexual trauma, PTSD severity or type (i.e., more severe PTSD symptoms at baseline, high combat exposure, trauma severity), greater number of stressors prior to trauma, other comorbid psychiatric disorders (e.g., mood and anxiety disorders, personality disorders), and social factors (e.g., lack of social support) [12–15]. When focusing on the specific population of patients with an AUD, studies have demonstrated that PTSD was associated with avoidance symptoms [16]. Childhood trauma, which is very prevalent in patients with an AUD [17,18], is strongly associated with the development of AUD and PTSD, and could play a central role in maintaining the association between the two disorders [19,20]. One possible explanation of the association between childhood trauma, PTSD, and AUD refers to Bowlby's theoretical framework and attachment theory [21]. According to Bowlby, attachment can be understood within an evolutionary context in that the caregiver (i.e., attachment figure) provides safety and security to the infant. Bowlby postulated that children who perceive their attachment figure as nearby, accessible, and attentive may be more likely to experience a secure attachment bond, while children who do not perceive their attachment figure as nearby, accessible, and attentive may be more likely to experience insecure attachment bond. Given that the existence of a childhood trauma may affect the attachment bond, the association between childhood trauma and AUD severity could be explained by a higher risk of insecure attachment (especially fearful attachment), which has been demonstrated to be strongly related to PTSD symptoms [22]. Studies investigating the potential differences in the course of PTSD between

AUD patients with and without childhood trauma could improve our ability to tailor evidence-based interventions for AUD patients.

In this study, we sought to identify the factors associated with poorer PTSD outcomes among AUD patients hospitalized in an addiction rehabilitation center, who have a more severe form of AUD and a higher prevalence of PTSD [23]. In addition, it is possible to screen for and treat PTSD among hospitalized patients and to observe the course of PTSD over the medium term, thus facilitating the study of predictors of PTSD outcomes. Although PTSD is highly comorbid with AUD in hospitalized patients, to the best of our knowledge there are no longitudinal data about the variables associated with the course of PTSD in this specific population.

The main objective of this study was to determine how many patients hospitalized for an AUD and with a comorbid PTSD remitted from their PTSD at the end of their hospitalization, and to identify the risk factors for non-remission (i.e., socio-demographic characteristics, baseline AUD or PTSD severity, and existence of traumatic life events, including those that occurred in childhood). We hypothesized that remission rates would be lower in patients with a history of childhood trauma, and that there would be no association with baseline AUD severity, PTSD severity, other types of trauma experienced, nor with age, gender or marital status.

2. Experimental Section

2.1. Participants and Procedure

We recruited all consecutive AUD patients admitted to the "Le Courbat" addiction rehabilitation center (Centre–Val de Loire region, France) between January 2016 and October 2017. "Le Courbat" is a national referral center for the treatment of people with AUD. In the last 10 years, it has been developing specific programs for patients with a co-occurring PTSD and AUD.

The study flow chart is presented in Figure 1. Patients were considered eligible for the study if they were aged at least 18 and if they were hospitalized for an AUD as diagnosed by an addiction specialist met at baseline ($n = 356$). Eligible patients were then proposed to participate to the study and we asked them to provide their informed and signed consent if they agreed (information was given by the person in charge of the data collection (P.A.) that the participation was free and that their decision would not modify their treatment protocol during their hospitalization). Out of these 356 patients, 53 refused to participate. Patients were then asked to complete self-administered questionnaires one week after admission (T1 = baseline) using digital tablets or computers provided specifically for this study and with the help of P.A. if they had difficulties in understanding the questions. The questionnaires were designed and completed online using Sphinx mobile iQ 2 software during a systematic visit with the person in charge of the data collection (P.A.). Out of these 303 patients, 298 had fully exploitable questionnaires at T1 (five patients had missing data for at least one questionnaire including the AUDIT (Alcohol Use Disorders Identification Test), PCL-5 (PTSD Checklist for DSM-5, i.e., Diagnostic and Statistical Manual for Mental Disorders, 5th edition), LEC-5 (Life Events Checklist for DSM-5), and CTQ-SF (Childhood Trauma Questionnaire, Short-Form); there was no significant difference between these five patients and the 298 others in terms of age, gender, AUDIT total score, number of traumatic events experiences, or CTQ sub-scores), including 149 patients who had a PTSD according to the LEC-5 and the PCL-5 (see the Measures subsection for the PTSD diagnostic criteria). Patients were then asked to complete again these self-administered questionnaires eight weeks after admission (T2; one week before discharge) using the same digital tablets or computers provided specifically for this study; this was proposed during a systematic visit conducted by the person in charge of the study collection (P.A.). We chose this eight-week period to match the length of stay in this rehabilitation center. Our final sample ($n = 91$; attrition rate was 38.9%) was composed of inpatients diagnosed with a co-occurring AUD and PTSD at baseline and who completed the self-administered questionnaires in full at both T1 and T2. Patients with PTSD who were included in this study ($n = 91$) did not differ from patients with PTSD who were lost to follow-up at T2 ($n = 58$) in terms of age, AUDIT total score, nor PCL-5 total score.

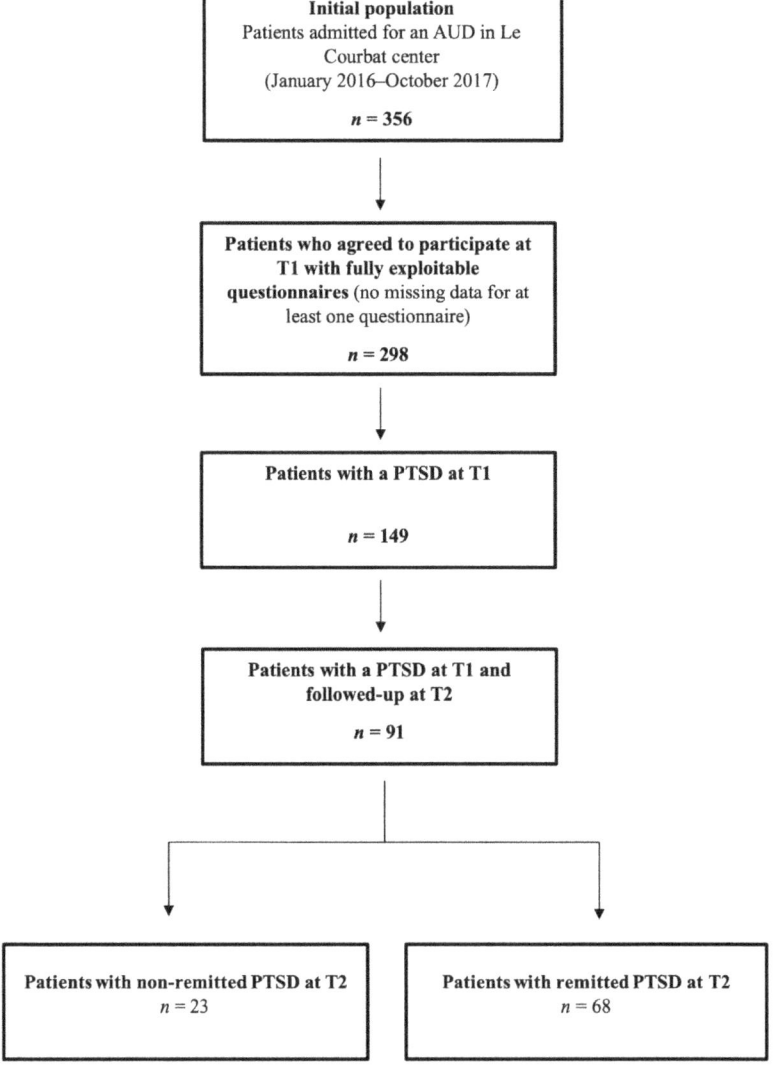

Figure 1. Study flow chart. Note: AUD, Alcohol Use Disorder; AUDIT, Alcohol Use Disorders Identification Test; PTSD, Post-Traumatic Stress Disorder. T1, Assessment one week after admission (baseline assessment); T2, Assessment eight weeks after initial assessment (one week before discharge).

All patients underwent the same treatment protocol during their hospitalization: a basic treatment protocol (i.e., systematic and regular consultations with a physician expert in addiction medicine and with a physician expert in sport medicine, as well as consultations with other health care professionals: nurse, psychologist, dietician, social worker, fitness trainer, and art therapist), and an additional PTSD module for patients who screened positive for PTSD. This PTSD module, that included group-sessions with a psychologist expert in PTSD, consisted of psycho-education and information about PTSD. There was no difference in terms of treatment protocol between patients who remitted from PTSD versus patients who did not remit from PTSD.

2.2. Measures

For each patient, we collected data regarding socio-demographic characteristics (age, gender, and marital status), PTSD, AUD severity, and different types of traumatic events, including those that occurred in childhood.

2.2.1. Childhood Trauma

History of childhood trauma was assessed at T1 using the Childhood Trauma Questionnaire, Short-Form (CTQ-SF; Bernstein et al., 2003 [24]; French validation by Paquette et al., 2004 [25]). The CTQ is a 28-item screening tool for a history of maltreatment during childhood. It measures five types of maltreatment: physical abuse (cut-off score ≥ 11), emotional abuse (cut-off score ≥ 16), sexual abuse (cut-off score ≥ 11), physical neglect (cut-off score ≥ 14), and emotional neglect (cut-off score ≥ 18). Participants answer items on a 5-point Likert scale, with responses ranging from "never true" to "very often true". The internal reliability of the CTQ-SF was excellent for the total score ($\alpha = 0.95$), good to excellent for four dimensions (Cronbach's alphas respectively 0.81–0.86, 0.84–0.89, 0.92–0.95, and 0.88–0.91), and acceptable for physical neglect (Cronbach's alpha ranging from 0.61–0.78) [24]. The 5-factor solution proved to be invariant across disordered-control comparison groups [26]. In this study, we used the CTQ-SF sub-scores as indicators of childhood trauma severity.

2.2.2. Lifetime Exposure to Traumatic Events

We assessed the history of traumatic events (lifetime exposure to 17 types of trauma) using the Life Event Checklist for DSM-5 (LEC-5; original version: Weathers et al., 2013 [27]; French adaptation by Montreal trauma study center, 2015). This tool screens for 17 potentially traumatic events in the respondent's lifetime, clustered in seven types: (1) natural disasters; (2) accidents; (3) physical aggressions; (4) sexual aggressions; (5) war-related trauma; (6) exposure to illness, injury, or death experiences; and (7) exposure to any other very stressful event or experience. In this study, in line with previous research, we combined these types of traumatic events into the following categories: (1) natural disasters or accidents; (2) physical or sexual aggression; (3) war-related trauma; (4) exposure to illness, injury, or death experiences; and (5) exposure to any other very stressful event or experience. The LEC-5 is often used in combination with other measures, such as the PCL-5, for the purpose of establishing exposure to a traumatic event corresponding to DSM-5 criterion A [27].

2.2.3. Post-Traumatic Stress Disorder

We assessed PTSD symptoms and severity at T1 and T2 with the PTSD Checklist for DSM-5 (PCL-5; Blevins et al., 2015 [28]; French validation: Ashbaugh et al., 2016 [29]). This 20-item self-administered questionnaire assesses PTSD symptoms using a Likert-type scale for each symptom, which can be divided into four sub-scales, with scores ranging from 0 (not at all) to 4 (extremely). It also assesses severity of symptoms (score 0 to 80; cut-off ≥ 31), with sub-scores for re-experiencing (0 to 20), avoidance (0 to 8), negative alteration in cognition and mood (0 to 24), and arousal (0 to 28) [28]. We asked the patients to refer to their worst traumatic event when completing the PCL-5.

In line with the DSM-5 diagnostic criteria, PTSD was diagnosed when participants had experienced at least one traumatic event (criterion A, as assessed by the LEC-5), indicated one or more of the intrusion symptoms (criterion B), one symptom of persistent avoidance of stimuli associated with the traumatic event (criterion C), two symptoms of negative alterations in cognitions and mood (criterion D), and two symptoms of marked alterations in arousal and reactivity (criterion E). We also assessed PTSD severity using the total PCL-5 score. PTSD was considered to be in remission when the PCL-5 score decreased by 30% or more between T1 and T2 [30–32].

2.2.4. Alcohol Use Disorder

In addition to the AUD diagnosis made by clinical assessment at baseline (T1), we assessed its severity at T1 and T2 using the Alcohol Use Disorders Identification Test (AUDIT; original version: Saunders et al., 1993 [33]; French validation: Gache et al., 2005 [34]). The AUDIT was developed in collaboration with the World Health Organization (WHO) and includes 10 questions about level of consumption, symptoms of dependence and alcohol-related consequences (cut-off ≥ 8). Its internal consistency was found to be high and test–retest data suggest good reliability ($\alpha = 0.86$) and sensitivity of 0.90 [33]. We used the AUDIT total score to assess AUD severity.

2.3. Statistical Analyses and Ethics

Analyses were conducted using SPSS® version 22 (IBM Corp. Released 2013. IBM SPSS Statistics for Windows, Version 22.0., IBM Corporation, Armonk, NY, USA). All analyses were two-tailed; p-values ≤ 0.05 were considered statistically significant.

Descriptive statistics included percentages for ordinal variables and means and standard deviations for continuous variables. We analyzed the correlations between our variables (Spearman's correlation tests). First, we determined the variables associated with PTSD status (remitted vs. non-remitted) using univariate analyses: either mean comparison tests (Mann–Whitney U test, when the distribution did not follow a normal distribution, with the corresponding z-value or Student's test with the corresponding t-value) or chi-squared tests (Pearson's chi-squared test or Fisher's exact test if expected frequencies were <5 in at least one cell), depending on the type of variable studied. We then used multivariate analyses (multiple linear regressions) to determine whether PTSD characteristics (each PCL-5 cluster), type of trauma encountered (including a history of childhood trauma) were significant predictors of remitted PTSD after adjusting for age (p was <0.20 in univariate analysis). For each dependent variable, we specified the beta regression coefficient, its 95% confidence interval, and its associated t-value and p-value.

This study obtained the approval of an institutional review board (Comité d'Éthique pour les Recherches Non Interventionnelles [CERNI] Tours-Poitiers) in July 2015, prior to the beginning of the study. All collected data were in line with the French recommendation regarding use of personal data, with the approval of the French Commission Nationale de l'Informatique et des Libertés (CNIL).

3. Results

3.1. Descriptive Statistics

Descriptive statistics for socio-demographic characteristics, AUD severity, PTSD severity, and different types of traumatic event (including those that occurred in childhood) at T1 are presented in Table 1. At baseline (T1), the majority of participants were male (82.4%), with a mean age of 42.8 ± 8.6 years; mean AUDIT score was 27.8 ± 7.7 (100% had an AUDIT score ≥8), and PCL-5 total score was 46.4 ± 10.9 (92.3% had a PCL-5 score ≥31). The most common categories of trauma were, in order of prevalence: accidents or natural disasters (87.9%; 82.4% experienced any accident and 46.2% experienced any natural disaster); physical or sexual aggression (82.4%; 82.4% experienced any physical aggression and 23.1% experienced any sexual aggression); any other very stressful event or experience (75.8%); exposure to illness, injury, or death experience (30.8%); and war-related trauma (6.6%). The most common categories of childhood traumatic experience were, in order of prevalence (as defined by a CTQ sub-score higher or equal to the corresponding cut-off): emotional abuse (33%); emotional negligence (29.7%); physical abuse (20.9%); physical negligence (13.2%); and sexual abuse (12.1%). Based on the LEC-5 and the CTQ, all patients experienced at least two traumatic experiences, i.e., all patients had multiple traumas. Based on the PCL-5 cutoffs, PTSD remission between T1 and T2 was observed in 74.7% of the sample. Mean total PCL-5 score dropped between T1 and T2 from 46.4 ± 10.9 to 22.6 ± 15.6 ($p < 0.001$).

Table 1. Descriptive statistics of the sample at baseline (T1; $n = 91$).

	Mean ± SD or Percentage (number)
Socio-Demographic Characteristics at T1	
Age (years)	42.9 ± 8.6
Gender (male)	82.4% (85)
Marital status (married or in a relationship)	36.3% (33)
Alcohol use disorder severity at T1 (AUDIT total score)	27.8 ± 7.7
PTSD severity at T1 (PCL-5 total score)	46.4 ± 10.9
Lifetime exposure to a traumatic event (LEC-5)	
At least one traumatic event	100% (91)
Natural disaster or/and accident (at least one)	87.9% (80)
Physical or/and sexual aggression (at least one)	82.4% (75)
War-related trauma (at least one)	6.6% (6)
Illness, injury, or death experience (at least one)	30.8% (28)
Any other traumatic event (at least one)	75.8% (69)
Childhood trauma (CTQ sub-scores)	
CTQ physical abuse score	8.3 ± 4.8
CTQ emotional abuse score	12.9 ± 5.9
CTQ sexual abuse score	6.8 ± 3.9
CTQ physical negligence score	8.9 ± 3.7
CTQ emotional negligence score	12.8 ± 5.0

Note: Descriptive data are presented as mean ± standard deviation (SD) or percentage (number). AUDIT, Alcohol Use Disorders Identification Test; CTQ, Childhood Trauma Questionnaire, short form; LEC-5, Life Event Checklist for DSM-5; PCL, PTSD Checklist for DSM-5; PTSD, Post-traumatic Stress Disorder; T1, Assessment at baseline (i.e., one week after admission).

3.2. Factors Associated with PTSD Remission in Univariate Analyses

Table 2 presents the baseline characteristics at T1 associated with PTSD remission at T2. Patients with non-remitted and remitted PTSD did not differ in terms of age, gender, or marital status. PTSD remission was not associated with the severity of AUD or PTSD at baseline. There was no difference between patients with and without remitted PTSD in terms of type of trauma encountered during lifetime (LEC-5). The only factors associated with lower remission rates were physical and emotional abuse during childhood, as assessed by the CTQ-SF.

Table 2. Baseline characteristics at T1 associated with PTSD remission at T2 in univariate analyses ($n = 91$).

	Non-Remitted PTSD at T2 ($n = 23$)	Remitted PTSD at T2 ($n = 68$)	Statistic Test
	Socio-demographic characteristics at T1		
Age (years)	40.0 ± 7.9	43.7 ± 8.7	$t = -1.83$
Gender (male)	73.9% (17)	85.3% (58)	$\chi^2 = 1.54$
Marital status (married or in a relationship)	26.1% (6)	39.7% (27)	$\chi^2 = 1.38$
Alcohol use disorder severity at T1 (AUDIT total score)	27.0 ± 7.3	28.0 ± 7.9	$t = -0.56$
PTSD severity at T1 (PCL-5 total score)	43.8 ± 8.8	47.3 ± 11.4	$t = 1.34$
	Lifetime exposure to a traumatic event (LEC-5)		
Natural disaster or/and accident (at least one)	91.3% (21)	86.8% (59)	$\chi^2 = 0.33$
Physical or/and sexual aggression (at least one)	78.3% (18)	83.8% (57)	$\chi^2 = 0.37$
War-related trauma (at least one)	8.6% (2)	5.9% (4)	$\chi^2 = 0.22$
Illness, injury, or death experience (at least one)	39.1% (9)	29.4% (20)	$\chi^2 = 0.75$
Any other traumatic event (at least one)	78.3% (18)	75% (51)	$\chi^2 = 0.10$
	Childhood trauma (CTQ sub-scores)		
CTQ physical abuse score *	10.7 ± 6.5	7.5 ± 3.8	$t = 2.22$
CTQ emotional abuse score *	15.1 ± 6.2	12.1 ± 5.6	$t = 2.16$
CTQ sexual abuse score	8.4 ± 6.1	6.2 ± 2.7	$t = 1.64$
CTQ physical negligence score	10.3 ± 3.8	8.4 ± 3.2	$t = 1.75$
CTQ emotional negligence score	13.7 ± 6.1	12.5 ± 4.6	$t = 0.99$

Note: Descriptive data are presented as mean ± standard deviation or percentage (number). We compared patients with remitted vs. non-remitted PTSD using mean comparison tests (Mann–Whitney U test or Student's test) and chi-squared tests. * indicates the variables significantly associated with PTSD remission. AUDIT, Alcohol Use Disorders Identification Test; CTQ, Childhood Trauma Questionnaire, short form; LEC-5, Life Event Checklist for DSM-5; PCL, PTSD Checklist for DSM-5; PTSD, Post-traumatic Stress Disorder; T1, Assessment at baseline (i.e., one week after admission); T2, Assessment eight weeks after admission (i.e., one week before discharge).

3.3. Factors Associated with PTSD Remission in Multivariate Analyses

Table 3 presents the multiple logistic regression model showing the baseline characteristics at T1 associated with PTSD remission at T2. After adjustment for age, the factors significantly associated with PTSD remission at T2 were physical abuse, emotional abuse, sexual abuse, and physical negligence during childhood, but not AUD severity, nor the other types of trauma experienced during lifetime (i.e., catastrophe, accident, physical assault, sexual assault, death, war, or any other kind of trauma). PTSD remission was not associated with baseline socio-demographic characteristics.

Table 3. Baseline T1 characteristics associated with PTSD remission at T2 in multiple logistic regressions after adjustment for age.

	Non-Remitted PTSD at T2 (n = 23)	Remitted PTSD at T2 (n = 68)	Chi-Squared	p-value	Odds-Ratio	CI 95%
	Socio-demographic characteristics					
Gender (male)	73.9% (17)	85.3% (58)	2.05	0.15	0.42	0.13–1.38
Marital status (married or in a relationship)	26.1% (6)	39.7% (27)	1.57	0.21	0.5	0.17–1.47
Alcohol use disorder severity at T1 (AUDIT total score)	27.0 ± 7.3	28.0 ± 7.9	0.46	0.5	1.02	0.96–1.09
PTSD severity at T1 (PCL-5 total score)	43.8 ± 8.8	47.3 ± 11.4	1.94	0.16	1.03	0.99–1.08
	Life events (LEC-5)					
Natural disaster or/and accident (at least one)	91.3% (21)	86.8% (59)	0.27	0.61	0.1.54	0.30–7.92
Physical or/and sexual aggression (at least one)	78.3% (18)	83.8% (57)	0.49	0.49	0.65	0.19–2.18
War-related trauma	8.6% (2)	5.9% (4)	1.2	0.27	2.98	0.42–20.99
Illness, injury, or death experience	39.1% (9)	29.4% (20)	1.77	0.18	2.05	0.71–5.91
Any other traumatic event	78.3% (18)	75% (51)	0.13	0.72	1.24	0.23–3.02
	Childhood trauma (CTQ sub-scores)					
CTQ physical abuse *	10.7 ± 6.5	7.5 ± 3.8	7.4	<0.001 *	0.8741	0.79–0.96
CTQ emotional abuse *	15.1 ± 6.2	12.1 ± 5.6	4.8	0.03 *	0.91	0.84–0.99
CTQ sexual abuse *	8.4 ± 6.1	6.2 ± 2.7	4.8	0.03 *	0.88	0.78–0.99
CTQ physical negligence *	10.3 ± 3.8	8.4 ± 3.2	4.05	0.05 *	0.88	0.78–0.99
CTQ emotional negligence	13.7 ± 6.1	12.5 ± 4.6	1.98	0.16	0.93	0.39–3.90

Note: Descriptive data are presented as mean ± standard deviation or percentage (number). We compared patients with remitted vs. non-remitted PTSD using multiple logistic regression adjusted for age. * indicates the variables significantly associated with PTSD remission. AUDIT, Alcohol Use Disorders Identification Test; CTQ, Childhood Trauma Questionnaire, short form; LEC-5, Life Event Checklist for DSM-5; PCL, PTSD Checklist for DSM-5; PTSD, Post-traumatic Stress Disorder; T1, Assessment at baseline (i.e., one week after admission); T2, Assessment eight weeks after admission (i.e., one week before discharge).

4. Discussion

The main objective of this study was to determine the baseline variables associated with PTSD remission among patients hospitalized for an AUD and with a comorbid PTSD. One of the key findings is that remission varied according to the existence of trauma during a particularly important period in one's life (i.e., childhood), but not in relation to baseline AUD severity, PTSD severity, or exposure to other types of traumatic event during lifetime.

Our results thus demonstrate that childhood traumas are predictors of non-remitted PTSD. First, our study confirms the high rate of childhood traumas in patients with AUD and PTSD, compared to all other types of trauma. In a study of AUD patients in an addiction rehabilitation center, Huang et al. found that the prevalence of childhood trauma was 55.1%, physical abuse 31.1%, emotional abuse 21.4%, sexual abuse 24%, physical neglect 19.9%, and emotional neglect 20.4% [18]. The relatively lower prevalence of sexual abuse observed in our study can be explained by the overrepresentation of men, who are less exposed to sexual abuse than women [35].

We also found that all types of childhood abuse (i.e., physical, emotional, and sexual) were associated with PTSD. In line with Bowlby's theoretical framework and attachment theory [21], this association could be explained by a higher risk of insecure attachment (especially fearful attachment), which has been demonstrated to be strongly related to PTSD symptoms [22]. Childhood trauma may also increase the risk of some high-risk personality traits (i.e., neuroticism or low extraversion) [36], and of psychiatric disorders such as bipolar disorder, anxiety disorders or treatment-resistant depression [18,37–39]. It could also lead to the possibility of more severe, earlier, and long-lasting psychiatric disorders, and thus higher risk for PTSD. Finally, early trauma may increase stress vulnerability through gene–environment interactions and impaired hypothalamic–pituitary–adrenal axis response [38]. A recent study by O'Hare et al. highlighted the increased risk for vasovagal syncope in patients with childhood trauma, which may be due to paradoxical parasympathetic overdrive in response to a sympathetic increase in heart rate, with a stress response being decoupled from the original acute stressor [40].

Contrary to the findings of a meta-analysis that some types of trauma were associated with better remission rates (i.e., natural disasters were associated with 60% remission rate vs. 31.4% when the trauma was related to physical health) [41], we found no evidence of association between the type of trauma and the course of PTSD. This could be explained by the fact that the patients in our sample had been exposed to more than one type of traumatic event, making it difficult to disentangle the effects of each specific trauma on PTSD outcome. Although PTSD symptoms at baseline were associated with AUD severity at baseline, the course of PTSD was surprisingly not associated with the baseline intensity of AUD or PTSD. The lack of association with AUD severity is in line with findings that improvements in PTSD had a greater positive impact on alcohol dependence symptoms than the reciprocal relationship [19]. The association between PTSD and AUD severity at baseline is in line with previous studies [42,43], and can be explained by the amnestic, anxiolytic, and sedative properties of alcohol that may help these patients to cope with and avoid the intrusive PTSD symptoms (self-medication hypothesis) [44]. On the other hand, the lack of association between PTSD outcome and at baseline might suggest that it is not the intensity of PTSD itself that affects outcome, but rather the fact that the trauma was experienced during a particularly important period in one's life (i.e., a trauma experienced during childhood could lead to earlier changes in personality traits or psychiatric disorders, and be associated with a long-established PTSD that could be harder to treat than a more recent one).

Another interesting finding of our study is the significant drop in the PTSD symptom score between baseline and eight weeks later. To our knowledge, this has not been assessed in previous longitudinal studies of patients with AUD and PTSD in an addiction rehabilitation center. A meta-analysis conducted by Morina et al., which focused on the course of PTSD and was not limited to AUD patients, found a spontaneous PTSD remission rate (without any specific treatment) of approximately 44% at 40-months follow-up [41]. Patients with co-occurring AUD and PTSD are an at-risk population, for whom inpatient treatment may be an interesting option when they do not respond to outpatient treatment. Addiction rehabilitation centers provide multidisciplinary care, offering patients new coping strategies, with beneficial effects on eating and sleeping habits, and reducing stress related to work or family. However, we cannot rule out the possibility that the positive PTSD outcome we observed was due to improvement in AUD, through the beneficial effects of prolonged withdrawal, or due to confounding factors associated with hospitalization (i.e., increased social support, improved physical activity, treatment of concurrent medical conditions). In addition, the study design (no control group) precludes us from demonstrating a beneficial effect of an inpatient rehabilitation program on PTSD. To demonstrate the potential beneficial effects of such programs, future studies should compare the evolution of inpatients with versus without a rehabilitation program (control-group).

At a practical level, our study highlights the importance of identifying those patients with AUD and PTSD who have a history of childhood trauma as a potential at-risk population requiring tailored treatment. These patients may have specific needs and expectations about treatment, given their psychological and psychiatric profile (more prevalent insecure attachment, more severe and earlier psychiatric disorders). Integrative psychological and psychosocial interventions focusing on trauma-related symptoms and alcohol dependence tailored to individual needs offer an interesting way to manage this vulnerable population and improve treatment outcomes [19]. One clinical implication of our study is that hospitalized AUD patients should be systematically screened for childhood abuse or neglect. Secondly, they should be assessed using different biological and psychological theoretical frameworks in order to better understand how these traumas may be linked to the co-occurring addictive disorder and PTSD. Our results also highlight the need for close and long-term follow-up of this at-risk population.

This study has several limitations. First, PTSD diagnosis and AUD severity were based on self-administered questionnaires, which increases the risk of false positives and possible recall bias. Given that the LEC-5 assesses lifetime exposure to trauma and the CTQ-SF assesses childhood trauma, there may be an overlap between the two measures. Although we knew if a trauma occurred during childhood, we did not assess the exact timing of the trauma during childhood or adulthood. Another limitation concerns the participants in our sample (AUD inpatients in a rehabilitation center), who may differ from other patients with AUD and comorbid PTSD (inpatients usually exhibit more severe AUD/PTSD). This selection bias and our small sample of patients with non-remitted PTSD may limit the generalizability of our findings. Finally, our study was conducted in a single center, where the other psychosocial interventions proposed concurrently may have impacted the course of PTSD.

5. Conclusions

We demonstrated that the main factor associated with poor PTSD outcome in patients with comorbid AUD and PTSD was a history of childhood trauma. We also found that neither the type of trauma experienced, nor the initial severity of AUD were associated with PTSD remission. These results highlight the importance of systematically assessing the history of childhood trauma in patients hospitalized for an AUD, and of tailoring evidence-based interventions for this high-risk population. Future studies should test the efficacy of trauma-focused interventions (i.e., EMDR or Cognitive and Behavioural Therapy) for treating both PTSD and AUD, and compare its efficacy in patients with and without a history of childhood trauma [45,46]. Tailored interventions for patients with AUD and PTSD could help us to meet the challenge of improving the therapeutic management of patients with these dual disorders [4].

Author Contributions: Conceptualization: F.I., D.B., R.C., N.B., and W.E.-H.; Data curation: P.A.; Formal analysis: P.B.; Investigation: K.L., F.I., D.M., P.A., S.B., G.B., R.C., H.E.A., M.G.-B., and C.H.; Project administration: W.E.-H.; Supervision: N.B. and W.E.-H.; Writing—original draft: P.B., K.L., F.I., D.M., P.A., S.B., G.B., R.C., H.E.A., M.G.-B., C.H., N.B., and W.E.-H.; Writing—review and editing: P.B., K.L., F.I., D.M., P.A., S.B., G.B., R.C., H.E.A., M.G.-B., C.H., N.B., and W.E.-H. All authors have read and agreed to the published version of the manuscript.

Funding: This study was conducted without specific funding. The University of Tours funded the open access option.

Acknowledgments: We thank Frédérique Yonnet and Sarah Trotet (head of Le Courbat rehabilitation center) who approved this study. We thank Elizabeth Yates for revising the English version of the manuscript.

Conflicts of Interest: N.B. reports personal fees from Lundbeck, Astra-Zeneca and D&A Pharma, unrelated to the submitted work. P.B. reports personal fees and non-financial support from Lundbeck, personal fees from Astra-Zeneca and D&A Pharma, unrelated to the submitted work. W.E.-H. reports personal fees from Lundbeck, Janssen-Cilag, Otsuka and UCB unrelated to this work. M.G.-B. declares that the Addictology and Psychiatry Department has received funding directly from the University Hospital of Nantes and gambling industry operators (FDJ and PMU); scientific independence in relation to gambling industry operators is assured; there were no constraints on publishing. M.G.-B. reports no financial or other relationship relevant to the subject of this article. K.L., F.I., D.M., H.E.A., P.A., S.B., G.B., C.H., and R.C. have nothing to disclose. The funders mentioned here had no role in the design of the study; in the collection, analyses, or interpretation of data; in the writing of the manuscript, or in the decision to publish the results.

References

1. Carvalho, A.F.; Heilig, M.; Perez, A.; Probst, C.; Rehm, J. Alcohol use disorders. *Lancet* **2019**, *394*, 781–792. [CrossRef]
2. American Psychiatric Association. *Diagnostic and Statistical Manual of Mental Disorders: Dsm-5*, 5th ed.; American Psychiatric Association Publishing: Washington, DC, USA, 2013; ISBN 978-0-89042-555-8.
3. Rehm, J.; Mathers, C.; Popova, S.; Thavorncharoensap, M.; Teerawattananon, Y.; Patra, J. Global burden of disease and injury and economic cost attributable to alcohol use and alcohol-use disorders. *Lancet* **2009**, *373*, 2223–2233. [CrossRef]
4. Torrens, M.; Rossi, P.C.; Martinez-Riera, R.; Martinez-Sanvisens, D.; Bulbena, A. Psychiatric Co-Morbidity and Substance Use Disorders: Treatment in Parallel Systems or in One Integrated System? *Subst. Use Misuse* **2012**, *47*, 1005–1014. [CrossRef] [PubMed]
5. Blanco, C.; Xu, Y.; Brady, K.; Pérez-Fuentes, G.; Okuda, M.; Wang, S. Comorbidity of posttraumatic stress disorder with alcohol dependence among US adults: Results from National Epidemiological Survey on Alcohol and Related Conditions. *Drug Alcohol Depend.* **2013**, *132*, 630–638. [CrossRef]
6. Kessler, R.C.; Sonnega, A.; Bromet, E.; Hughes, M.; Nelson, C.B. Posttraumatic stress disorder in the National Comorbidity Survey. *Arch. Gen. Psychiatry* **1995**, *52*, 1048–1060. [CrossRef]
7. Khoury, L.; Tang, Y.L.; Bradley, B.; Cubells, J.F.; Ressler, K.J. Substance use, childhood traumatic experience, and Posttraumatic Stress Disorder in an urban civilian population. *Depress. Anxiety* **2010**, *27*, 1077–1086. [CrossRef]
8. Norman, S.B.; Haller, M.; Hamblen, J.L.; Southwick, S.M.; Pietrzak, R.H. The burden of co-occurring alcohol use disorder and PTSD in U.S. Military veterans: Comorbidities, functioning, and suicidality. *Psychol. Addict. Behav.* **2018**, *32*, 224–229. [CrossRef]
9. Dore, G.; Mills, K.; Murray, R.; Teesson, M.; Farrugia, P. Post-traumatic stress disorder, depression and suicidality in inpatients with substance use disorders. *Drug Alcohol Rev.* **2012**, *31*, 294–302. [CrossRef]
10. Drapkin, M.L.; Yusko, D.; Yasinski, C.; Oslin, D.; Hembree, E.A.; Foa, E.B. Baseline functioning among individuals with posttraumatic stress disorder and alcohol dependence. *J. Subst. Abus. Treat.* **2011**, *41*, 186–192. [CrossRef]
11. Back, S.E.; Brady, K.T.; Sonne, S.C.; Verduin, M.L. Symptom Improvement in Co-Occurring PTSD and Alcohol Dependence. *J. Nerv. Ment. Dis.* **2006**, *194*, 690–696. [CrossRef]
12. Chapman, C.; Mills, K.; Slade, T.; McFarlane, A.C.; Bryant, R.A.; Creamer, M.; Silove, D.; Teesson, M. Remission from post-traumatic stress disorder in the general population. *Psychol. Med.* **2012**, *42*, 1695–1703. [CrossRef]
13. Müller, M.; Ajdacic-Gross, V.; Rodgers, S.; Kleim, B.; Seifritz, E.; Vetter, S.; Egger, S.T.; Rössler, W.; Castelao, E.; Preisig, M.; et al. Predictors of remission from PTSD symptoms after sexual and non-sexual trauma in the community: A mediated survival-analytic approach. *Psychiatry Res.* **2018**, *260*, 262–271. [CrossRef]
14. Rosellini, A.J.; Liu, H.; Petukhova, M.V.; Sampson, N.A.; Aguilar-Gaxiola, S.; Alonso, J.; Borges, G.; Bruffaerts, R.; Bromet, E.J.; de Girolamo, G.; et al. Recovery from DSM-IV post-traumatic stress disorder in the WHO World Mental Health surveys. *Psychol. Med.* **2018**, *48*, 437–450. [CrossRef]

15. Steinert, C.; Hofmann, M.; Leichsenring, F.; Kruse, J. The course of PTSD in naturalistic long-term studies: High variability of outcomes. A systematic review. *Nord. J. Psychiatry* **2015**, *69*, 483–496. [CrossRef]
16. Dworkin, E.R.; Wanklyn, S.; Stasiewicz, P.R.; Coffey, S.F. PTSD symptom presentation among people with alcohol and drug use disorders: Comparisons by substance of abuse. *Addict. Behav.* **2018**, *76*, 188–194. [CrossRef] [PubMed]
17. Grundmann, J.; Lincoln, T.M.; Lüdecke, D.; Bong, S.; Schulte, B.; Verthein, U.; Schäfer, I. Traumatic Experiences, Revictimization and Posttraumatic Stress Disorder in German Inpatients Treated for Alcohol Dependence. *Subst. Use Misuse* **2017**, 1–9. [CrossRef] [PubMed]
18. Huang, M.-C.; Schwandt, M.L.; Ramchandani, V.A.; George, D.T.; Heilig, M. Impact of multiple types of childhood trauma exposure on risk of psychiatric comorbidity among alcoholic inpatients. *Alcohol. Clin. Exp. Res.* **2012**, *36*, 1099–1107. [CrossRef]
19. Brady, K.T.; Back, S.E. Childhood trauma, posttraumatic stress disorder, and alcohol dependence. *Alcohol Res.* **2012**, *34*, 408–413.
20. Müller, M.; Vandeleur, C.; Rodgers, S.; Rössler, W.; Castelao, E.; Preisig, M.; Ajdacic-Gross, V. Posttraumatic stress avoidance symptoms as mediators in the development of alcohol use disorders after exposure to childhood sexual abuse in a Swiss community sample. *Child Abus. Negl.* **2015**, *46*, 8–15. [CrossRef]
21. Bowlby, J. *Attachment: Attachment and Loss Volume One (Basic Books Classics)*, 2nd ed.; Basic Books: New York, NY, USA, 1983; ISBN 978-0-465-00543-7.
22. Woodhouse, S.; Ayers, S.; Field, A.P. The relationship between adult attachment style and post-traumatic stress symptoms: A meta-analysis. *J. Anxiety Disord.* **2015**, *35*, 103–117. [CrossRef]
23. Schäfer, I.; Najavits, L.M. Clinical challenges in the treatment of patients with posttraumatic stress disorder and substance abuse. *Curr. Opin. Psychiatry* **2007**, *20*, 614–618. [CrossRef] [PubMed]
24. Bernstein, D.P.; Stein, J.A.; Newcomb, M.D.; Walker, E.; Pogge, D.; Ahluvalia, T.; Stokes, J.; Handelsman, L.; Medrano, M.; Desmond, D.; et al. Development and validation of a brief screening version of the Childhood Trauma Questionnaire. *Child Abus. Negl.* **2003**, *27*, 169–190. [CrossRef]
25. Paquette, D.; Laporte, L.; Bigras, M.; Zoccolillo, M. [Validation of the French version of the CTQ and prevalence of the history of maltreatment]. *Sante Ment. Que.* **2004**, *29*, 201–220. [CrossRef] [PubMed]
26. Spinhoven, P.; Penninx, B.W.; Hickendorff, M.; van Hemert, A.M.; Bernstein, D.P.; Elzinga, B.M. Childhood Trauma Questionnaire: Factor structure, measurement invariance, and validity across emotional disorders. *Psychol. Assess.* **2014**, *26*, 717. [CrossRef]
27. Weathers, F.W.; Blake, D.D.; Schnurr, P.P.; Kaloupek, D.G.; Marx, B.P.; Keane, T.M. The life events checklist for DSM-5 (LEC-5). 2013. Available online: https://www.ptsd.va.gov/professional/assessment/te-measures/life_events_checklist.asp (accessed on 29 June 2020).
28. Blevins, C.A.; Weathers, F.W.; Davis, M.T.; Witte, T.K.; Domino, J.L. The Posttraumatic Stress Disorder Checklist for DSM-5 (PCL-5): Development and Initial Psychometric Evaluation. *J. Trauma. Stress* **2015**, *28*, 489–498. [CrossRef]
29. Ashbaugh, A.R.; Houle-Johnson, S.; Herbert, C.; El-Hage, W.; Brunet, A. Psychometric Validation of the English and French Versions of the Posttraumatic Stress Disorder Checklist for DSM-5 (PCL-5). *PLoS ONE* **2016**, *11*, e0161645. [CrossRef]
30. Zohar, J.; Amital, D.; Miodownik, C.; Kotler, M.; Bleich, A.; Lane, R.M.; Austin, C. Double-blind placebo-controlled pilot study of sertraline in military veterans with posttraumatic stress disorder. *J. Clin. Psychopharmacol.* **2002**, *22*, 190–195. [CrossRef]
31. Brady, K.; Pearlstein, T.; Asnis, G.M.; Baker, D.; Rothbaum, B.; Sikes, C.R.; Farfel, G.M. Efficacy and safety of sertraline treatment of posttraumatic stress disorder: A randomized controlled trial. *JAMA* **2000**, *283*, 1837–1844. [CrossRef]
32. Dunlop, B.W.; Kaye, J.L.; Youngner, C.; Rothbaum, B. Assessing treatment-resistant posttraumatic stress disorder: The Emory treatment resistance interview for PTSD (E-TRIP). *Behav. Sci.* **2014**, *4*, 511–527. [CrossRef]
33. Saunders, J.B.; Aasland, O.G.; Babor, T.F.; de la Fuente, J.R.; Grant, M. Development of the Alcohol Use Disorders Identification Test (AUDIT): WHO Collaborative Project on Early Detection of Persons with Harmful Alcohol Consumption–II. *Addiction* **1993**, *88*, 791–804. [CrossRef]

34. Gache, P.; Michaud, P.; Landry, U.; Accietto, C.; Arfaoui, S.; Wenger, O.; Daeppen, J.-B. The Alcohol Use Disorders Identification Test (AUDIT) as a screening tool for excessive drinking in primary care: Reliability and validity of a French version. *Alcohol. Clin. Exp. Res.* **2005**, *29*, 2001–2007. [CrossRef] [PubMed]
35. Dragan, M.; Lis-Turlejska, M. Prevalence of posttraumatic stress disorder in alcohol dependent patients in Poland. *Addict. Behav.* **2007**, *32*, 902–911. [CrossRef] [PubMed]
36. Ozen, S.; Dalbudak, E.; Topcu, M. The Relationship of Posttraumatic Stress Disorder with Childhood Traumas, Personality Characteristics, Depression and Anxiety Symptoms in Patients with Diagnosis of Mixed Anxiety-Depression Disorder. *Psychiatr. Danub.* **2018**, *30*, 340–347. [CrossRef] [PubMed]
37. Etain, B.; Mathieu, F.; Henry, C.; Raust, A.; Roy, I.; Germain, A.; Leboyer, M.; Bellivier, F. Preferential association between childhood emotional abuse and bipolar disorder. *J. Trauma. Stress* **2010**, *23*, 376–383. [CrossRef]
38. Gottschalk, M.G.; Domschke, K. Genetics of generalized anxiety disorder and related traits. *Dialogues Clin. Neurosci.* **2017**, *19*, 159–168.
39. Yrondi, A.; Aouizerate, B.; Bennabi, D.; Richieri, R.; D'Amato, T.; Bellivier, F.; Bougerol, T.; Horn, M.; Camus, V.; Courtet, P.; et al. Childhood maltreatment and clinical severity of treatment-resistant depression in a French cohort of outpatients (FACE-DR): One-year follow-up. *Depress. Anxiety* **2020**, *37*, 365–374. [CrossRef]
40. O'Hare, C.; McCrory, C.; O'Leary, N.; O'Brien, H.; Kenny, R.A. Childhood trauma and lifetime syncope burden among older adults. *J. Psychosom. Res.* **2017**, *97*, 63–69. [CrossRef]
41. Morina, N.; Wicherts, J.M.; Lobbrecht, J.; Priebe, S. Remission from post-traumatic stress disorder in adults: A systematic review and meta-analysis of long term outcome studies. *Clin. Psychol. Rev.* **2014**, *34*, 249–255. [CrossRef]
42. Hingray, C.; Cohn, A.; Martini, H.; Donné, C.; El-Hage, W.; Schwan, R.; Paille, F. Impact of trauma on addiction and psychopathology profile in alcohol-dependent women. *Eur. J. Trauma Dissociation* **2018**, *2*, 101–107. [CrossRef]
43. Walton, J.L.; Raines, A.M.; Cuccurullo, L.-A.J.; Vidaurri, D.N.; Villarosa-Hurlocker, M.C.; Franklin, C.L. The relationship between DSM-5 PTSD symptom clusters and alcohol misuse among military veterans. *Am. J. Addict.* **2018**, *27*, 23–28. [CrossRef]
44. Hruska, B.; Pacella, M.L.; George, R.L.; Delahanty, D.L. The association between daily PTSD symptom severity and alcohol-related outcomes in recent traumatic injury victims. *Psychol. Addict. Behav.* **2017**, *31*, 326–335. [CrossRef] [PubMed]
45. Sannibale, C.; Teesson, M.; Creamer, M.; Sitharthan, T.; Bryant, R.A.; Sutherland, K.; Taylor, K.; Bostock-Matusko, D.; Visser, A.; Peek-O'Leary, M. Randomized controlled trial of cognitive behaviour therapy for comorbid post-traumatic stress disorder and alcohol use disorders. *Addiction* **2013**, *108*, 1397–1410. [CrossRef] [PubMed]
46. Schäfer, I.; Chuey-Ferrer, L.; Hofmann, A.; Lieberman, P.; Mainusch, G.; Lotzin, A. Effectiveness of EMDR in patients with substance use disorder and comorbid PTSD: Study protocol for a randomized controlled trial. *BMC Psychiatry* **2017**, *17*, 95. [CrossRef] [PubMed]

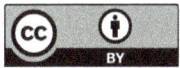

© 2020 by the authors. Licensee MDPI, Basel, Switzerland. This article is an open access article distributed under the terms and conditions of the Creative Commons Attribution (CC BY) license (http://creativecommons.org/licenses/by/4.0/).

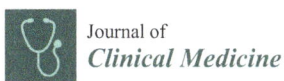

Article

Traumatic Events in Dual Disorders: Prevalence and Clinical Characteristics

Laura Blanco [1,2], Albert Sió [1], Bridget Hogg [3,4], Ricard Esteve [5], Joaquim Radua [6,7,8,9], Aleix Solanes [6], Itxaso Gardoki-Souto [3,4], Rosa Sauras [5], Adriana Farré [5], Claudio Castillo [5], Alicia Valiente-Gómez [3,4,5,9,10], Víctor Pérez [4,5,9,10], Marta Torrens [4,5,9,10,11], Benedikt L. Amann [3,4,5,9,10,*] and Ana Moreno-Alcázar [3,4,9]

1. Benito Menni Complex Assistencial en Salut Mental, Sant Boi de Llobregat, 08830 Barcelona, Spain; lbpresas@gmail.com (L.B.); asioeroles@gmail.com (A.S.)
2. Department of Personality, Evaluation and Psychological Treatments, University of Barcelona, 08007 Barcelona, Spain
3. Centre Fòrum Research Unit, Institut de Neuropsiquiatria i Addiccions, Parc de Salut Mar, 08019 Barcelona, Spain; bridget.hogg@e-campus.uab.cat (B.H.); itxasogardoki@gmail.com (I.G.-S.); avaliente@parcdesalutmar.cat (A.V.-G.); amoreno.centreforum@gmail.com (A.M.-A.)
4. Hospital del Mar Medical Research Institute (IMIM), 08003 Barcelona, Spain; VPerezSola@parcdesalutmar.cat (V.P.); MTorrens@parcdesalutmar.cat (M.T.)
5. Institut de Neuropsiquiatria i Addiccions, Parc de Salut Mar, 08003 Barcelona, Spain; restevevila@gmail.com (R.E.); rsauras@parcdesalutmar.cat (R.S.); adrianaf2@hotmail.com (A.F.); CCastillo@parcdesalutmar.cat (C.C.)
6. Imaging of Mood and Anxiety-Related Disorders (IMARD) group, Institut d'Investigacions Biomèdiques August Pi i Sunyer (IDIBAPS), 08036 Barcelona, Spain; quimradua@gmail.com (J.R.); al.solanes@gmail.com (A.S.)
7. Early Psychosis: Interventions and Clinical-detection (EPIC) Laboratory, Department of Psychosis Studies, Institute of Psychiatry, Psychology & Neuroscience, King's College London, London WC2R2LS, UK
8. Department of Clinical Neuroscience, Centre for Psychiatry Research, Karolinska Institutet, Solna, 17177 Stockholm, Sweden
9. Centro de Investigación Biomédica en Red de Salud Mental (CIBERSAM), 28029 Madrid, Spain
10. Department of Psychiatry, Universitat Autònoma de Barcelona, Bellaterra, 08193 Barcelona, Spain
11. RETICS-Redes Temáticas de Investigación Cooperativa en Salud en Trastornos Adictivos, 08003 Barcelona, Spain
* Correspondence: benedikt.amann@gmail.com; Tel.: +34-933-268-500 (ext. 8527); Fax: +34-933-268-560

Received: 6 July 2020; Accepted: 31 July 2020; Published: 6 August 2020

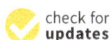

Abstract: Psychological trauma has been identified in substance use disorders (SUD) as a major etiological risk factor. However, detailed and systematic data about the prevalence and types of psychological trauma in dual disorders have been scarce to date. In this study, 150 inpatients were recruited and cross-sectionally screened on their substance use severity, psychological trauma symptoms, comorbidities, and clinical severity. One hundred patients fulfilled criteria for a dual disorder, while 50 patients were diagnosed with only SUD. Ninety-four percent of the whole sample suffered from at least one lifetime traumatic event. The prevalence rates of Posttraumatic Stress Disorder diagnosis for dual disorder and only SUD was around 20% in both groups; however, patients with dual disorder presented more adverse events, more childhood trauma, more dissociative symptoms, and a more severe clinical profile than patients with only SUD. Childhood maltreatment can also serve as a predictor for developing a dual disorder diagnosis and as a risk factor for developing a more complex and severe clinical profile. These data challenge our current clinical practice in the treatment of patients suffering from dual disorder or only SUD diagnosis and favor the incorporation of an additional trauma-focused therapy in this population. This may improve the prognosis and the course of the illness in these patients.

Keywords: psychological trauma; posttraumatic stress disorder; substance use disorders; dual diagnosis; prevalence

1. Introduction

Substance use disorder (SUD) is a psychiatric condition that affects judgement and alters cognitive functions, such as learning, memory, and impulse control [1]. SUD has a multifactorial etiology, resulting from the combination of different genetic [2] and environmental [3] factors. Moreover, like in many other psychiatric pathologies, a better or worse evolution is associated with multiple biological and socio-demographical variables, such as age of onset, access to drugs, social environment, race, and presence of external stressors [2–4]. Out of all these variables, psychological trauma has gained importance in clinical research studies, due to the strong negative impact it has on the onset, course, and prognosis of many psychiatric pathologies [5]. More than 70% of the adult population worldwide have experienced at least one psychological trauma event in their life, and 31% have suffered from four or more traumatic events. The majority recover from them without any external intervention [6]. However, those who do continue to experience symptoms related to psychological trauma are at risk of developing post-traumatic stress disorder (PTSD). Of note, in SUD samples, Posttraumatic Stress Disorder (PTSD) prevalence rates over the last 12 months vary from 15% to 41%, and lifetime rates vary from 26% to 52% [7]. These results are striking when compared to prevalence rates of current PTSD of 0.2–3.8% and lifetime prevalence of 1.3–12.3% in the general population [6]. There appears to be a greater vulnerability to develop, in general, somatic and/or psychiatric disorders when the traumatic event is experienced during childhood [8,9].

The relation between PTSD and SUD is a source of controversy. Briefly, the most accepted view is the "self-medication model" hypothesis, which means the traumatic event occurred prior to the substance use [10]. The "high-risk hypothesis" argues that substance abuse comes first, and this increases the probability of being exposed to more traumatic events, and in consequence to PTSD [11]. Thirdly, there is the "shared liability model", which considers that both disorders develop simultaneously after the traumatic event due to a common biopsychosocial process [12–14]. Finally, the "susceptibility model" posits high anxiety and arousal as a consequence of chronic substance use, which in turn leads to a higher risk of PTSD [15]. Besides the lack of consensus between the different explanatory models, there does seem to be an agreement that SUD increases the severity of PTSD presentation, and PTSD seems to be an independent risk factor for an unfavorable outcome of SUD [4,16,17]. Specifically, patients with both disorders present a worse prognosis and evolution [4], a greater number of further comorbid somatic and psychiatric disorders [18], a higher number of detoxification treatment admissions and relapses [19], an earlier start to substance use [20], greater number of years of use [21], a poly-substance consumption pattern [22], a greater severity of PTSD symptoms [23], and a higher number, as well as a greater severity and intensity, of dissociative symptoms in those with poly-substance SUD [24]. In summary, patients with SUD and PTSD have a more severe and complex clinical profile [7].

In the last decade, epidemiological and clinical research has increasingly focused on the importance of detecting and treating the comorbidity of severe mental disorders and SUD, the so-called dual disorder [25]. Dual disorder patients, in comparison to only SUD patients, present a worse prognosis and a more severe and complex clinical profile, characterized by a greater number of further comorbid disorders [18], more associated medical and psychological problems, a higher number of detoxification treatment admissions [26], an earlier start to substance use [20], and a poly-substance consumption pattern [22]. However, despite the clear and strong association between PTSD and SUD, specific data about the prevalence and clinical characterization of psychological trauma in patients with dual disorders, and especially in comparison with SUD patients, are scarce so far.

Therefore, the present study aims to evaluate the prevalence and detailed characterization of traumatic psychological trauma and life events and PTSD and their relation to clinical variables in hospitalized dual disorder patients versus patients with only SUD. Our hypothesis was that patients with dual disorder would suffer from more adverse events, more childhood trauma, have more dissociative symptoms, and have a more severe clinical profile than patients with only SUD. Furthermore, we hypothesized that patients with dual disorder would have a higher prevalence of a PTSD diagnosis than patients with only SUD.

2. Materials and Methods

2.1. Participants

This multicenter collaborative study was conducted from 2017 to 2019 and involved the participation of three different dual pathology inpatient units (one at Hospital Benito Menni, Sant Boi and two at the Hospital Parc de Salut Mar) from the Barcelona catchment area, Spain. Our study sample is representative and a random representation of typical SUD patients with or without psychiatric comorbidity due to the nature of the two units. One is in the centre of Barcelona city (Hospital Parc de Salut Mar), in a mainly low and middle-class sociodemographic area and connected to the University, while the other one (Hospital Benito Menni, Sant Boi) is a community hospital, based in the outskirts of Barcelona in a mainly rural middle-class social catchment area, which widens the representativeness of our sample. The criteria for admission are the same in both centres, namely a clinical decompensation due to SUD and a comorbid psychiatric disorder. This means that there are no exclusion criteria (unless in the case of a severe somatic disorder) and patients cannot be rejected as long as they belong to the corresponding sector. Participants were selected for the following inclusion criteria: (1) admitted to an inpatient dual pathology unit; (2) aged between 18–65 years; (3) fulfilling Diagnostic and Statistical Manual of Mental Disorders, fifth edition, (DSM-5) criteria for SUD, based on a revised version for DSM-5 of the Spanish version of Psychiatric Research Interview for Substance and Mental Disorders (PRISM) [27] and (4) capable of speaking Spanish. Exclusion criteria were: (1) severe cognitive impairment; (2) organic brain syndrome; (3) suicidal thoughts; and (4) an acute psychotic state. Of the 517 eligible patients, 220 did not meet the inclusion criteria due to the following reasons: 199 were either in an acute psychotic state, clinically too unstable, or presented suicidal thoughts; 18 had marked cognitive impairment, and three did not speak and understand the Spanish language. Furthermore, 32 refused to participate, 62 requested early voluntary discharge and could not be evaluated, 36 were readmissions to the same unit, and 17 patients were not evaluated for other reasons. The final sample therefore consisted of 150 patients. Evaluation of the patients was carried out by clinical psychologists after an initial detoxification period during which clinical symptoms were stabilized. This was approximately two weeks from the day of admission.

The ethics committees of both hospitals approved the study (Benito Menni CASM: PR-2017-24 and Hospital Parc de Salut Mar: 2017/7650/I) and all participants signed written informed consent prior to enrollment. Participants did not receive any compensation for participation in the study.

2.2. Measures

Sociodemographic and some clinical variables were collected through an interview using a specific Case Report Form (CRF) designed for the study. The CRF collected data on sex, age, race, educational level, personal and family background, current pharmacological treatment, and drug use pattern. The latter included age of onset, quantity, frequency, and whether drug consumption started before or after experiencing a traumatic event.

Severity of addiction was assessed using the following scale:

1. Severity of Dependence Scale (SDS) [28]: The SDS is a 5-item questionnaire which evaluates the degree of dependence on different types of drugs. Each item can be rated from 0 to 3, and higher scores mean greater dependence.

Psychological trauma symptoms were evaluated using the following tools:

1. Global Assessment of Posttraumatic Stress Questionnaire (EGEP-5) [29]: The EGEP-5 is a 58-item questionnaire which evaluates current PTSD based on DSM-5 criteria. This questionnaire contains three different sections: (1) presence of traumatic events; (2) intensity of symptoms related to intrusion, avoidance, disturbances in cognition and mood, as well as activation and reactivity; (3) functionality in different areas of the person's life.
2. Childhood Trauma Questionnaire (CTQ) [30], Spanish validation [31]: The CTQ is a self-administered 28-item scale that measures five types of childhood maltreatment: emotional, physical, and sexual abuse, and emotional or physical neglect. A 5-point Likert scale is used for the responses, ranging from "Never True" to "Very Often True".
3. Dissociative Experiences Scale (DES) [32], Spanish validation [33]: This scale consists of a 28-item self-report questionnaire that measures different experiences related to dissociation. A total score higher than or equal to 30 indicates the presence of dissociation.
4. The Holmes-Rahe Life Stress Inventory [34], Spanish validation [35]: This scale assesses the frequency of 43 common stressful life events over the last year. Scores below 150 reflect low levels of stress, scores between 150 and 299 represent a 50% risk of a stress-related illness in the near future, and scores above 300 represent an 80% risk of suffering from stress.

Comorbid disorders and clinical severity were assessed using the following instruments:

1. Dual Diagnosis Screening Interview (DDSI) [36]: The DDSI is a 63-item screening interview used to identify different psychiatric comorbidity in substance users, such as panic disorders, social phobia, agoraphobia, simple phobias, generalized anxiety, depression, dysthymia, mania, psychosis, attention deficit hyperactivity disorder, and PTSD.
2. The diagnoses of any psychiatric comorbidity were confirmed using the corresponding module of the Spanish version of the Psychiatric Research Interview for Substance and Mental Disorders, revised for the DSM-5 (PRISM) [27].
3. Hamilton Depression Rating Scale (HDRS) [37], Spanish validation [38]: This scale is a 17-item clinician-administered scale designed to identify depressive symptoms over the last week. Each item is scored on a 3- or 5-point scale, depending on the item, with a maximum score of 52. Scores are interpreted as follows: no depression (0–7), mild depression (8–16), moderate depression (17–23), and severe depression ($\geq$ 24).
4. Young Mania Rating Scale (YMRS) [39], Spanish validation [40]: The YMRS is an 11-item clinician-administered scale to evaluate hypomanic and manic symptoms over the last 48 h. Four items are scored from 0 to 8, while the remaining seven items are scored from 0 to 4. Higher scores mean greater severity.
5. Brief Psychiatric Rating Scale (BPRS) [41], Spanish validation [42]: The BPRS is an 18-item clinician-administered scale which measures psychiatric symptoms, such as depression, anxiety, hallucinations, and unusual behavior. Each item is scored from 1 (not present) to 7 (extremely severe).

2.3. Statistical Analysis

For the purpose of this study, the sample of patients was divided into patients with a dual disorder diagnosis, and patients with only a SUD diagnosis. To describe the sample, we reported the means and standard deviations of the age, number of years of education, age of onset, number of substances used in the last year, and the scores of the clinical scales (HDRS, YMRS, BPRS, DES, SDS, CTQ). We reported the total number and percentage of the different groups of gender, nationality, relationship status, employment status, patient diagnosis, previous traumatic event, life events, axis 1 diagnosis, family background, and suicide attempts.

To investigate the clinical correlates of a dual diagnosis, we first assessed whether it was associated with increased depressive (HDRS), manic (YMRS), psychotic (BPRS), or dissociative symptoms (DES), whether childhood maltreatment (CTQ scores) was associated with having a dual diagnosis, and whether dual diagnosis was associated with the severity of the substance use disorders. Additionally, we repeated the same analysis to investigate the clinical correlates of gender differences.

To investigate the mental health consequences of childhood maltreatment in adults with substance use disorders, we assessed whether CTQ scores were associated with increased depressive (HDRS), manic (YMRS), or psychotic symptoms (BPRS), with an increased number of suicide attempts, and with the severity of the substance use disorders.

Finally, we conducted an analysis to study the association between the severity of the SUD and dissociative, intrusive, avoidance, and reactivity symptoms.

When the dependent variable was binary (e.g., having a dual diagnosis), we used logistic regressions covarying by age and sex. When the dependent variable was numeric (e.g., PRISM), we conducted standard regressions covarying by age and sex, but we found the statistical significance using the Freedman Lane permutation algorithm, which is very robust to violations of normality [https://doi.org/10.1016/j.neuroimage.2014.01.060]. This was necessary because most independent variables did not show a normal distribution and standard transformations to approximate normality were unsuccessful. All statistics were conducted in R Core Team (2020).

3. Results

3.1. Sample Characteristics

Sociodemographic data are shown in Table 1, and clinical data are presented in Table 2.

Table 1. Sociodemographic characteristics of the sample. Data are presented as mean (SD) or number (%).

	Total Sample ($n = 150$)	Dual Disorders ($n = 100$)	Only SUD ($n = 50$)
Age	44 (10)	44.4 (10)	43.2 (10)
Gender			
Female	57 (38%)	44 (44%)	13 (26%)
Male	93 (62%)	66 (66%)	37 (74%)
Nationality			
Spanish	134 (89.3%)	86 (86%)	48 (96%)
Latin	8 (5.3%)	8 (8%)	0 (0%)
Moroccan	3 (2%)	3 (3%)	0 (0%)
Other	5 (3.3%)	3 (3%)	2 (4%)
Education (years of studies)	11.2 (3.4)	11.2 (3.5)	11.2 (3.2)
Relationship status			
Single	58 (38.7%)	35 (35%)	23 (46%)
Married	39 (26%)	28 (28%)	11 (22%)
Separate/divorce	49 (32.6%)	35 (35%)	14 (28%)
Widowed	4 (2.7%)	2 (2%)	2 (4%)
Employment status			
Student	1 (0.07%)	1 (1%)	0 (0%)
Full time employment	11 (7.3%)	3 (3%)	8 (16%)
Part-time employment	1 (0.07%)	1 (1%)	0 (0%)
Sick leave	55 (36.7%)	37 (37%)	18 (36%)
Unemployed	46 (30.7%)	28 (28%)	18 (36%)
Work incapacity by mental health problems	26 (17.3%)	24 (24%)	2 (4%)
Work incapacity by other reasons	10 (6.6%)	6 (6%)	4 (8%)

Table 2. Clinical characteristics of the sample. Data are presented as mean (SD) and/or number (%).

	Total Sample (n = 150)	Dual Disorder (n = 100)	Only SUD (n = 50)
Age of onset			
Nicotine	15.3 (3.7) n = 141 *	15 (4) n = 94 *	15.7 (3) n = 47 *
Alcohol	15.1 (3.8) n = 143 *	15.4 (4.1) n = 95 *	14.7 (3.3) n = 48 *
Cannabis	16.8 (5) n = 80 *	17.2 (5.7) n = 52 *	16.1 (3.2) n = 28 *
Cocaine	20.9 (7.8) n = 97 *	21.2 (7.6) n = 66 *	20.3 (8.2) n = 31 *
Heroin	29.1 (8.9) n = 11 *	29 (9.3) n = 10 *	30 (-) n = 1 *
Stimulants	19 (5.3) n = 14 *	20.3 (6.9) n = 7 *	17.7 (2.9) n = 7 *
Sedatives	34.4 (10.1) n = 24 *	34.6 (10.9) n = 19 *	33.6 (7.4) n=5 *
Number of drugs in the last year	2.28 (0.93)	2.29 (0.93)	2.26 (0.94)
Previous traumatic event			
No	9 (6%)	3 (3%)	6 (12%)
Yes	141 (94%)	97 (97%)	44 (88%)
PTSD diagnosis	31 (20.67%)	21 (21%)	10 (20%)
Non-PTSD diagnosis	110 (73.33%)	76 (76%)	34 (68%)
Live events (last 12 months)			
From 1 to 5 events	42 (28%)	29 (29%)	13 (26%)
From 6 to 10 events	62 (41.3%)	40 (40%)	22 (44%)
From 11 to 15 events	33 (22%)	22 (22%)	11 (22%)
From 16 to 20 events	8 (5.3%)	6 (6%)	2 (4%)
From 21 to 25 events	4 (2.7%)	2 (2%)	2 (4%)
>26 events	1 (0.7%)	1 (1%)	0 (0%)
Comorbid diagnosis axis 1			
Mood disorders	37 (24.7%)	37 (37%)	0 (0%)
Anxiety disorders	4 (2.7%)	4 (4%)	0 (0%)
Psychotic disorders	7 (4.7%)	7 (7%)	0 (0%)
Induced psychotic or mood disorders	18 (12%)	2 (2%)	16 (32%)
Eating disorders	1 (0.7%)	1 (1%)	0 (0%)
Family history			
Father			
None	107 (71.3%)	72 (72%)	35 (70%)
SUD	34 (22.7%)	21 (21%)	13 (26%)
Mood disorders	4 (2.7%)	3 (3%)	1 (2%)
SUD + other	5 (3.3%)	4 (4%)	1 (2%)
Mother			
None	111 (74%)	72 (72%)	39 (78%)
SUD	6 (4%)	3 (3%)	3 (6%)
Mood disorders	25 (16.7%)	17 (17%)	8 (16%)
SUD + other	6 (4%)	6 (6%)	0 (0%)
Sibling			
None	97 (64.7%)	58 (58%)	39 (78%)
SUD	33 (22%)	24 (24%)	9 (18%)
Mood disorders	12 (8%)	11 (11%)	1 (2%)
SUD + other	6 (4%)	6 (6%)	0 (0%)
Suicide attempts			
None	72 (48%)	38 (38%)	34 (68%)
One	33 (22%)	23 (23%)	10 (20%)
Two	20 (13.3%)	15 (15%)	5 (10%)
Three or more	43 (28.7%)	37 (37%)	6 (12%)

SUD: Substance Use Disorder; PTSD: Posttraumatic Stress Disorder; * Number of patients who consume the substance.

Of the whole study sample, 100 patients fulfilled the diagnosis of a dual disorder, and 50 patients fulfilled only SUD diagnoses, according to DSM-5 criteria by PRISM. The most frequently used substances in the last month prior to the current admission included alcohol (n = 115), cocaine (n = 59), cannabis (n = 31), benzodiazepines (n = 20), opioids (n = 5), hallucinogens (n = 3), and amphetamines (n = 1). In the whole sample, 24 patients used one substance (16%), 67 patients used two substances

(44.67%), and 58 patients three more substances (38.67%). The following types of medication were described in our sample: antipsychotics ($n = 90$), anticonvulsants ($n = 58$), antidepressants ($n = 93$), hypnotics ($n = 46$), and drugs for SUD ($n = 17$). Four patients (2.7%) did not take any medication.

With regard to traumatic experiences, in the whole sample, 141 patients (94%) reported at least one traumatic event in the EGEP-5 questionnaire. The death of a family member or close friend was the most prevalent (18%) event, followed by psychological abuse (15%), physical violence (13%), sexual violence (11%), severe accident (6%), and other adverse events (3%). Of those patients, 31 met criteria for current PTSD, following criteria of the EGEP-5. Dual disorder patients had a prevalence of PTSD diagnosis of 21%, and only SUD patients of 20%. In terms of adverse life events of the last year, all patients reported at least one of them. Finally, regarding childhood maltreatment, the results showed the subjects, on average, had experienced low-to-moderate levels of all types of child abuse and neglect in the CTQ, with both emotional abuse and neglect being the most frequent maltreatment reported by the patients (See Table 3). Minimization and denial in the CTQ were controlled for.

Table 3. Clinical differences between patients with dual disorder diagnosis and only Substance Use Disorder (SUD) diagnosis. Data are presented as mean (SD).

	All Sample ($n = 150$)	Dual Disorder ($n = 100$)	Only SUD ($n = 50$)	p-Value (a)
HDRS	7 (5.2)	7.7 (5.4)	5.6 (5.4)	0.04
YMRS	1.3 (2.7)	1.5 (2.9)	0.6 (2.9)	0.109
BPRS	24.3 (5)	25.1 (5.2)	22.8 (5.2)	0.005
DES				
Total score	10.8 (9.4)	11.9 (10.3)	8.4 (10.3)	0.02
Amnesia	6.9 (8.2)	7.4 (9.1)	5.8 (9.1)	0.25
Dissociation	16.1 (12.7)	17.7 (13.5)	12.9 (13.5)	0.014
Depersonalization	6.4 (8.6)	7.6 (9.8)	3.9 (9.8)	0.009
SDS-Nicotine	8.6 (3.8)	8.5 (4)	8.9 (4)	0.67
SDS-Alcohol	9.5 (3.4)	9.6 (3.3)	9.4 (3.3)	0.81
SDS-Cocaine	9.8 (4.1)	9.7 (4.3)	9.8 (4.3)	0.64
SDS-Cannabis	8.4 (4.2)	8.6 (4.6)	7.7 (4.6)	0.42
CTQ				
Total score	44.4 (17)	47.3 (18.7)	38.8 (18.7)	0.003
Emotional abuse	10.4 (5.3)	11.4 (5.5)	8.6 (5.5)	0.001
Physical abuse	7.6 (4.1)	8.1 (4.5)	6.7 (4.5)	0.067
Sexual abuse	6.8 (3.9)	7.5 (4.6)	5.5 (4.6)	0.009
Emotional neglect	11.7 (5)	12.2 (5.2)	10.8 (5.2)	0.12
Physical neglect	7.7 (3.3)	8.1 (3.5)	7 (3.5)	0.042
PTSD	31 (20.7%)	21 (21%)	10 (20%)	0.82

HDRS: Hamilton Depression Rating Scale; YMRS: Young Mania Rating Scale; BPRS: Brief Psychiatric Rating Scale; DES: Dissociative Experiences Scale; SDS: Severity of Dependence Scale; CTQ: Childhood Trauma Questionnaire; (a) p-value derived from the comparisons between individuals with dual diagnosis and individuals with no dual diagnosis via logistic regressions or Freedman-Lane permutation tests covarying for age and sex.

3.2. Clinical Differences between Patients with Dual Disorder Diagnosis and Only SUD Diagnosis

Patients with dual disorder diagnosis showed significantly higher scores in terms of depressive and psychotic symptoms in comparison with patients with a diagnosis of only SUD. Regarding the trauma variables, the results showed that dissociative symptoms and total CTQ score, as well as emotional abuse, sexual abuse, and physical neglect scores from the CTQ subscales, were also all statistically significantly higher in the dual disorder group than in the group with only SUD diagnosis. No significant differences were found between groups in terms of manic symptoms, nor in the severity of dependence on nicotine, alcohol, cannabis, and cocaine (see Table 3).

3.3. Association Between Clinical Symptoms and Childhood Maltreatment

In Table 4, the relationship between childhood maltreatment and depressive, manic, and psychotic symptoms, as well as the number of suicide attempts, can be seen. The HMDS and the BPRS scales showed an association with all variables of the CTQ, except for physical abuse. In contrast, the YMRS scale did not show any significant correlations with any variable of the CTQ. Finally, the number of suicide attempts showed only a significant correlation with emotional neglect.

Table 4. Freedman Lane analysis to evaluate the relation between the childhood trauma questionnaire scores and clinical variables from the HDRS, YMRS, BPRS, and the suicide attempts.

CTQ	HDRS	YMRS	BPRS	SA
Total score	R = 0.28, t = 3.54, $p \leq 0.01$	R = 0.04, t = 0.53, $p = 0.53$	R = 0.23, t = 2.91, $p = 0.01$	R = 0.16, t = 2.00, $p = 0.06$
Emotional abuse	R = 0.17, t = 2.06, $p = 0.03$	R = 0.006, t = 0.08, $p = 0.91$	R = 0.17, t = 2.11, $p = 0.03$	R = 0.14, t = 1.75, $p = 0.09$
Physical abuse	R = 0.16, t = 2.02, $p = 0.06$	R = 0.08, t = 0.95, $p = 0.33$	R = 0.15, t = 1.88, $p = 0.06$	R = 0.07, t = 0.88, $p = 0.2$
Sexual abuse	R = 0.23, t = 2.86, $p = 0.01$	R = 0.14, t = 1.71, $p = 0.12$	R = 0.18, t = 2.17, $p = 0.03$	R = 0.11, t = 1.32, $p = 0.24$
Emotional neglect	R = 0.28, t = 3.61, $p \leq 0.01$	R = −0.06, t = 0.79, $p = 0.39$	R = 0.21, t = 2.55, $p = 0.01$	R = 0.16, t = 2.02, $p = 0.04$
Physical neglect	R = 0.24, t = 3.04, $p = 0.01$	R = 0.05, t = 0.65, $p = 0.49$	R = 0.19, t = 2.32, $p = 0.02$	R = 0.16, t = 2.00, $p = 0.13$

HDRS: Hamilton Depression Rating Scale; YMRS: Young Mania Rating Scale; BPRS: Brief Psychiatric Rating Scale; SA: suicide attempts; R converted from the t obtained in the Freedman-Lane linear model.

3.4. Association Between Severity of Substance Dependence and Childhood Maltreatment and other Trauma-Related Variables

No significant correlations were found between the severity of dependence on nicotine, alcohol, cannabis, cocaine and childhood maltreatment or dissociative, intrusive, avoidance, and reactivity symptoms.

3.5. Childhood Maltreatment as Predictor of Dual Disorder Diagnosis

Using logistic regression, we found that childhood maltreatment can serve as a predictor for developing a dual disorder diagnosis (CTQ total score: z = 2.70; $p = 0.006$), with both emotional and sexual abuse being the most significant predictors (CTQ EA: z = 2.89; $p = 0.003$; CTQ SA: z = 2.36; $p = 0.01$).

3.6. Gender Differences of Clinical Variables

The sample consisted of 57 female and 93 male patients. We detected statistically higher scores for female patients in the total CTQ score and in the sexual abuse CTQ score in the total sample, when compared to male patients. We did not find any further sex-specific differences in clinical variables (see Table 5).

Table 5. Clinical differences by gender. Data are presented as mean (SD).

	All Sample (n = 150)	Women (n = 57)	Men (n = 93)	p-Value (a)
HDRS	7.03 (5.25)	8.05 (5.18)	6.41 (5.22)	0.086
YMRS	1.28 (2.67)	1.3 (2.76)	1.27 (2.63)	0.884
BPRS	24.33 (4.97)	24.11 (4.02)	24.46 (5.5)	0.604
DES				
Total score	10.76 (9.37)	10.87 (10.43)	10.7 (8.71)	0.822
Amnesia	6.88 (8.24)	7 (9.34)	6.81 (7.55)	0.872
Dissociation	16.12 (12.72)	15.72 (13.23)	16.37 (12.47)	0.856
Depersonalization	6.37 (8.63)	6.75 (9.74)	6.13 (7.93)	0.588
SDS-Alcohol	9.5 (3.4)	9.82 (2.97)	9.31 (3.64)	0.438
SDS-Cocaine	9.76 (4.14)	9.45 (4.41)	9.89 (4.06)	0.788
SDS-Cannabis	8.37 (4.22)	7.83 (4.34)	8.65 (4.23)	0.67
SDS-Nicotine	8.63 (3.82)	8.23 (4.43)	8.86 (3.45)	0.37
CTQ				
Total score	44.44 (16.9)	48.05 (20.64)	42.23 (13.79)	**0.034**
Emotional abuse	10.45 (5.26)	11.28 (5.89)	9.94 (4.79)	0.078
Physical abuse	7.64 (4.12)	8.3 (5.11)	7.24 (3.35)	0.124
Sexual abuse	6.82 (3.95)	8.65 (5.46)	5.7 (1.94)	**<0.001**
Emotional neglect	11.73 (5.05)	12.14 (5.2)	11.48 (4.96)	0.448
Physical neglect	7.75 (3.32)	7.68 (3.69)	7.78 (3.1)	0.946

HDRS: Hamilton Depression Rating Scale; YMRS: Young Mania Rating Scale; BPRS: Brief Psychiatric Rating Scale; DES: Dissociative Experiences Scale; SDS: Severity of Dependence Scale; CTQ: Childhood Trauma Questionnaire; (a) p-value derived from the comparisons between individuals with PTSD diagnosis and non-PTSD diagnosis via logistic regressions or Freedman-Lane permutation tests covarying for age and sex.

4. Discussion

To the best of our knowledge, this is one of the few studies to evaluate, in detail and systematically, the prevalence of psychological trauma and its association with clinical symptoms in a well-described and diagnosed sample of dual disorder patients versus only SUD patients. Additionally, we compared clinical variables in the whole sample dividing patients by gender.

The main analysis showed that two thirds of the whole sample fulfilled a diagnosis of dual disorder, all patients had an early onset of nicotine, alcohol, cannabis, and cocaine, and approximately one third had a positive family history of mood and SUD disorders. As expected, psychiatric symptoms were, in general, higher in the dual disorder sample than in the only SUD group. Regarding psychological trauma, the first overall result is that 94% of the whole sample suffered from at least one lifetime traumatic event, mainly related to deaths of relatives or friends and psychological, physical, and sexual abuse. These data are beyond the 70% of lifetime prevalence of one psychological trauma event found in the world-wide adult population [6], indicating that this population is vulnerable to suffering a greater number of negative life experiences than the general population [43]. Furthermore, our sample presented an overwhelming number of stressful life events in the 12 months prior to evaluation, supporting again the evidence of a high exposure to adverse events in both groups, which is similar to other psychiatric disorders, such as depression, bipolar disorder, or schizoaffective disorders [44–47].

Remarkably, of the whole sample, 20.67% met criteria for current PTSD. Dual disorder patients had a prevalence rate of 21%, and only SUD patients of 20%. These data are higher than the prevalence rates of current PTSD of 0.2–3.8% in the general population [6], and within the range of prior data for only SUD patients with current PTSD, which range from 15% to 41% [7]. Despite our results being consistent with prior studies, which have shown that an important proportion of patients with only SUD have suffered from traumatic events and present marked PTSD symptomatology, our findings do not support our previous hypothesis that dual disorder patients will show a higher PTSD prevalence rate than patients with only SUD. However, patients with dual disorder presented more adverse events, more childhood trauma, more dissociative symptoms, and a more severe clinical profile than patients with only SUD. Specifically, total scores and scores of emotional and sexual abuse and physical neglect in the CTQ were higher in the dual disorder group when compared with the only SUD group. These results support previous research that have found that early traumatic experiences, especially childhood maltreatment, are not only a risk factor for developing several mental health problems in adulthood, including SUD, psychosis, depression, or bipolar disorder [48–50], among others, but that they represent also a risk factor for developing a more severe clinical presentation in dual disorder patients [51]. As a matter of fact, we also found that childhood maltreatment can serve as a predictor for developing a dual disorder diagnosis, with both emotional and sexual abuse being the most significant predictors. These data are similar to the results found by Fetzner et al. (2011), which suggested that childhood maltreatment is a predictor for the course of SUD, even in the absence of comorbid PTSD [52]. However, interestingly, while both groups of patients scored more highly across subtypes in the CTQ than the general population, their scores were in the low–moderate range, which is not in line with prior literature in only SUD populations (e.g., [53]). One possible explanation could be the predominance of male patients in our sample, as the prevalence of childhood adversity is higher in women with SUD than in men [54,55]. In fact, we detected that women specifically showed higher scores in the total score and sexual abuse score in the CTQ as compared to men. We also did not include in our analysis patients with an acute psychotic episode. This might have influenced these results, as adversity in childhood is an etiological risk factor for developing psychosis and might therefore be more prevalent in dual disorder than in patients with mood or anxiety disorders [56].

The dual disorder sample also presented higher scores in depressive and psychotic symptoms compared to patients with only SUD. This can be expected, due to the nature of a comorbid psychiatric disorder, but it might also indicate a more severe and complex clinical profile in a dual disorder, as suggested in a study by Sells et al., 2016 [18]. Moreover, dual disorder patients also showed higher scores in dissociation and depersonalization, but not in amnesia when compared to the only SUD group, which also underlines a more complex clinical picture and a higher trauma load in this sample. Interestingly, dissociative scores of our sample were, in general, also in the lower range. These data are consistent with a recent meta-analysis which assessed dissociation in several mental disorders and reported that the largest dissociation scores were found for dissociative disorders, followed by PTSD, borderline personality disorder, and conversion disorder, and the lower range of scores included substance-related and addictive disorders, schizophrenia, anxiety disorder, and affective disorders, amongst others [57]. Regarding the severity of dependence on nicotine, alcohol, cannabis, and cocaine, both groups showed a similar pattern of consumption, which is surprising due to prior evidence that dual disorder patients have an earlier start to substance use [20], and a poly-substance consumption pattern [22].

With respect to the relationship between psychiatric symptoms and the number of suicide attempts and childhood maltreatment, we found that the HDRS and the BPRS scales showed an association with all variables of the CTQ, except for physical abuse. This points towards the influence of childhood maltreatment as a risk factor for developing a variety of psychiatric symptoms in adult life, as also suggested in prior literature [58–60]. In contrast, the YMRS scale interestingly did not show any significant correlations with any variable of the CTQ. This is of interest, as, for example, the Kessler et al. study from 1995 detected, in a large PTSD sample, a high risk, especially in men, of developing manic episodes in the long-term. However, psychopathological scores were, in general, low in our sample, as patients were evaluated once their clinical symptoms were stabilized, meaning these results must be interpreted with caution.

Finally, the number of suicide attempts showed a significant correlation with emotional neglect in the CTQ. This finding is in line with a recent meta-analysis, which showed a two- to three-fold increased risk for suicide attempts and suicidal ideation in adults who experienced childhood adversities compared with adults who have not experienced maltreatment during childhood [61]. Therefore, these data support previous studies which suggest that childhood maltreatment can aggravate the clinical symptoms of existing psychopathologies [49–51].

Our work includes various limitations. One is the cross-sectional nature of our study and the lack of a longer stabilization phase. Furthermore, we did not clearly define a stabilization phase using a determined score range in psychopathological scales during a longer period of time to evaluate our patients. This was not planned as such due to a possible low adherence and short admission duration in this clinically complex population. However, both aspects might have possibly influenced our results. There was also a slight predominance of male patients, meaning results cannot be completely generalized to female patients. Furthermore, dual disorder patients with acute psychotic states were excluded, meaning the dual disorder sample consisted mainly of comorbid mood and anxiety disorders. This limits its representativeness across the wide psychiatric diagnostic spectrum, including schizoaffective disorder and schizophrenia. The main reason for this was that we considered that psychotic states needed more time for stabilization beyond the median duration of a stay of 20 days in both units. We considered that psychopathological instability would influence the evaluation. We also excluded a smaller number of patients with cognitive impairment, as this was highly likely to have also influenced the quality of our evaluation. Patients with suicidal thoughts were also not included, as the evaluation of traumatic events might have worsened suicidal thoughts when no trauma-focused therapy was offered. Our hypothesis is that, if these exclusion criteria did influence results in any way, it would have led to a lower estimation of prevalence rates. There is, for example, compelling evidence that one major etiological factor of psychosis is childhood trauma [56] Broadening the diagnoses in future studies might overcome this limitation.

Strengths of our work include the systematic investigation of psychological trauma and life events in a large sample of patients using established and validated scales in Spanish. Furthermore, we used a gold-standard clinical structured interview, the PRISM, following DSM-5 criteria, to establish SUD or dual disorder diagnosis together with the DDSI. Therefore, our level of confidence in diagnosis, and especially in the prevalence estimate is high.

5. Conclusions

In conclusion, we found a high rate of traumatization in the form of negative life events or PTSD throughout the sample, with some types of childhood maltreatment as a predictor of a dual diagnosis and as a risk factor to develop a more complex and severe clinical profile. The prevalence rates of PTSD in dual disorder and only SUD patients were around 20%, which means that one in five dual disorder patients actually have a triple diagnosis. Our data therefore challenge our current clinical practice in the treatment of patients suffering from dual or only SUD diagnosis, and favor the incorporation of an additional trauma-focused strategy in this population, such as trauma-focused psychological interventions, namely cognitive behavioural therapy [62] or Eye Movement Desensitization Reprocessing (EMDR) therapy [63,64]. This may improve the prognosis of the often. complex course of illness in individuals suffering from dual disorder or only SUD.

Author Contributions: A.M.A., L.B. and B.L.A. had the idea of the project; C.C., A.V.-G., V.P., and M.T. contributed to the design of the study; R.S. and A.F. recruited the patients and did the screening evaluations; L.B., A.S. (Albert Sió), B.H., R.E., I.G.-S., and E.B. evaluated the included participants; J.R. and A.S. (Aleix Solanes) carried out all statistical analysis; A.M.-A. and L.B. wrote the first draft of the manuscript with the supervision of B.L.A.; A.S. (Albert Sió), B.H., R.E., J.R., A.S. (Aleix Solanes), I.G.-S., E.B., R.S., A.F., C.C., A.V.-G., V.P., and M.T. contributed to the revisions and modifications of the manuscript. All authors have read and agreed to the published version of the manuscript.

Funding: This research was funded by the Catalonia Government with a PERIS Grant (SLT006/17/00038) to BLA, which is highly appreciated.

Acknowledgments: MT is grateful for the support by the ISCIII-Red de Trastornos Adictivos-RTA-FEDER (RD16/0017/0010). AMA and BLA want to thank also to the "Secretaria d'Universitats i Recerca del Departament d'Economia i Coneixement (2017 SGR 46 to "Unitat de Recerca del Centre Fòrum"), Generalitat de Catalunya (Government of Catalonia)" for the recognition as an emerging research group. VP wants to thank unrestricted research funding from "Secretaria d'Universitats i Recerca del Departament d'Economia i Coneixement (2017 SGR 134 to "Mental Health Research Group"), Generalitat de Catalunya (Government of Catalonia)". We also acknowledge the continuous support by the CIBERSAM (Centro de Investigación Biomédica en Red de Salud Mental). The sources of funding have no influence on the design and the conducting and the reporting of the trial.

Conflicts of Interest: The authors declare that the research was conducted in the absence of any commercial or financial relationships that could be construed as a potential conflict of interest.

References

1. Volkow, N.D.; Baler, R.D.; Goldstein, R.Z. Addiction: Pulling at the neural threads of social behaviors neuroview. *Neuron* **2011**, *69*, 599–602. [CrossRef] [PubMed]
2. Yu, C.; Mcclellan, J. Genetics of substance use disorders. *Child Adolesc. Psychiatry Clin. N. Am.* **2016**, *25*, 377–385. [CrossRef] [PubMed]
3. Mennis, J.; Stahler, G.J.; Mason, M.J. Risky substance use environments and addiction: A new frontier for environmental justice research. *Int. J. Environ. Res. Public Health* **2016**, *13*, 607. [CrossRef] [PubMed]
4. Driessen, M.; Schulte, S.; Luedecke, C.; Schaefer, I.; Sutmann, F.; Kemper, U.; Koesters, G.; Chodzinski, C.; Schneider, U.; Dette, C.; et al. Trauma and PTSD in patients with alcohol, drug, or dual dependence: A multi-center study. *Alcohol. Clin. Exp. Res.* **2008**, *32*, 481–488. [CrossRef]
5. Mauritz, M.W.; Goossens, P.J.J.; Draijer, N.; van Achterberg, T. Prevalence of interpersonal trauma exposure and trauma-related disorders in severe mental illness. *Eur. Child Adolesc. Psychiatry* **2013**, *4*. [CrossRef]
6. Shalev, A.; Liberzon, I.; Marmar, C. Post-traumatic stress disorder. *N. Engl. J. Med.* **2017**, *376*, 2459–2469. [CrossRef]
7. Schäfer, I.; Najavits, L.M. Clinical challenges in the treatment of patients with posttraumatic stress disorder and substance abuse. *Curr. Opin. Psychiatry* **2007**, *20*, 614–618. [CrossRef]
8. Gradus, J.L. Prevalence and prognosis of stress disorders: A review of the epidemiologic literature. *Clin. Epidemiol.* **2017**, *9*, 251–260. [CrossRef]
9. Lippard, E.T.C.; Nemeroff, C.B. The devastating clinical consequences of child abuse and neglect: Increased disease vulnerability and poor treatment response in mood disorders. *Am. J. Psychiatry* **2020**, *177*, 20–36. [CrossRef]
10. Khantzian, E.J. The self medication hypothesis of addictive disorders: Focus on heroin and cocaine dependence. *Am. J. Psychiatry* **1985**, *142*, 1259–1264. [CrossRef]
11. Chilcoat, H.D.; Breslau, N. Investigations of causal pathways between PTSD and drug use disorders. *Addict. Behav.* **1998**, *23*, 827–840. [CrossRef]
12. Breslau, N.; Davis, C.; Peterson, E.L.; Schulz, L. Psychiatric sequelae of posttraumatic stress disorder in women. *Arch. Gen. Psychiatry* **1997**, *54*, 81–87. [CrossRef] [PubMed]
13. Krueger, R.F.; Markon, K.E. Reinterpreting comorbidity: A model-based approach to understanding and classifying psychopathology. *Annu. Rev. Clin. Psychol.* **2006**, *2*, 111–133. [CrossRef]
14. Wolf, E.J.; Miller, M.W.; Krueger, R.F.; Lyons, M.J.; Tsuang, M.T.; Koenen, K.C. Posttraumatic stress disorder and the genetic structure of comorbidity. *J. Abnorm. Psychol.* **2010**, *119*, 320–330. [CrossRef]
15. Jacobsen, L.K.; Southwick, S.M.; Kosten, T.R. Substance use disorders in patients with posttraumatic stress disorder: A review of the literature. *Am. J. Psychiatry* **2001**, *158*, 1184–1190. [CrossRef]
16. Guina, J.; Nahhas, R.W.; Goldberg, A.J.; Farnsworth, S. PTSD symptom severities, interpersonal traumas, and benzodiazepines are associated with substance related problems in trauma patients. *J. Clin. Med.* **2016**, *5*, 70. [CrossRef] [PubMed]
17. Kok, T.; De Haan, H.; Van Der Meer, M.; Najavits, L.; De Jong, C. Assessing traumatic experiences in screening for PTSD in substance use disorder patients: What is the gain in addition to PTSD symptoms? *Psychiatry Res.* **2015**, *226*, 328–332. [CrossRef]
18. Sells, J.R.; Waters, A.J.; Schwandt, M.L.; Kwako, L.E.; Heilig, M.; George, D.T.; Ramchandani, V.A. Characterization of comorbid PTSD in treatment-seeking alcohol dependent inpatients: Severity and personality trait differences. *Drug Alcohol Depend.* **2016**, *163*, 242–246. [CrossRef]
19. Najavits, L.M.; Gastfriend, D.R.; Barber, J.P.; Reif, S.; Muenz, L.R.; Blaine, J.; Frank, A.; Crits-Christoph, P.; Thase, M.; Weiss, R.D. Cocaine dependence with and without PTSD among subjects in the national institute on drug abuse collaborative cocaine treatment study. *Am. J. Psychiatry* **1998**, *155*, 214–219. [CrossRef]
20. Johnson, S.D.; Striley, C.; Cottler, L.B. The association of substance use disorders with trauma exposure and PTSD among African American drug users. *Addict. Behav.* **2006**, *31*, 2063–2073. [CrossRef]
21. Read, J.P.; Brown, P.J.; Kahler, C.W. Substance use and posttraumatic stress disorders: Symptom interplay and effects on outcome. *Addict. Behav.* **2004**, *29*, 1665–1672. [CrossRef] [PubMed]

22. Dragan, M.; Lis-Turlejska, M. Prevalence of posttraumatic stress disorder in alcohol dependent patients in poland. *Addict. Behav.* **2007**, *32*, 902–911. [CrossRef] [PubMed]
23. Saladin, M.E.; Brady, K.T.; Dansky, B.S.; Kilpatrick, D.G. Understanding comorbidity between PTSD and substance use disorders: Two preliminary investigations. *Addict. Behav.* **1995**, *20*, 643–655. [CrossRef]
24. Schäfer, I.; Langeland, W.; Hissbach, J.; Luedecke, C.; Ohlmeier, M.D.; Chodzinski, C.; Kemper, U.; Keiper, P.; Wedekind, D.; Havemann-reinecke, U.; et al. Childhood trauma and dissociation in patients with alcohol dependence, drug dependence, or both—A multi-center study. *Drug Alcohol Depend.* **2010**, *109*, 84–89. [CrossRef]
25. Torrens, M.; Mestre-Pintó, J.I.; Montanari, L.; Vicente, J.; Domingo-Salvany, A. Patología dual: Una perspectiva Europea. *Adicciones* **2017**, *29*, 3–5. [CrossRef]
26. Ouimette, P.C.; Brown, P.J.; Najavits, L.M. Course and treatment of patients with both substance use and posttraumatic stress disorders. *Addict. Behav.* **1998**, *23*, 785–795. [CrossRef]
27. Torrens, M.; Serrano, D.; Astals, M.; Pérez-Domínguez, G.; Martín-Santos, R. Diagnosing comorbid psychiatric disorders in substance abusers: Validity of the Spanish versions of the psychiatric research interview for substance and mental disorders and the structured clinical interview for DSM-IV. *Am. J. Psychiatry* **2004**, *161*, 1231–1237. [CrossRef]
28. Gossop, M.; Darke, S.; Griffiths, P.; Hando, J.; Powis, B.; Hall, W.S.J. The Severity of Dependence Scale (SDS): Psychometric properties of the SDS in English and Australian samples of heroin, cocaine and amphetamine users. *Addiction* **1995**, *90*, 607–614. [CrossRef]
29. María Crespo y Mª Mar Gómez. Posttraumatic stress assessment: Introducing the global assessment of posttraumatic stress questionnaire. *Clín. y Salud* **2012**, *23*, 25–41.
30. Bernstein, D.P.; Fink, L.; Handelsman, L.; Foote, J.; Lovejoy, M.; Wenzel, K.; Sapareto, E.; Ruggiero, J. Initial reliability and validity of a new retrospective measure of child abuse and neglect. *Am. J. Psychiatry* **1994**, *151*, 1132–1136. [CrossRef]
31. Hernandez, A.; Gallardo-Pujol, D.; Pereda, N.; Arntz, A.; Bernstein, D.P.; Gaviria, A.M.; Labad, A.; Valero, J.; Gutiérrez-Zotes, J.A. Initial validation of the Spanish childhood trauma questionnaire-short form: Factor structure, reliability and association with parenting. *J. Interpers. Violence* **2013**, *28*, 1498–1518. [CrossRef] [PubMed]
32. Bernstein, E.M.; Putnam, F.W. Development, reliability, and validity of a dissociation scale. *J. Nerv. Ment. Dis.* **1986**, 727–735. [CrossRef] [PubMed]
33. Icaran, E.; Colom, R.; Orengo Garcia, F. Dissociative experiences: A measurement scale. *Exp. Disociativas Una Escala Medida* **1996**, *70*, 69–84.
34. Holmes, T.H.; Rahe, R.H. The social readjustment rating scale. *J. Psychosom. Res.* **1967**, *11*, 213–218. [CrossRef]
35. González de Rivera, J.L.; Morera Fumero, A. La valoración de sucesos vitales: Adaptación española de la escala de holmes y rahe. *Psiquis* **1983**, *4*, 7–11.
36. Mestre-Pintó, J.I.; Domingo-Salvany, A.; Martín-Santos, R.; Torrens, M.; Group, T.P. Dual diagnosis screening interview to identify psychiatric comorbidity in substance users: Development and validation of a brief instrument. *Eur. Addict. Res.* **2014**, *20*, 41–48. [CrossRef]
37. Hamilton, M.C. Hamilton depression rating scale (HAM-D). *Redloc* **1960**, *23*, 56–62. [CrossRef]
38. Ramos-Brieva, J.A.; Cordero-Villafafila, A. A new validation of the hamilton rating scale for depression. *J. Psychiatr. Res.* **1988**, *22*, 21–28. [CrossRef]
39. Young, R.C.; Biggs, J.T.; Ziegler, V.E.; Meyer, D.A. A rating scale for mania: Reliability, validity and sensitivity. *Br. J. Psychiatry* **1978**, *133*, 429–435. [CrossRef]
40. Colom, F.; Vieta, E.; Martínez-Arán, A.; Garcia-Garcia, M.; Reinares, M.; Torrent, C.; Goikolea, J.M.; Banös, S.; Salamero, M. Spanish version of a scale for the assessment of mania: Validity and reliability of the young mania rating scale. *Med. Clin.* **2002**, *119*, 366–371. [CrossRef]
41. Overall, J.E.; Gorham, D.R. The brief psychiatric rating scale. *Psychol. Rep.* **1962**, *10*, 799–812. [CrossRef]
42. Sánchez, R.; Ibáñez, M.A. PA factor analysis and validation of a Spanish version of the brief psychiatric rating scale in Colombia. *Biomedica* **2005**, *25*, 120–128. [CrossRef] [PubMed]
43. Brady, K.T.; Back, S.E.; Coffey, S.F. Substance abuse and posttraumatic stress disorder. *Curr. Dir. Psychol. Sci.* **2004**, *14*, 206–209. [CrossRef]
44. Aldinger, F.; Schulze, T.G. Environmental factors, life events, and trauma in the course of bipolar disorder. *Psychiatry Clin. Neurosci.* **2017**, *71*, 6–17. [CrossRef] [PubMed]
45. Vardaxi, C.C.; Gonda, X.; Fountoulakis, K.N. Life events in schizoaffective disorder: A systematic review. *J. Affect. Disord.* **2018**, *227*, 563–570. [CrossRef]

46. Pemberton, R.; Fuller Tyszkiewicz, M.D. Factors contributing to depressive mood states in everyday life: A systematic review. *J. Affect. Disord.* **2016**, *200*, 103–110. [CrossRef]
47. Cerdá, M.; Sagdeo, A.; Johnson, J.; Galea, S. Genetic and environmental influences on psychiatric comorbidity: A systematic review. *J. Affect. Disord.* **2010**, *126*, 14–38. [CrossRef]
48. Agnew-Blais, J.; Danese, A. Childhood maltreatment and unfavourable clinical outcomes in bipolar disorder: A systematic review and meta-analysis. *Lancet Psychiatry* **2016**, *3*, 342–349. [CrossRef]
49. Nanni, V.; Uher, R.; Danese, A. Childhood maltreatment predicts unfavorable course of illness and treatment outcome in depression: A meta-analysis. *Am. J. Psychiatry* **2012**, *169*, 141–151. [CrossRef]
50. Thomas, S.; Höfler, M.; Schäfer, I.; Trautmann, S. Childhood maltreatment and treatment outcome in psychotic disorders: A systematic review and meta-analysis. *Acta Psychiatr. Scand.* **2019**, *140*, 295–312. [CrossRef]
51. Mergler, M.; Driessen, M.; Havemann-Reinecke, U.; Wedekind, D.; Lüdecke, C.; Ohlmeier, M.; Chodzinski, C.; Teunißen, S.; Weirich, S.; Kemper, U.; et al. Differential relationships of PTSD and childhood trauma with the course of substance use disorders. *J. Subst. Abuse Treat.* **2018**, *93*, 57–63. [CrossRef] [PubMed]
52. Fetzner, M.G.; McMillan, K.A.; Sareen, J.; Asmundson, G.J.G. What is the association between traumatic life events and alcohol abuse/dependence in people with and without PTSD? Findings from a nationally representative sample. *Depress. Anxiety* **2011**, *28*, 632–638. [CrossRef] [PubMed]
53. Douglas, K.R.; Chan, G.; Gelernter, J.; Arias, A.J.; Anton, R.F.; Weiss, R.D.; Brady, K.; Poling, J.; Farrer, L.; Kranzler, H.R. Adverse childhood events as risk factors for substance dependence: Partial mediation by mood and anxiety disorders. *Addict. Behav.* **2010**, *35*, 7–13. [CrossRef]
54. Medrano, M.A.; Desmond, D.P.; Zule, W.A.; Hatch, J.P. Histories of childhood trauma and the effects on risky HIV behaviors in a sample of women drug users. *Am. J. Drug Alcohol Abuse* **1999**, *25*, 593–606. [CrossRef] [PubMed]
55. Huang, M.-C.; Schwandt, M.L.; Ramchandani, V.A.; George, D.T.; Heilig, M. Impact of multiple types of childhood trauma exposure on risk of psychiatric comorbidity among alcoholic inpatients. *Alcohol. Clin. Exp. Res.* **2012**, *36*, 598–606. [CrossRef] [PubMed]
56. Varese, F.; Smeets, F.; Drukker, M.; Lieverse, R.; Lataster, T.; Viechtbauer, W.; Read, J.; Van Os, J.; Bentall, R.P. Childhood adversities increase the risk of psychosis: A meta-analysis of patient-control, prospective-and cross-sectional cohort studies. *Schizophr. Bull.* **2012**, *38*, 661–671. [CrossRef]
57. Lyssenko, L.; Schmahl, C.; Bockhacker, L.; Vonderlin, R.; Bohus, M.; Kleindienst, N. Dissociation in psychiatric disorders: A meta-analysis of studies using the dissociative experiences scale. *Am. J. Psychiatry* **2018**, *175*, 37–46. [CrossRef]
58. Felitti, V.J.; Anda, R.F.; Nordenberg, D.; Williamsom, D.F.; Spitz, A.M.; Edwards, V.; Koss, M.P.; Marks, J.S. Relationship of childhood abuse and household dysfunction to many of the leading causes of death in adults the Adverse Childhood Experiences (ACE) study. *Am. J. Prev. Med.* **1998**, *14*, 245–258. [CrossRef]
59. Nelson, J.; Klumparendt, A.; Doebler, P.; Ehring, T. Childhood maltreatment and characteristics of adult depression: Meta-analysis. *Br. J. Psychiatry* **2017**, *210*, 96–104. [CrossRef]
60. Dvir, Y.; Denietolis, B.; Frazier, J.A. Childhood trauma and psychosis. *Child Adolesc. Psychiatr. Clin. N. Am.* **2013**, *22*, 629–641. [CrossRef]
61. Angelakis, I.; Gillespie, E.L.; Panagioti, M. Childhood maltreatment and adult suicidality: A comprehensive systematic review with meta-analysis. *Psychol. Med.* **2019**, *49*, 1057–1078. [CrossRef] [PubMed]
62. Mueser, K.T.; Rosenberg, S.D.; Xie, H.; Jankowski, M.K.; Bolton, E.E.; Lu, W.; Hamblen, J.L.; Rosenberg, H.J.; McHugo, G.J.; Wolfe, R. A randomized controlled trial of cognitive-behavioral treatment for posttraumatic stress disorder in severe mental illness. *J. Consult. Clin. Psychol.* **2008**, *76*, 259–271. [CrossRef] [PubMed]
63. Valiente-Gómez, A.; Moreno-Alcázar, A.; Treen, D.; Cedrón, C.; Colom, F.; Pérez, V.; Amann, B.L. EMDR beyond PTSD: A systematic literature review. *Front. Psychol.* **2017**, *8*, 1–10. [CrossRef] [PubMed]
64. Valiente-Gómez, A.; Moreno-Alcázar, A.; Radua, J.; Hogg, B.; Blanco, L.; Lupo, W.; Pérez, V.; Robles-Martínez, M.; Torrens, M.; Amann, B.L. A multicenter phase ii rater-blinded randomized controlled trial to compare the effectiveness of eye movement desensitization reprocessing therapy vs. treatment as usual in patients with substance use disorder and history of psychological trauma: A study design and protocol. *Front. Psychiatry* **2019**, *10*, 108. [CrossRef]

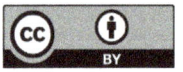

© 2020 by the authors. Licensee MDPI, Basel, Switzerland. This article is an open access article distributed under the terms and conditions of the Creative Commons Attribution (CC BY) license (http://creativecommons.org/licenses/by/4.0/).

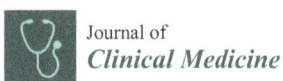

Article

The Relevance of Dual Diagnoses among Drug-Dependent Patients with Sleep Disorders

Carlos Roncero [1,2,3,*], Llanyra García-Ullán [1,2,3], Alberto Bullón [1,3], Diego Remón-Gallo [3], Begoña Vicente-Hernández [1,3], Ana Álvarez [1,3], Amaya Caldero [3,4], Andrea Flores [2] and Lourdes Aguilar [1,2,3]

[1] Psychiatry Service, University of Salamanca Health Care Complex, Paseo de San Vicente 58-182, 37007 Salamanca, Spain; mlullan@saludcastillayleon.es (L.G.-U.); abullons@saludcastillayleon.es (A.B.); bvicenteh@saludcastillayleon.es (B.V.-H.); aialvarez@saludcastillayleon.es (A.Á.); maguilar@saludcastillayleon.es (L.A.)
[2] Psychiatry Unit, School of Medicine, University of Salamanca, Campus Miguel de Unamuno C/ Alfonso X El Sabio s/n, 37007 Salamanca, Spain; afc@usal.es
[3] Institute of Biomedicine, University of Salamanca, Paseo de San Vicente, 58-182, 37007 Salamanca, Spain; diego_biscab@hotmail.com (D.R.-G.); amayacaldero@hotmail.com (A.C.)
[4] Psychiatry Service, Zamora University Health Care Complex, Hernán Cortés Street, 40, 49071 Zamora, Spain
* Correspondence: croncero@saludcastillayleon.es

Received: 30 July 2020; Accepted: 1 September 2020; Published: 4 September 2020

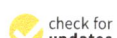

Abstract: Background: Sleep disorders are often associated with drug use. Nearly 70% of patients admitted for detoxification report sleep problems. Dual disorder (DD) is the comorbidity between mental disorders in general and disorders related to psychoactive substance use. The association between substance use and sleep disorders (SD) appears to be bidirectional. Our objective is to analyze the association between sleep disturbance history and drug use pattern (alcohol, cannabis, opioids, and cocaine). Methods: Analysis of data in the first interview at the Addictions Unit of the Department of Psychiatry at the University of Salamanca Health Care Complex between October 2017 and January 2020. The sample consists of 398 patients. We studied the association between different variables: origin of patients (Inpatient Dual Diagnosis Detoxification Unit (IDDDU) vs. Outpatient Drug Clinic (ODC), presence of affective disorder, psychotic disorder, type of drug used, and treatment. Results: Of patients with DD, 62% had more delayed sleep induction, sleep fragmentation, early awakening, and nightmares. Outpatients had more difficulty falling asleep because, in many cases, they had not previously sought any medical assistance. On the other hand, 67% of the patients with insomnia presented depression. Conclusions: There is evidence of a harmful association between DD and SD.

Keywords: dual disorders (DD); insomnia; sleep disorders (SD); benzodiazepine use disorder (BUD)

1. Introduction

Sleep disorders are associated with drug use. Almost 70% of all the patients who are admitted for detoxification have sleep disorders [1,2]. The association between the use of substances and insomnia (here used as sleep disorders in general) seems to be bidirectional [3], since sleep disorders increase the risk of developing substance use disorders [4], and the use of substances causes sleep disorders [5]. Long-term abstinence may reverse some sleep disorders [6]. On the other hand, drugs are known to be used as self-medication to relieve some sleep disorders [7]. Sleep disorders may also be a risk factor for a relapse in substance abuse [8]. Insomnia, and particularly delayed sleep induction (DSI), is related to a relapse in alcohol use [9]. It has also been associated with relapses in the use of cocaine [10], and there is evidence showing that improvements in sleep disorders may predict abstinence in opioid-dependent patients [11].

Insomnia is present in several stages of alcohol use [12]. In turn, alcohol is used by 45% of patients with substance use disorders, as self-medication for their sleep disorders [8]. As the alcohol consumption becomes chronic, it decreases its hypnotic effect. The rates of insomnia among alcoholics range between 35 and 70% [13]. These rates are higher than those observed for the general population (15–30%) [13]. Patients report difficulty falling asleep, sleep fragmentation, daytime sleepiness, bad quality of sleep and, sometimes, hypersomnia [14]. Knowing the changes in circadian rhythms caused by alcohol can help us in its treatment. After a single acute intake of alcohol, changes in biological rhythms are reflected in melatonin and cortisol secretions and central body temperature (CBT) rhythms. These alterations are more severe during alcohol use disorder (AUD) and persist over time. Opposite patterns of the physiological relationship of melatonin between daytime and night-time discharge have been observed (N/D < 1 ratio). Resynchronization of circadian cortisol and CBT rhythms occurs approximately one month after leaving alcohol. Disruption of circadian melatonin rhythms may persist for 3–12 weeks [15].

Sleeping problems associated with alcohol use disorder are some of the most refractory disorders [9]. Cognitive behavioral therapy for insomnia (CBT-I) has been described as the first line treatment. On the other hand, mirtazapine, gabapentin, and quetiapine have a moderate level of evidence. Benzodiazepines should be avoided [16].

As in the case of alcohol, the use of cannabis improves insomnia, particularly when used over a short period of time [17]. However, the chronic consumption of cannabis is associated with negative effects on sleep that are more visible during abstinence. These effects are present during the interruption of cannabis use, particularly in habitual cannabis users, but also in people exposed to low doses [18,19].

Cocaine abstinence is behind many complaints related to sleep. During the first week of abstinence, patients may show insomnia, nightmares and, sometimes, hypersomnia. They also report depressive symptoms, fatigue, increased appetite, and agitation episodes [20]. Eighty percent of the people with an increased need for sleep during cocaine abstinence in the early stages self-medicate with alcohol and opioids [21]. When the patients remain abstinent, the quality of sleep improves [22], and sleeping routines return to normal after several weeks [21].

There are a limited number of studies on the effects of abstinence and chronic use of opioids. Asaad et al. described alterations including insomnia, hypersomnia, increased latency, and decreased duration of sleep after three weeks of abstinence [23]. The quality of sleep was studied in patients 5 days after starting treatment with methadone. Patients without previous sleep disorders obtained lower scores in the Pittsburgh Sleep Quality Index (PSQI) and showed daytime sleepiness in the Epworth Sleepiness Scale (ESS) [24].

On the other hand, during the first stages of methadone detoxification [25] patients reported inadequate quality and quantity of sleep, as well as difficulties falling asleep [26]. After long periods of treatment with methadone, it was observed that this difficulty falling asleep lasted from 6 to 12 months [27].

Among the anti-depressants that can cause insomnia are those that inhibit the reuptake of serotonin and noradrenaline (SNRIs), noradrenaline reuptake inhibitors (NRIs), monoamine oxidase inhibitors (MAOIs), selective serotonin reuptake inhibitors (SSRIs), and tricyclic antidepressant activators (TCAs). In contrast, antihistamine-active antidepressants, such as the sedative tricyclic antidepressants, mirtazapine, mianserin, and serotonin 5-HT2 receptor antagonists, such as trazodone and nefazodone, rapidly improve sleep. Some patients already show an improvement in sleep quality after the first dose of the drug [28], which was observed with mirtazapine in relation to the faster onset of antidepressant action [29].

On the other hand, antidepressants can cause sleep disorders or worsen existing ones. Mianserin and mirtazapine can induce restless leg syndrome in up to 28% of patients. It has also been described for SSRIs as well as venlafaxine [30]. SSRIs, SNRIs, and ACTs induce or exacerbate sleep bruxism and alter the regulation of muscle tone during REM sleep [31,32]. In addition, although antidepressants are recommended for the treatment of post-traumatic sleep disorder, they can induce nightmares, especially with mirtazapine.

The relationship between insomnia, psychiatric disorders (mainly depression and anxiety), and drug use disorder has already been described [33–35]. Winkour et al. observed that 100% of the patients in a sample of 1257 people with depression also presented comorbid insomnia [36]. The relationship between sleep disorders and psychiatric disorders is gaining increased attention, particularly as evidence shows that insomnia is not just a typical symptom of depression or other psychiatric disorders, but that it may actually be a predictive factor (or an independent risk factor) for the development of other psychiatric disorders, including substance use [37].

Our objective is to analyze whether patients with dual disorder present more sleep alterations than non-dual addicts, and to assess the types of sleep disorders (DSI, sleep fragmentation, early awakening, and nightmares) depending on the accompanying disorder, consumed substance, or both. We will also study the presence of sleep disorders based on whether the patients are receiving outpatient or inpatient care.

2. Materials and Methods

The study included patients diagnosed with substance use disorder based on the Diagnostic and Statistical Manual of Mental Disorders (DSM)-criteria who visited the Outpatient Drug Clinic (ODC) or were admitted into the Inpatient Dual Diagnoses Detoxification Unit (IDDDU) of the Salamanca Health Care University Complex from October 2017 to January 2020. Dual disorder (DD) is the comorbidity between mental disorders in general and disorders related to psychoactive substance use [38]. Patients who requested voluntary discharge on the first day of admission were excluded from the study, as well as those who had difficulties answering the questions due to cognitive or language alterations, and those who only cooperated partially when being assessed.

The research was approved by the Ethical Committee of Salamanca University Health Care Complex according to the Declaration of Helsinki (2075/A/19). Figure 1 shows gender and the origin (ODC/IDDU) of the study sample.

The assessment included a structured interview with 16 items, some of which had yes/no answers: presence of a dual disorder being treated in a program; presence of non-addictive mental disorder; affective disorder; psychotic disorder; patient from the ODC; patient from the IDDDU; type of addiction (alcohol, cannabis, cocaine, and heroin); alcohol withdrawal score ≥ 10 in the CIWA-AR scale (Revised Clinical Institute Withdrawal Assessment for Alcohol Scale) [39]; cannabis withdrawal syndrome; delayed sleep induction; sleep fragmentation; early awakening; and nightmares. Other items showed multiple options: occupational status (working, unemployed, on leave, or retired); treatment in the first interview; age; amount of cannabis consumed; amount of alcohol consumed; amount of cocaine consumed; amount of opioids consumed; and amount of benzodiazepines consumed. Multiple drug-users are codified when abuse or dependence on more than one drug exists (not including tobacco).

The diagnosis of insomnia is made when the patient reports dissatisfaction with sleep (difficultly to sleep or to remain asleep, when the sleep was fragmented, when there was an early awakening or nightmares) and other daytime symptoms (e.g., fatigue, decreased energy, mood disturbances and reduced cognitive functions such as impaired attention, concentration, and memory) for at least 3 nights per week and that lasts for more than 3 months [40]; all the data were collected and analyzed with SPSS version 25. The comparative analysis was carried out with the nonparametric chi-squared test.

Binomial logistic regression was used, including the variables that were significantly associated with insomnia: origin of the patient (ODC/IDDDU), presence of dual disorders; previous treatment in a different center; occupational status, pharmacological treatment in the first interview, and amount of benzodiazepines consumed.

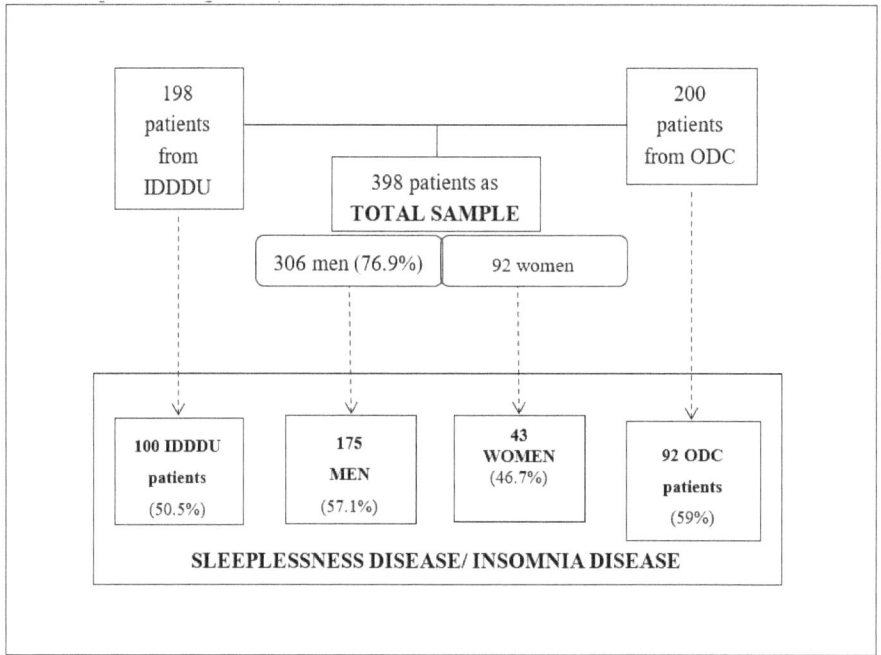

Figure 1. Flowchart of gender and origin characteristics from the sample. Abbreviations; IDDDU: Inpatient Dual Diagnoses Detoxification Unit; ODC: Outpatient Drug Clinic.

3. Results

The sample included 398 patients (76.9% men; mean age: 47 years). Of these, 198 patients (49.7%) came from the IDDDU, and 200 (50.3%) came from the ODC. Men presented more sleep disorders, represented in the column labeled "Insomnia/Any sleep disorder" (57.1%), than women (46.7%) (Table 1). The highest rate of Insomnia/Any Sleep Disorder was observed in the 48–57 age group (35.8%). Patients who consumed 1–5 units of cannabis had the most sleep disorders, particularly DSI and sleep fragmentation (Table 2). The same was true for patients with alcohol use disorder: those who consumed up to 20 alcohol units per day presented more sleep disorders than those who consumed 41 alcohol units per day or more. That is, lower consumption rates were correlated with higher rates of sleep disorder.

Delayed sleep induction ($\chi^2 = 10.48$; $p = 0.01$), early awakening ($\chi^2 = 5.598$; $p = 0.018$), and nightmares ($\chi^2 = 3.898$; $p = 0.048$) were more common in outpatients (Table 3). In our sample, 61.6% of the patients had dual disorders and presented more sleep disorders than non-dual patients: insomnia ($\chi^2 = 4.267$; $p = 0.039$), difficulty falling asleep ($\chi^2 = 2.877$; $p = 0.09$), sleep fragmentation ($\chi^2 = 4.862$; $p = 0.027$), early awakening ($\chi^2 = 7.554$; $p = 0.006$), and nightmares ($\chi^2 = 12.988$; $p = 0.000$).

With regard to cocaine use, those who consumed 1 g per week showed higher sleep disorder rates (12.3% of nightmares group) than those that consumed more cocaine. Opioid consumers represent between 21.2 and 26.7% of sleep disorders groups, particularly conciliation insomnia.

Similarly, patients with a dual disorder who had been treated in a different program (N = 172) showed higher rates of delayed sleep induction ($\chi^2 = 9.291$; $p = 0.02$), sleep fragmentation ($\chi^2 = 4.180$; $p = 0.041$), early awakening ($\chi^2 = 9.913$; $p = 0.02$), and nightmares ($\chi^2 = 10.814$; $p = 0.001$) than non-dual patients.

Table 1. Descriptive representation of demographic, clinical, and psychiatric variables in each sleep disorder and in the total sample. N and percentages are represented for each variable. Abbreviations: IDDDU: Inpatient Dual Diagnoses Detoxification Unit; ODC: Outpatient Drug Clinic.

Characteristics		Sample	Insomnia/Any Sleep Disorder	Delayed Sleep Induction	Sleep Fragmentation	Early Awakening	Nightmares
		N = 398	N = 218	N = 150	N = 137	N = 85	N = 80
Sex	Men	306 (76.9%)	175 (80.3%)	121 (80.7%)	107 (78.1%)	65 (76.5%)	53 (66.2%)
	Women	92 (23.1%)	43 (19.7%)	29 (19.3%)	30 (21.9%)	20 (23.5%)	27 (33.8%)
Age 18–27 years		22 (5.5%)	11 (5.0%)	9 (6.0%)	7 (5.1%)	4 (4.7%)	4 (5.0%)
28–37 years		60 (15.0%)	32 (14.7%)	23 (15.4%)	22 (16.1%)	8 (9.4%)	12 (15.0%)
38–47 years		128 (32.2%)	67 (30.7%)	45 (30.0%)	44 (32.1%)	28 (32.9%)	28 (35.0%)
48–57 years		138 (34.7%)	78 (35.8%)	57 (38.0%)	51 (37.2%)	37 (43.5%)	32 (40.0%)
58–67 years		39 (9.8%)	24 (11.0%)	14 (9.3%)	10 (7.3%)	7 (8.3%)	4 (5.0%)
≥68 years		11 (2.8%)	6 (2.8%)	2 (1.3%)	3 (2.2%)	1 (1.2%)	0 (0.0%)
Origin	IDDDU	198 (49.7%)	100 (45.9%)	58 (38.7%)	58 (42.3%)	32 (37.6%)	31 (38.8%)
	ODC	200 (50.3%)	118 (54.1%)	92 (61.3%)	79 (57.7%)	53 (62.4%)	49 (61.3%)
Dual Disorder		245 (61.6%)	146 (67.0%)	102 (68%)	96 (70.1%)	64 (75.3%)	64 (80%)
Affective disorder		154 (40.8%)	91 (42.7%)	65 (43.3%)	60 (44.1%)	42 (50.6%)	41 (51.9%)
Psychotic disorder		48 (12.7%)	26 (12.2%)	20 (13.3%)	19 (14.0%)	10 (12%)	13 (16.5%)
Personality disorder		86 (22.3%)	53 (24.3%)	40 (26.7%)	39 (28.5%)	24 (28.2%)	30 (37.5%)
Previous treatment		172 (43.2%)	103 (49.5%)	81 (55.9%)	69 (53.1%)	49 (61.3%)	48 (62.3%)
Multiple drug-users		193 (48.5%)	117 (53.7%)	88 (58.7%)	78 (57.0%)	49 (57.6%)	50 (62.5%)
Occupational status							
Working		75 (18.8%)	31 (14.2%)	22 (14.7%)	18 (13.1%)	10 (11.8%)	6 (7.5%)
Unemployed		151 (37.9%)	96 (44.0%)	68 (45.3%)	66 (48.2%)	45 (52.9%)	46 (57.5%)
On leave		43 (10.8%)	19 (8.7%)	11 (7.3%)	11 (8.0%)	5 (5.9%)	6 (7.5%)
Retired		108 (27.1%)	61 (28.0%)	40 (26.7%)	24 (17.5%)	19 (22.3%)	20 (25.0%)
Other conditions		21 (5.4%)	11 (5.1%)	9 (6.0%)	18 (13.1%)	6 (7.1%)	2 (2.5%)
Pharmacological treatment on first interview							
Alprazolam		17 (4.3%)	9 (4.1%)	7 (4.7%)	8 (5.8%)	4 (4.7%)	2 (2.5%)
Disulfiram		13 (3.3%)	3 (1.4%)	2 (1.3%)	2 (1.5%)	1 (1.2%)	2 (3.4%)
Clorazepate		7 (1.8%)	3 (1.4%)	2 (1.3%)	0 (0.0%)	0 (0.0%)	1 (1.3%)
Diazepam		13 (3.3%)	3 (1.4%)	1 (0.7%)	1 (0.7%)	0 (0.0%)	1 (1.3%)
Lorazepam		24 (6.0%)	15 (6.9%)	10 (6.7%)	8 (5.8%)	8 (9.4%)	6 (7.5%)
Lormetazepam		1 (0.3%)	5 (2.3%)	4 (2.7%)	2 (1.5%)	3 (3.5%)	2 (2.5%)
Methadone		2 (0.5%)	1 (0.6%)	1 (0.7%)	2 (1.5%)	0 (0.0%)	0 (0.0%)
Mirtazapine		8 (2.0%)	6 (2.8%)	6 (4.0%)	3 (2.2%)	3 (3.5%)	3 (3.8%)
Olanzapine		9 (2.3%)	7 (3.2%)	4 (2.7%)	5 (3.6%)	2 (2.4%)	3 (3.8%)

Table 1. Cont.

Characteristics	Sample N = 398	Insomnia/Any Sleep Disorder N = 218	Delayed Sleep Induction N = 150	Sleep Fragmentation N = 137	Early Awakening N = 85	Nightmares N = 80
Pregabalin	4 (1.0%)	4 (1.8%)	3 (2.0%)	3 (2.2%)	0 (0.0%)	2 (2.5%)
Quetiapine	12 (3.0%)	4 (1.8%)	2 (1.3%)	1 (0.7%)	2 (2.4%)	2 (2.5%)
Tiapride	12 (3.0%)	7 (3.2%)	5 (3.3%)	4 (2.9%)	4 (4.7%)	4 (5.0%)
Trazodone	10 (2.5%)	7 (3.2%)	5 (3.3%)	5 (3.6%)	4 (4.7%)	3 (3.8%)

Table 2. Use and quantity of cannabis, cocaine, alcohol, opioids, and benzodiazepines consumed. Data for total sample and subgroups associated with sleep disorders appear in different columns. For alcohol and cannabis users there is an extra variable related with withdrawal. Abbreviations: CWA-Ar ≥ 10; Revised Clinical Institute Withdrawal Assessment for Alcohol Scale, upper 10 score.

Type of Consumers	Sample N = 398 N (%)	Insomnia/any Sleep Disorder N = 218 N (%)	Delayed Sleep Induction N = 150 N (%)	Sleep Fragmentation N = 137 N (%)	Early Awakening N = 85 N (%)	Nightmares N = 80 N (%)
Cannabis Consumers	115 (28.9%)	65 (29.8%)	50 (33.3%)	43 (31.4%)	23 (27.0%)	25 (31.2%)
Quantity of Cannabis						
1–5 U	95 (23.9%)	55 (25.2%)	42 (28.0%)	36 (26.3%)	20 (23.5%)	22 (27.5%)
6–10 U	2 (0.5%)	1 (0.5%)	0 (0.0%)	0 (0.0%)	0 (0.0%)	0 (0.0%)
11–15 U	0 (0.0%)	0 (0.0%)	0 (0.0%)	0 (0.0%)	0 (0.0%)	0 (0.0%)
16–30 U	0 (0.0%)	0 (0.0%)	0 (0.0%)	0 (0.0%)	0 (0.0%)	0 (0.0%)
31 U or more	18 (4.5%)	9 (4.1%)	8 (5.3%)	7 (5.1%)	3 (3.5%)	3 (3.8%)
Cannabis withdrawal	38 (9.9%)	22 (10.1%)	17 (11.3%)	18 (13.1%)	7 (8.2%)	9 (11.3%)
Cocaine consumers	113 (28.4%)	83 (38.1%)	67 (44.7%)	49 (64.2%)	30 (35.3%)	36 (45.0%)
Quantity of Cocaine						
1 g/week	30 (7.5%)	19 (9.5%)	13 (9.6%)	13 (10.1%)	6 (7.6%)	9 (12.3%)
2 g/week	21 (5.3%)	13 (6.5%)	11 (8.1%)	9 (7.0%)	3 (3.8%)	3 (4.1%)
3 g/week	9 (2.3%)	7 (3.5%)	6 (4.4%)	4 (3.1%)	4 (5.1%)	4 (5.5%)
4 g/week	11 (2.8%)	6 (3.0%)	5 (1.5%)	1 (0.8%)	1 (1.3%)	3 (5.5%)
5 g/week	7 (1.0%)	4 (2.0%)	2 (1.5%)	4 (3.1%)	3 (3.8%)	1 (1.4%)
6 g/week or more	35 (8.8%)	17 (8.8%)	15 (11.1%)	10 (7.8%)	7 (8.9%)	9 (12.3%)
Alcohol consumers	236 (66.1%)	142 (65.1%)	93 (62.0%)	87 (63.5%)	57 (67.1%)	47 (58.7%)
Quantity of Alcohol						
1–20 units/day	220 (55.3%)	117 (53.7%)	77 (53.1%)	71 (51.8%)	47 (55.3%)	38 (47.5%)
21–40 units/day	36 (9.0%)	21 (9.6%)	14 (9.3%)	14 (10.2%)	8 (9.4%)	8 (10.0%)

Table 2. Cont.

Type of Consumers	Sample N = 398	Insomnia/any Sleep Disorder N = 218	Delayed Sleep Induction N = 150	Sleep Fragmentation N = 137	Early Awakening N = 85	Nightmares N = 80
	N (%)	N (%)	N (%)	N (%)	N (%)	N (%)
41 units/day or more	7 (1.8%)	3 (1.4%)	2 (1.3%)	2 (1.5%)	2 (2.4%)	1 (1.3%)
CIWA-Ar ≥ 10	169 (44.1%)	94 (43.1%)	58 (38.7%)	55 (40.1%)	30 (35.3%)	25 (31.3%)
Opioids consumers	72 (18.1%)	48 (22.0%)	40 (26.7%)	32 (23.4%)	21 (24.7%)	17 (21.2%)
Quantity of Opioids						
1–10 g/week	72 (18.1%)	48 (22.0%)	40 (26.7%)	32 (23.4%)	21 (24.7%)	17 (21.2%)
Benzodiazepines consumers	93 (23.7%)	61 (28.0%)	48 (32.0%)	46 (33.6%)	30 (35.3%)	31 (38.7%)
1–10 mg/day	47 (11.8%)	32 (14.7%)	24 (16.0%)	23 (16.8%)	15 (17.6%)	15 (12.4%)
11–21 mg/day	12 (3.0%)	8 (3.7%)	7 (4.7%)	8 (5.8%)	5 (5.9%)	4 (5.0%)
22–31 mg/day	1 (0.3%)	1 (0.5%)	1 (0.7%)	1 (0.7%)	1 (1.2%)	0 (0.0%)
32 mg or more	33 (8.3%)	20 (9.2%)	16 (10.7%)	14 (10.2%)	9 (10.6%)	12 (15.0%)

Table 3. Relationships between variables analyzed with non-parametric test chi-square and p-values. Abbreviations; IDDDU: Inpatient Dual Diagnoses Detoxification Unit; ODC: Outpatient Drug Clinic. *: significant values with $p < 0.05$.

Characteristics	Insomnia/Any Sleep Disorder (n = 218)		Delayed Sleep Induction (n = 150)		Sleep Fragmentation (n = 216)		Early Awakening (n = 85)		Nightmares (n = 80)	
	χ^2	p	χ^2	p	χ^2	p	χ^2	p	χ^2	p
Sex	3.023	0.082	1.781	0.182	0.121	0.728	0.016	0.898	7.069	0.008 *
Age	2.585	0.764	2.758	0.737	1.322	0.93	5.313	0.379	5.346	0.375
IDDDU/ODC	2.092	0.148	10.48	0.010 *	3.456	0.063	5.598	0.018 *	3.898	0.048 *
Dual Disorder	4.267	0.039 *	2.877	0.090	4.862	0.027 *	7.554	0.006 *	12.988	0.000 *
Previous treatment	2.442	0.118	9.291	0.002 *	4.180	0.041 *	9.913	0.002 *	10.814	0.001 *
Affective disorder	1.935	0.380	1.365	0.505	1.579	0.454	4.640	0.098	5.598	0.061
Psychotic disorder	0.122	0.727	0.056	0.813	247	0.619	0.033	0.855	1.353	0.254
Personality disorder	1.592	0.207	1.84	0.175	4.475	0.034 *	2.183	0.140	13.596	0.000 *
Multiple drug- users	4.254	0.039 *	9.368	0.002 *	5.469	0.019 *	3.532	0.060	7.603	0.006 *
Unemployed	13.557	0.019 *	8.867	0.14 *	12.438	0.029 *	12.823	0.025 *	25.732	0.000 *
Pharmacological treatment on first interview	29.55	0.009 *	24.06	0.064	28.737	0.017 *	19.306	0.2	13.295	0.579
Amount of cannabis consumed	16.935	0.390	22.760	0.120	11.728	0.762	7.919	0.951	19.666	0.236
Cannabis withdrawal	0.016	0.898	0.490	0.484	2.345	0.126	0.401	0.527	0.255	0.614
Amount of alcohol consumed	1.447	0.695	2.018	0.569	1.491	0.684	0.589	0.899	2.827	0.419
CIWA-Ar ≥ 10	0.208	0.649	2.805	0.094	1.257	0.262	3.511	0.061	6.488	0.011 *
Amount of cocaine consumed	3.852	0.697	9.53	0.16	7.294	0.294	5.99	0.424	8.41	0.21
Amount of opioids consumed	0.122	0.727	0.056	0.813	0.247	0.619	0.33	0.855	1.353	0.245
Amount of benzodiazepines consumed	9.848	0.043 *	15.21	0.04 *	16.924	0.002 *	13.316	0.010 *	18.980	0.001 *

The most commonly used drug for insomnia in the initial interview was alprazolam (4.3%), followed by diazepam (3.3%). The use of benzodiazepines was clearly associated with all types of insomnia ($\chi^2 = 9.848$; $p = 0.043$), delayed sleep induction ($\chi^2 = 15.21$; $p = 0.04$), sleep fragmentation ($\chi^2 = 16.924$; $p = 0.002$), early awakening ($\chi^2 = 13.316$; $p = 0.010$), and nightmares ($\chi^2 = 18.980$; $p = 0.001$). Consuming a larger quantity of benzodiazepines was associated with all types of sleep disorder.

The presence of nightmares during sleep is significantly associated with an ambulatory treatment ($\chi^2 = 3.898$; $p = 0.0048$), being a woman ($\chi^2 = 7.069$; $p = 0.008$), having a dual disorder ($\chi^2 = 10.814$; $p = 0.001$), being treated with benzodiazepines ($\chi^2 = 18.980$; $p = 0.001$), and alcohol abstinence ($\chi^2 = 6.488$; $p = 0.011$).

Finally, multivariate analysis is depicted in Table 4. Benzodiazepine use disorder ($p = 0.029$; OR = 0.354), treatment with trazodone ($p = 0.031$; OR = 0.129), and treatment with pregabalin ($p = 0.031$; OR = 0.129) were protector factors for insomnia. Having a concomitant psychiatric disorder ($p = 0.039$; OR = 1.553) and the origin of the patients were risk factors for some sleep disorders, such as conciliation insomnia ($p = 0.01$; OR = 1.991), early awakening ($p = 0.019$; OR = 1.80), and nightmares ($p = 0.050$; OR = 1.656).

Table 4. Several binomial logistic regression analyses with the dependent variable varying among sleep disorder subgroups. Abbreviations; IDDDU: Inpatient Dual Diagnoses Detoxification Unit; ODC: Outpatient Drug Clinic.

Dependent Variable	Wald	p	OR	IC 95%
Insomnia/any sleep disorder				
Benzodiazepine use disorder	4.779	0.029	0.354	0.140–0.898
Dual Disorder	4.246	0.039	1.553	1.022–2.361
Treatment with trazodone	4.626	0.031	0.129	0.020–0.834
Treatment with pregabalin	4.626	0.031	0.129	0.020–0.834
Delayed sleep induction				
Origin: ODC/IDDDU	10.364	0.001	1.991	1.309–3.027
Previous treatment	9.198	0.002	0.519	0.34–0.793
Benzodiazepine use disorder	7.189	0.007	0.319	0.138–0.735
Treatment with pregabalin	3.857	0.05	0.091	0.008–0.995
Sleep fragmentation				
Dual Disorder	4.824	0.028	0.606	0.388–0.948
Previous treatment	4.158	0.041	0.639	0.515–0.983
Benzodiazepine use disorder	4.567	0.033	0.423	0.192–0.931
Treatment with pregabalin	3.857	0.05	0.091	0.008–0.995
Personality disorder	4.426	0.035	0.590	0.361–0.965
Early awakening				
Dual Disorder	7.353	0.007	0.470	0.273–0.811
Origin: ODC/IDDDU	5.519	0.019	1.810	1.103–2.970
Previous treatment	9.657	0.002	0.447	0.269–0.743
Benzodiazepine use disorder	3.900	0.048	0.433	0.189–0.994
Nightmares				
Origin: ODC/IDDDU	3.856	0.050	1.656	1.001–2.741
Previous treatment	10.490	0.001	0.425	0.254–0.714
Dual Disorder	12.256	0.000	0.346	0.191–0.627
Benzodiazepine use disorder	9.455	0.002	0.278	0.123–0.629
Personality disorder	4.426	0.035	0.590	0.361–0.965

4. Discussion

In our sample, 62% of the patients had dual disorders and presented more sleep disorders than non-dual patients: insomnia, difficulty falling asleep, sleep fragmentation, early awakening, and nightmares. Occupational status and consuming larger amounts of benzodiazepines were associated with the presence of sleep disorders; while being a woman, symptoms of alcohol withdrawal, and personality disorders were associated with the presence of nightmares. On the other hand, 67.3% of the patients who reported insomnia had a dual disorder, and this rate is much higher than that of the general population (9–12%) [34,41].

The most common disorders in the dual population were affective and psychotic disorders, which is in line with what was reported in previous studies [2,35,42,43]. Approximately 20% of all addict patients with sleep disorders present some symptom of depression [44–47]. Staner et al. already observed that having a psychiatric disorder, and particularly depression, was the most important risk factor for insomnia [47]. Therefore, it may be said that the relationship between insomnia and depression in addict patients is bidirectional.

With regard to personality disorders, these were associated with sleep fragmentation and, more notably, nightmares. This last finding coincides with what has been observed in other studies that described a higher number of admissions of addict patients with sleep disorders and a comorbid personality disorder [2].

The presence of nightmares was also associated with being a woman. This finding had already been observed in women with alcohol and other drug disorders. They did not only report having nightmares, but had in many cases been diagnosed with depression, personality disorders, and psychosis [48]. It is important to highlight that the main type of drug that was used had an influence on the results. In this regard, in patients with alcohol use disorders, the most common alterations were sleep fragmentation and delayed sleep induction (62%). In the same vein, in most of the previous studies, the prevalence of insomnia in patients with an alcohol use disorder ranged between 35 and 75% [12], because the patients often used alcohol as self-medication to sleep [7,49,50]. Patients with a cannabis use disorder presented lower rates of insomnia (29.8%) than those who did not consume it (70.2%), although the chronic use of cannabis is known to be associated with negative effects on sleep, particularly during periods of abstinence. Cannabis may improve subjective complaints about sleep when used over short periods of time [51,52]. Nightmares are generally the most common sleep disorders during abstinence [53]. They usually start 1–3 days after stopping consumption [53–55], they reach their peak after 2–6 days, and they last for 4–14 days [53]. Other studies report that difficulties in falling asleep last around 43 days [56] and nightmares may last up to 45 days [53]. As a consequence, there are generally relapses in the use of alcohol and cannabis to fall asleep [56].

In patients with cocaine use disorder, delayed sleep induction was the most common disorder, with the highest rates among patients who consumed over 6 g/week (11.1%). Eighty percent of the patients who wanted to sleep more during a period of abstinence from cocaine self-medicated in the early stages with alcohol and opioids [57–59]. No differences were observed regarding the type of insomnia in patients with opioid use disorder. Although there is little evidence on this topic, an association has been described between heroin use and sleep disorders [60–62], particularly falling asleep and maintaining sleep during the first stages of detoxification with methadone [62].

Some authors have described that multiple admissions to detoxification units are associated with more sleep disorders, with promotes substance use and relapses [1,2] and leads to a worse evolution of the addiction [2]. However, in our case, outpatients reported more difficulties falling asleep, and the sleep was of poorer quality than in hospitalized patients.

Benzodiazepines are the most widely sold group of drugs for sleep disorders, as has already been described in other series of addict patients [2] and mental health patients [63]. Benzodiazepine use disorder is common in patients who are being treated for a different addiction. It is associated with complications such as overdoses and suicide attempts. Although these drugs may modulate sleep disorders, they are not recommended for the treatment of insomnia in addict patients [64–66], and the risk and possibilities of their misuse must be taken into consideration [1].

This study must be analyzed considering its limitations, since it is a cross-sectional analysis that does not make it possible to establish causal associations regarding the influence of drug abstinence or the psychopathological evolution of the patients. We may highlight that the assessment of the presence of insomnia did not include electrophysiological tests such as polysomnography and actigraphy. However, electrophysiological tests are recommended as a second choice, because the diagnosis of insomnia is mainly clinical, and it is based on the history of the patient.

Nevertheless, this study has some strengths, since it includes a large sample of unselected real-world outpatients and inpatients who required treatment. In this regard, it is important to highlight that there are very few analyses that describe the prevalence of insomnia in dual patients and that specify the type of sleep disorder [67]. Most of the studies published in the literature only include alcohol-dependent patients.

5. Conclusions

Patients with a dual disorder present sleep disorders (delayed sleep induction, sleep fragmentation, early awakening, and nightmares) with a significantly higher rate than non-dual patients. On the other hand, 67.3% of the patients who reported insomnia had an associated psychiatric disorder, mostly affective disorders, with psychopathology as the most common one.

The main drug associated with sleep disorders was alcohol (65.1%), and nightmares showed a significant association with alcohol withdrawal syndrome.

An association was found between sleep disorders and the origin of the patients, and outpatients showed more difficulties falling asleep.

The presence of a dual disorder is relevant for the appearance of sleep disorders in addict patients and vice versa. In patients with sleep disorders and substance use disorders, the existence of a dual pathology must be taken into account.

Benzodiazepine use disorder was significantly associated with all the types of sleep disorders. An association was also observed between insomnia and the use of trazodone and pregabalin.

Sleep disorders are a severity marker in patients who use drugs and have an associated psychopathological disorder. It is necessary to continue researching the influence of insomnia in the severity of the psychopathology and relapses. Sleep disorders must be considered a "clinical marker" of the presence of a dual pathology in addict patients and, therefore, it is necessary to thoroughly assess the presence of other mental disorders in patients who consume drugs and report insomnia.

Author Contributions: C.R., L.A., and A.Á. conceptualized, designed, and supervised the study; B.V.-H., A.B., and L.G.-U. collected the data and performed data processing and statistical analysis; D.R.-G., A.C., and A.F. wrote the manuscript. C.R. and L.A. supervised the project; A.B. and L.G.-U. critically revised and edited the manuscript. All authors have read and agreed to the published version of the manuscript.

Funding: This research project was supported by Castile and León's (Spain) Regional Management of Health (GRS 2075/A/2019) Scholarship for the project "Clinical characterization of psychotic symptoms and their relationship with addiction severity among patients consulting for alcohol and cocaine intake and alcohol intake." This 12-month scholarship was awarded to C. Roncero (main researcher) and his research team.

Acknowledgments: The author would like to thank the Medical Association of Salamanca for the translation of this article; the University Health Care Complex of Salamanca for their support to the ODC and the IDDDU; and the following professionals from the ODC of the University Health Care Complex of Salamanca: Joaquina Recio, Eulalia Fraile, Manuela Rodríguez Ruano, Maria Ángeles Garzón, Ana Pérez-Madruga and Pablo Gutiérrez, who collaborated on the clinical assessment of the patients.

Conflicts of Interest: Carlos Roncero declares that, over the last years, he has been paid for his participation as a speaker in events organized by Janssen-Cilag, Indivior, Lundbeck, Otsuka, Servier, GSK, Astra, Gilead, MSD, Sanofi, Exceltis, Abbvie, Takeda Rubio and Casein. He has been paid for his services as an advisor in meetings by Gilead, MSD, Mundipharm, INDIVIOR, Exeltis, Martindale, Camurus, Gebro and Abbive. He received funding for the Proteus and the COSTEDOPIA projects from Indivior. He has received medical training scholarships from Gilead. Begoña Vicente-Hernández declares that over the last years she has been paid for her participation as a speaker by Janssen-Cilag and Lundbeck. The rest of the authors declare no conflict of interests.

References

1. Roncero, C.; Grau-López, L.; Díaz-Morán, S.; Miquel, L.; Martínez-Luna, N.; Casas, M. Evaluación de las alteraciones del sueño en pacientes drogodependientes hospitalizados (Evaluation of sleep disorders in hospitalized drug-dependent patients). *Med. Clin.* **2012**, *138*, 332–335. [CrossRef] [PubMed]
2. Grau-López, L.; Daigre, C.; Grau-López, L.; Rodriguez-Cintas, L.; Egido, Á.; Casas, M.; Roncero, C. Administrative prevalence of insomnia and associated clinical features in patients with addiction during active substance use. *Actas Esp. Psiquiatr.* **2016**, *44*, 64–71. [PubMed]
3. Johnson, E.O.; Breslau, N. Sleep problems and substance use in adolescence. *Drug Alcohol Depend.* **2001**, *64*, 1–7. [CrossRef]
4. Haario, P.; Rahkonen, O.; Laaksonen, M.; Lahelma, E.; Lallukka, T. Bidirectional associations between insomnia symptoms and unhealthy behaviours. *J. Sleep Res.* **2013**, 2289–2295. [CrossRef] [PubMed]
5. Burke, C.K.; Peirce, J.M.; Kidorf, M.S.; Neubauer, D.; Punjabi, N.M.; Stoller, K.B.; Hursh, S.; Brooner, R.K. Sleep problems reported by patients entering opioid agonist treatment. *J. Subst. Abuse Treat.* **2008**, *35*, 328–333. [CrossRef]
6. Brower, K.J.; Krentzman, A.; Robinson, E.A. Persistent insomnia, abstinence, and moderate drinking in alcohol-dependent individuals. *Am. J. Addict.* **2011**, *20*, 435–440. [CrossRef]
7. Brower, K.J.; Aldrich, M.S.; Robinson, E.A.; Zucker, R.A.; Greden, J.F. Insomnia, self-medication, and relapse to alcoholism. *Am. J. Psychiatry* **2001**, *158*, 399–404. [CrossRef]
8. Brower, K.J.; Perron, B.E. Sleep disturbance as a universal risk factor for relapse in addictions to psychoactive substances. *Med. Hypotheses* **2010**, *74*, 928–933. [CrossRef]
9. Brower, K.J.; Aldrich, M.S.; Hall, J.M. Polysomnographic and subjective sleep predictors of alcoholic relapse. *Alcoholism Clin. Exp. Res.* **1998**, *22*, 1864–1871. [CrossRef]
10. Morgan, P.T.; Angarita, G.A.; Canavan, S.; Pittman, B.; Oberleitner, L.; Malison, R.T.; Mohsenin, V.; Hodges, S.; Easton, C.; McKee, S.; et al. Modafinil and sleep architecture in an inpatient-outpatient treatment study of cocaine dependence. *Drug Alcohol Depend.* **2016**, *160*, 49–56. [CrossRef]
11. Dijkstra, B.A.; De Jong, C.A.; Krabbe, P.F.; van der Staak, C.P. Prediction of abstinence in opioid-dependent patients. *J. Addict. Med.* **2008**, *2*, 194–201. [CrossRef] [PubMed]
12. Vitiello, M. Sleep, alcohol and alcohol abuse. *Addict. Biol.* **1997**, *2*, 151–158. [CrossRef] [PubMed]
13. Brower, K.J. Alcohol's effects on sleep in alcoholics. *Alcohol Res. Health* **2001**, *25*, 110–125. [PubMed]
14. Arnedt, J.T.; Conroy, D.A.; Armitage, R.; Brower, K.J. Cognitive-behavioral therapy for insomnia in alcohol dependent patients: A randomized controlled pilot trial. *Behav. Res. Ther.* **2011**, *49*, 227–233. [CrossRef] [PubMed]
15. Meyrel, M.; Rolland, B.; Geoffroy, P.A. Alterations in circadian rhythms following alcohol use: A systematic review. *Prog. Neuropsychopharmacol. Biol. Psychiatry* **2020**, *99*, 109831. [CrossRef] [PubMed]
16. Geoffroy, P.A.; Lejoyeuxa, M.; Rolland, B. Management of insomnia in alcohol use disorder. *Expert. Opin. Pharmacother.* **2020**, *21*, 297–306. [CrossRef]
17. Conroy, D.A.; Arnedt, J.T. Sleep and substance use disorders: An update. *Curr. Psychiatry Rep.* **2014**, *16*, 487. [CrossRef]
18. Haney, M.; Ward, A.S.; Comer, S.D.; Foltin, R.W.; Fischman, M.W. Abstinence symptoms following oral THC administration to humans. *Psychopharmacology* **1999**, *141*, 385–394. [CrossRef]
19. Crowley, T.J.; Macdonald, M.J.; Whitmore, E.A.; Mikulich, S.K. Cannabis dependence, withdrawal, and reinforcing effects among adolescents with conduct symptoms and substance use disorders. *Drug Alcohol Depend.* **1998**, *50*, 27–37. [CrossRef]
20. Brower, K.J.; Maddahian, E.; Blow, F.C.; Beresford, T.P. A comparison of self-reported symptoms and DSM-III-R criteria for cocaine withdrawal. *Am. J. Drug Alcohol Abuse* **1988**, *14*, 347–356. [CrossRef]
21. Gawin, F.H.; Kleber, H.D. Abstinence symptomatology and psychiatric diagnosis in cocaine abusers. Clinical observations. *Arch. Gen. Psychiatry* **1986**, *43*, 107–113. [CrossRef] [PubMed]
22. Weddington, W.W.; Brown, B.S.; Haertzen, C.A.; Cone, E.J.; Dax, E.M.; Herning, R.I.; Michaelson, B.S. Changes in mood, craving, and sleep during short-term abstinence reported by male cocaine addicts. A controlled, residential study. *Arch. Gen. Psychiatry* **1990**, *47*, 861–868. [CrossRef] [PubMed]

23. Asaad, T.A.; Ghanem, M.H.; Abdel Samee, A.M.; El–Habiby, M.M. Sleep Profile in Patients With Chronic Opioid Abuse: A Polysomnographic Evaluation in an Egyptian Sample. *Addict. Disord. Treat.* **2011**, *10*, 21–28. [CrossRef]
24. Wang, D.; Teichtahl, H.; Drummer, O.; Goodman, C.; Cherry, G.; Cunnington, D.; Kronborg, I. Central sleep apnea in stable methadone maintenance treatment patients. *Chest* **2005**, *128*, 1348–1356. [CrossRef]
25. Oyefeso, A.; Sedgwick, P.; Ghodse, H. Subjective sleep-wake parameters in treatment-seeking opiate addicts. *Drug Alcohol Depend.* **1997**, *48*, 9–16. [CrossRef]
26. Kay, D.C. Human sleep and EEG through a cycle of methadone dependence. *Electroencephalogr. Clin. Neurophysiol.* **1975**, *38*, 35–43. [CrossRef]
27. Peles, E.; Schreiber, S.; Hamburger, R.B.; Adelson, M. No change of sleep after 6 and 12 months of methadone maintenance treatment. *J. Addict. Med.* **2011**, *5*, 141–147. [CrossRef]
28. Schmid, D.A.; Wichniak, A.; Uhr, M.; Ising, M.; Brunner, H.; Held, K.; Weikel, J.C.; Sonntag, A.; Steiger, A. Changes of sleep architecture, spectral composition of sleep EEG, the nocturnal secretion of cortisol, ACTH, GH, prolactin, melatonin, ghrelin, and leptin, and the DEX-CRH test in depressed patients during treatment with mirtazapine. *Neuropsychopharmacology* **2006**, *31*, 832–844. [CrossRef]
29. Thompson, C. Onset of action of antidepressants: Results of different analyses. *Hum. Psychopharmacol.* **2002**, *17*, S27–S32. [CrossRef]
30. Narowska, D.; Bozek, M.; Krysiak, K.; Antczak, J.; Holka-Pokorska, J.; Jernajczyk, W.; Wichniak, A. Frequent difficulties in the treatment of restless legs syndrome—Case report and literature review. *Psychiatr. Pol.* **2015**, *49*, 921–930. [CrossRef]
31. Wichniak, A.; Wierzbicka, A.; Jernajczyk, W. Sleep and antidepressant treatment. *Curr. Pharm. Des.* **2012**, *18*, 5802–5817. [CrossRef] [PubMed]
32. Wilson, S.; Argyropoulos, S. Antidepressants and sleep: A qualitative review of the literature. *Drugs* **2005**, *65*, 927–947. [CrossRef]
33. Johnson, E.O.; Roth, T.; Breslau, N. The association of insomnia with anxiety disorders and depression: Exploration of the direction of risk. *J. Psychiatr. Res.* **2006**, *40*, 700–708. [CrossRef] [PubMed]
34. Taylor, D.J.; Lichstein, K.L.; Durrence, H.H.; Reidel, B.W.; Bush, A.J. Epidemiology of insomnia, depression, and anxiety. *Sleep* **2005**, *28*, 1457–1464. [CrossRef]
35. Tsuno, N.; Besset, A.; Ritchie, K. Sleep and Depression. *J. Clin. Psychiatry* **2005**, *66*, 1254–1269. [CrossRef] [PubMed]
36. Winokur, G.; Clayton, P.J.; Reich, T. *Manic Depressive Illness*; Mosby: St. Louis, MO, USA, 1969; p. 165.
37. Riemann, D.; Berger, M.; Voderholzer, U. Sleep and depression—Results from psychobiological studies: An overview. *Biol. Psychol.* **2001**, *57*, 67–103. [CrossRef]
38. Torrens, M.; Mestre-Pintó, J.I.; Montanari, L.; Vicente, J.; Domingo-Salvany, A. Dual diagnosis: An European perspective. *Adicciones* **2017**, *29*, 3–5. [CrossRef]
39. Stuppaeck, C.H.; Barnas, C.; Falk, M.; Guenther, V.; Hummer, M.; Oberbauer, H.; Pycha, R.; Whitworth, A.B.; Fleischhacker, W.W. Assessment of the alcohol withdrawal syndrome—Validity and reliability of the translated and modified Clinical Institute Withdrawal Assessment for Alcohol scale (CIWA-A). *Addiction* **1994**, *89*, 1287–1292. [CrossRef]
40. *International Classification of Sleep Disorders: Diagnostic and Coding Manual*, 3rd ed.; American Academy of Sleep Medicine: Darien, IL, USA, 2014.
41. Leger, D.; Guilleminault, C.; Dreyfus, J.P.; Delahaye, C.; Paillard, M. Prevalence of insomnia in a survey of 12,778 adults in France. *J. Sleep Res.* **2000**, *9*, 35–42. [CrossRef]
42. Soldatos, C.R. Insomnia in relation to depression and anxiety: Epidemiologic considerations. *J. Psychosom. Res.* **1994**, *38*, 3–8. [CrossRef]
43. Riemann, D. Insomnia and comorbid psychiatric disorders. *Sleep Med.* **2007**, *8*, 20. [CrossRef]
44. Ohayon, M.M.; Caulet, M.; Lemoine, P. Comorbidity of mental and insomnia disorders in the general population. *Compr. Psychiatry* **1998**, *39*, 185–197. [CrossRef]
45. Quera-Salva, M.A.; Orluc, A.; Goldenberg, F.; Guilleminault, C. Insomnia and use of hypnotics: Study of a French population. *Sleep* **1991**, *14*, 386–391. [CrossRef]
46. Weissman, M.M.; Greenwald, S.; Niño-Murcia, G.; Dement, W.C. The morbidity of insomnia uncomplicated by psychiatric disorders. *Gen. Hosp. Psychiatry* **1997**, *19*, 245–250. [CrossRef]
47. Staner, L. Comorbidity of insomnia and depression. *Sleep Med. Rev.* **2010**, *14*, 35–46. [CrossRef]

48. Cernovsky, Z.Z. MMPI and nightmare reports in women addicted to alcohol and other drugs. *Percept. Mot. Skills* **1986**, *62*, 717–718. [CrossRef]
49. Ford, D.E.; Kamerow, D.B. Epidemiologic study of sleep disturbances and psychiatric disorders. An opportunity for prevention? *JAMA* **1989**, *262*, 1479–1484. [CrossRef]
50. Dijk, D.J. Slow-wave sleep deficiency and enhancement: Implications for insomnia and its management. *World J. Biol. Psychiatry* **2010**, *11*, 22–28. [CrossRef]
51. Chait, L.D.; Zacny, J.P. Reinforcing and subjective effects of oral delta 9-THC and smoked marijuana in humans. *Psychopharmacology* **1992**, *107*, 255–262. [CrossRef]
52. Budney, A.J.; Moore, B.A.; Vandrey, R.G.; Hughes, J.R. The time course and significance of cannabis withdrawal. *J. Abnorm. Psychol.* **2003**, *112*, 393–402. [CrossRef]
53. Budney, A.J.; Hughes, J.R.; Moore, B.A.; Vandrey, R. Review of the validity and significance of cannabis withdrawal syndrome. *Am. J. Psychiatry* **2004**, *161*, 1967–1977. [CrossRef] [PubMed]
54. Vandrey, R.; Smith, M.T.; McCann, U.D.; Budney, A.J.; Curran, E.M. Sleep disturbance and the effects of extended-release zolpidem during cannabis withdrawal. *Drug Alcohol Depend.* **2011**, *117*, 38–44. [CrossRef] [PubMed]
55. Copersino, M.L.; Boyd, S.J.; Tashkin, D.P.; Huestis, M.A.; Heishman, S.J.; Dermand, J.C.; Simmons, M.S.; Gorelick, D.A. Cannabis withdrawal among non-treatment-seeking adult cannabis users. *Am. J. Addict.* **2006**, *15*, 8–14. [CrossRef] [PubMed]
56. Schierenbeck, T.; Riemann, D.; Berger, M.; Hornyak, M. Effect of illicit recreational drugs upon sleep: Cocaine, ecstasy and marijuana. *Sleep Med. Rev.* **2008**, *12*, 381–389. [CrossRef] [PubMed]
57. Garcia, A.N.; Salloum, I.M. Polysomnographic sleep disturbances in nicotine, caffeine, alcohol, cocaine, opioid, and cannabis use: A focused review. *Am. J. Addict.* **2015**, *24*, 590–598. [CrossRef]
58. Angarita, G.A.; Emadi, N.; Hodges, S.; Morgan, P.T. Sleep abnormalities associated with alcohol, cannabis, cocaine, and opiate use: A comprehensive review. *Addict. Sci. Clin. Pract.* **2016**, *11*, 9. [CrossRef]
59. Liao, Y.; Tang, J.; Liu, T.; Chen, X.; Luo, T.; Hao, W. Sleeping problems among Chinese heroin-dependent individuals. *Am. J. Drug Alcohol Abuse* **2011**, *37*, 179–183. [CrossRef]
60. Kay, D.C.; Pickworth, W.B.; Neidert, G.L.; Falcone, D.; Fishman, P.M.; Othmer, E. Opioid effects on computer-derived sleep and EEG parameters in nondependent human addicts. *Sleep* **1979**, *2*, 175–191. [CrossRef]
61. Lewis, S.A.; Oswald, I.; Evans, J.I.; Akindele, M.O.; Tompsett, S.L. Heroin and human sleep. *Electroencephalogr. Clin. Neurophysiol.* **1970**, *28*, 374–381. [CrossRef]
62. Trksak, G.H.; Jensen, J.E.; Plante, D.T.; Penetar, D.M.; Tartarini, W.L.; Maywalt, M.A.; Brendel, M.; Dorsey, C.M.; Renshaw, P.F.; Lukas, S.E. Effects of sleep deprivation on sleep homeostasis and restoration during methadone-maintenance: A ^{31}P MRS brain imaging study. *Drug Alcohol Depend.* **2010**, *106*, 79–91. [CrossRef]
63. de la Iglesia-Larrad, J.I.; Barral, C.; Casado-Espada, N.M.; de Alarcón, R.; Maciá-Casas, A.; Vicente Hernandez, B.; Roncero, C. Benzodiazepine abuse, misuse, dependence, and withdrawal among schizophrenic patients: A review of the literature. *Psychiatry Res.* **2020**, *284*, 112660. [CrossRef] [PubMed]
64. Kaplan, K.A.; McQuaid, J.; Batki, S.L.; Rosenlicht, N. Behavioral treatment of insomnia in early recovery. *J. Addict. Med.* **2014**, *8*, 395–398. [CrossRef] [PubMed]
65. Ruiz, C. Revisión de los diversos métodos de evaluación del trastorno de insomnio (Review of some methods of evaluation for insomnia disorder). *Anales Psicol.* **2007**, *23*, 109–117.
66. Vorspan, F.; Barré, T.; Pariente, A.; Montastruc, F.; Tournier, M. Should the Duration of Treatment Be Limited Using Benzodiazepines? *Presse Med.* **2018**, *47*, 892–898. [CrossRef]
67. Grau-López, L.; Grau-López, L.; Daigre, C.; Palma-Álvarez, R.F.; Rodriguez-Cintas, L.; Ros-Cucurull, E.; Roncero, C. Pharmacological Treatment of Insomnia Symptoms in Individuals with Substance Use Disorders in Spain: A Quasi-Experimental Study. *Subst. Use Misuse* **2018**, *53*, 1267–1274. [CrossRef]

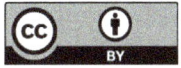

© 2020 by the authors. Licensee MDPI, Basel, Switzerland. This article is an open access article distributed under the terms and conditions of the Creative Commons Attribution (CC BY) license (http://creativecommons.org/licenses/by/4.0/).

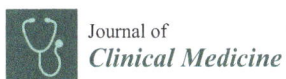

Article

Sleep Quality and Sleep Disturbance Perception in Dual Disorder Patients

Gianina Luca and Lola Peris *

CNP-Centre Neuchâtelois de Psychiatrie, 2074 Marin, Switzerland; gianina.luca@cnp.ch
* Correspondence: lola.peris@cnp.ch

Received: 28 April 2020; Accepted: 25 June 2020; Published: 26 June 2020

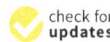

Abstract: Background: Sleep problems are particularly frequent in psychiatric disorders, but their bidirectional intersection is poorly clarified. An especial link between substance use and sleep seems to exist. While dual disorder patients are certainly at higher risk of experiencing sleep problems, very limited research is available today. Methods: Forty-seven dual disorder hospitalized patients were included in this first study. A complete psychiatric evaluation was performed, and sleep habits, patterns and potential disorders were evaluated with specific sleep scales, as well as anxiety. Results: The global prevalence of insomnia symptoms was considerably higher compared with the general population. Different abuse patterns as a function of concurrent psychiatric diagnosis were found, with no significant gender differences. The association between the investigated sleep parameters and any specific substance of abuse was minor. The addict behavior started in more than half of the patients prior to the main psychiatric diagnosis and close to the beginning of sleep problems. Men had a higher prevalence of insomnia symptoms, together with a higher incidence of anxiety. Overall, subjective daytime functioning was not altered as a consequence of poor sleep. Conclusion: Dual disorder patients face significant sleep disturbances, with low sleep quality. The role of sleep in addiction and dual disorders deserves greater research.

Keywords: dual disorders; addiction; sleep; risk factors

1. Introduction

Sleep problems are especially frequent in psychiatric disorders, but their complex bidirectional interactions are still poorly understood and, although several common neurobiological abnormalities may explain why sleep disorders are related to the risk of developing different psychiatric disorders, the causal relationships have not been clearly identified [1,2]. Xue Gao et al. noted the work of Charrier et al., stressing that the single-nucleotide polymorphisms in the core circadian genes are associated with psychiatric disorders [3], and of Akers et al., proposing methods for using sleep as a therapy for psychiatric disorders after evaluating the regulation of sleep and epigenetic modifications of adult neurogenesis and memory consolidation [2,4].

In a large community study with a one-year follow-up interview evaluating sleep disturbances and psychiatric disorders, Ford and Kamerow noted a much higher prevalence of psychiatric disorders in those with sleep complaints, as well as a greater rate of new psychiatric disorders one year later, also among those with sleep complaints [5]. A cross-sectional (six-month) association between sleep disturbances and major depression, anxiety disorders and substance use disorders is reported in this study. Similar findings were described by Breslau et al. in a longitudinal epidemiological study of young adults [6], while Xue Gao et al. suggested the causal role of insomnia in autism spectrum disorder and bipolar disorder [2] and Acker et al. stated the relevance of psychiatric comorbidities in the treatment of patients with obstructive sleep apnea syndrome, focusing their research on depression [7].

The relationship with addiction and dual disorders is probably the strongest example of this interaction. It has long been known that sleep problems are more prevalent among persons with use of or dependence on substances and that those with sleep problems have a higher risk of developing substance use problems than the general population [5,8]. Nevertheless, although evidence links sleep and substance use, little research exists on this topic.

Overall, it is estimated that between 50% and 80% of the treatment-seeking psychiatric population is affected by insomnia. People with substance use disorders (SUD) are at an especially high risk of suffering sleep problems. For example, between 36% and 72% of alcohol-dependent patients treated in addiction facilities report significant sleep problems [9,10].

Sleep problems in SUD may appear as direct effects of the substance or as a result of withdrawal, but pre-existing sleep problems may also provoke the development of addiction [10,11].

In a cross-sectional study utilizing retrospective self-reported sleep disturbance and substance use, Dolsen and Harvey found that a lifetime history of insomnia and hypersomnia was associated with a higher frequency of all substance use at treatment entry and higher rates of cocaine use at 12-month post-treatment assessment, although the characteristics of the study did not allow it to define if sleep disturbances were caused by substance use, if substance use caused sleep disturbances or if other variables could influence these relationships [12].

Most of the drugs of abuse are disruptive to sleep and/or daytime alertness, but such disturbances are not major criteria for SUD in current psychiatric classifications [13]. Cannabis, sedative hypnotics and alcohol may become reinforcers and lead to substance use given their capacity to induce sleep in persons with insomnia. Further, risky patterns of substance use are associated with poor sleep, potentially inducing a risk of future mood or other psychiatric disorders and/or poor levels of functioning [14]. The alerting effects of stimulants are reinforcing for individuals who experience sleepiness, fatigue or have difficulty functioning at a "normal" level. Rotating shift workers and night workers report a disproportionate use of sedative drugs, especially alcohol to improve their sleep and stimulants, and especially caffeine to improve their alertness: this kind of substance use may increase risks of misuse. Similarly, acute rapid eye movement (REM) sleep deprivation by awakening enhances pain sensitivity, according to studies. As opiates suppress REM, their analgesic effect may be reduced. Whether this hypothesized reduction leads to a need for higher doses or to the development of physical dependence is also a critical issue [13].

Abnormal sleep patterns can persist for up to three years in alcohol dependence. However, while it is tempting to attribute these sleep abnormalities to excessive alcohol drinking, sleep problems could precede the development of dependence, or they could be secondary to the development of other medical or psychiatric disorders related to excessive alcohol drinking. Some studies suggest that a slow wave sleep deficiency may be associated with the development of alcohol dependence (it is known that alcohol enhances slow wave sleep with acute use) [13].

It has been hypothesized that continued substance use, difficulty reducing use and relapse may reflect "self-medication" to reverse the excessive sleepiness when abstaining from some substances. Both the objective and subjective measures of sleep after acute abstinence predict the likelihood of relapse during long-term abstinence better than variables such as age, employment, marital status, severity of alcoholism, hepatic enzymes or depression ratings. In cocaine-dependent individuals, total sleep time was positively related to days of abstinence over a six-week study. These data raise the question whether insomnia-focused treatment would have a beneficial effect on substance use treatment. Although the role of sleep/alertness disturbances in SUD is not fully understood, the need for clinical trials that focus on the treatment of sleep complaints in substance use is clearly evident. Sleep disturbance seems to be causally related to alcohol and drug use, either as the precipitant or the consequence. Sleep disturbance may be comorbid (as suggested in the literature), and treatment must be directed at both disorders, independent, or related to a third common factor [13,15].

Insomnia and SUD may share common neurobiological disturbances. Data suggest that insomnia is a disorder of "hyperarousal", which constitutes, in part, HPA-axis dysfunction involving corticotropin releasing hormone (CRF) and norepinephrine (NE). Many theories of addiction hypothesize that stress increases one's vulnerability to drug use. The activation of the brain circuits involved in stress lead to CRF/NE activation, which also activates the dopaminergic brain motivational pathways known to be engaged by drugs of abuse [13]. Alterations in the dopaminergic neurons have long been associated with alcohol and drug use but also with other disorders like post-traumatic sleep disorder and autism. The causal role of mesocorticolimbic dopaminergic activity in sleep and wakefulness has been described by authors like Eban-Rotschild et al. [16].

The orexin system is thought to have a role in the rewarding effects of drugs, in addition to its role in arousal. It has been suggested that orexin is specifically engaged in substance use during elevated motivational states, such as when the effort to obtain the drug is high or when stress exists. Orexin antagonists like suvorexant, which is currently approved for the treatment of insomnia, are being evaluated for the treatment of SUD, as the effect of orexin could be of help in attenuating drug rewards and improving sleep disturbances by preventing the potentiation of reward and arousal [17,18].

To fully identify how the circuits and substrates that regulate sleep and arousal intersect with those that mediate rewards and how they are targeted by drugs should be the "first step" to advance in this field. However, although the neurobiological links between sleep dysfunction and substance use behavior are well accepted, the research is still in its nascent stages. Moreover, how the interaction between sleep and substance use is modulated by genetics, life events, sex and circadian rhythms remains largely unknown [16]. Nevertheless, research is increasingly showing that sleep disturbances experienced early in life may precede and/or predispose an individual to develop SUD, and a growing number of studies support the bidirectional component of the relationship between sleep patterns and substance use [19].

Roncero et al. [20] found that almost 70% of drug-dependent in-patients reported sleep problems prior to admission and that 80% of those patients related such problems to their substance use. Nevertheless, according to Arnedt et al. [8], in clinical settings, there may be a failure to appreciate the importance of sleep, especially in the early stages of recovery from addiction. Untreated sleep problems substantially increase the likelihood of relapse for those addicted to drugs.

Gender and age are the most important demographic variables related to the prevalence of insomnia, with women experiencing a higher rate of insomnia than men and complaints of insomnia increasing with age (although this association seems not to be robust when more severe criteria of insomnia are applied) [21,22]. Medical and psychiatric status influence the frequency of insomnia, which is more frequent among patients with psychiatric disorders. Moreover, very few studies address the question of the interaction between addiction, sleep and sex. One of them, evaluating problematic internet use and risk of sleep disturbances in adolescents, found a greater association in girls [23]. In addition, according to the study of Ogeil et al. [24], women reporting risky alcohol and cannabis use had the highest global Pittsburgh Sleep Quality Index scores, reflecting the poorest sleep quality.

Gender differences in mental disorders are well documented. However, although some studies have detected differences for dual disorders (DD) [25,26], little published research is available to establish clear conclusions. However, prevention, treatment, and prognosis would undoubtedly benefit the individualization of each gender characteristic for DD.

Published studies in this field have mainly referred to psychiatric patients or substance use disorder patients, indicating only marginally the possibility of co-occurring disorders among some of those patients. Evidence suggests that DD are the rule rather than the exception. The interaction between a sleep problem, a substance use disorder and another psychiatric disorder certainly adds more complexity.

Bearing this problem in mind, we decided to develop the first observational study to characterize potential sleep problems in a sample of hospitalized dual disorder patients. Although several studies have focused globally on sleep and SUD, this preliminary cross-sectional study was directly focused on sleep and DD patients, aiming to investigate the frequency and severity of sleep disturbances one month prior to admission for on-demand controlled withdrawal.

2. Materials and Methods

2.1. Sample

Forty-seven patients with dual diagnosis hospitalized in our dual disorders unit (Préfargier Hospital, Marin-Epagnier, Switzerland) were randomly invited to take part in the study after obtaining their informed consent. Four of them (2 men, 2 women) refused to participate. The project was approved by the hospital and was carried out according to the directives of the Swiss Federal Office of Public Health and following the rules of the Declaration of Helsinki.

Patients were admitted electively, at their request, for controlled withdrawal. A tailored treatment plan was discussed with the participants prior to hospitalization. This project included treatment settings, discussion of psychopharmacologic approach, participation in different groups and assessment of personal needs (social services, family or couple therapy, occupational therapy, long term rehabilitation institution projects, etc.).

A complete psychiatric evaluation was performed at admission by the medical team of the unit. Psychiatric diagnoses were established according to the International Classification of Diseases, ICD-10 criteria [27]. None of the patients presented an acute exacerbation of their main psychiatric disorder.

Beside the specific complete psychiatric evaluation, after the resolution of withdrawal symptoms, patients were invited to complete a comprehensive set of self-administered questionnaires (Supplementary Figure S1) evaluating their sleep habits and sleep patterns, as well as specific sleep disorder questionnaires.

The Pittsburgh Sleep Quality Index (PSQI) is a validated, effective, self-administered questionnaire used to evaluate sleep quality over the last 30 days. It has seven domains (regrouped from 19 questions), each rated from 0 to 3 (sleep duration, sleep efficiency, sleep latency, sleep disturbance, daytime dysfunction, frequency of sleep medications and subjective sleep quality), where 3 is the negative extreme. The cut-off score of 5 allows the distinction between healthy controls and persons with poor sleep quality. [28]

The Insomnia Severity Index (ISI) is a 7-item self-report questionnaire assessing perceived insomnia severity over the last month. This questionnaire evaluates the severity of sleep onset, sleep maintenance and early morning awakening problems, as well as the impact of these disturbances on daytime functioning. The total score ranging from 0 to 28 includes four categories: absence of insomnia (0–7), sub-threshold insomnia (8–14), moderate insomnia (15–21) and severe insomnia (22–28) [29].

Regarding PSQI and ISI, patients were asked to consider the month before admission, in order to avoid the bias of sleep disturbances during the withdrawal process.

The Epworth sleepiness scale (ESS) is widely used to assess sleepiness (in the general population and in subjects with sleep disorders). This scale rates the chance of falling asleep in eight different situations. A score higher than 10 is associated with excessive daytime sleepiness [30].

In order to evaluate the presence of an intrinsic sleep disorder as central hypersomnia, obstructive sleep apnea syndrome or restless legs syndrome, the clinical interview focused on related symptoms. The set of questions was derived from the International Classification of Sleep Disorders, third edition [31]. The presence of insomnia was based on actual diagnostic criteria: difficulties initiating or maintaining sleep impacting daytime functioning (fatigue, impaired social, family, occupational or academic performance, daytime sleepiness, etc.) [32] which cannot be explained purely by inadequate opportunity; the sleep disturbance and associated daytime symptoms occur at least three times per week and have been present for at least 3 months.

Furthermore, the potential existence of anxiety was evaluated with the GAD-7 [33], a valid and efficient tool for screening generalized anxiety disorder and assessing its severity in clinical practice and research. Mild, moderate and severe anxiety are established based on the three cut-off scores of 5, 10 or 15 points out of a maximum of 21.

2.2. Sleep Disturbances

The presence of sleep disturbances was considered based on the results obtained in the above-described questionnaires: PSQI > 5 or ISI > 14 or ESS > 10. One patient was previously diagnosed and successfully treated for respiratory disturbances during sleep.

2.3. Other Variables

Data on demographic and functional variables were obtained: ethnicity (Caucasian/other, with Caucasian group as reference) marital status (married, divorced, never married, with "married" group as reference), employment status (employed/unemployed, with "employed" group as reference) and academic achievement.

Less than 9 years of school was considered low academic achievement, normal academic achievement was considered completing high school and high academic achievement meant a bachelor's degree or higher. For the analysis, we used "normal academic achievement" as the reference group.

These data were obtained from admission records and confirmed through the addressed questionnaires.

Patients gave detailed information regarding the primary drug of concern. We also collected data about the patients' comorbid psychiatric and medical conditions, actual medications and duration of the admission.

2.4. Statistical Analysis

Data collected from each patient were completely anonymized. All statistical tests were performed using SPSS 22.0, (IBM SPSS Statistics, Armonk, NY, USA). Gender differences in the distribution of sleep disturbances and sleep quality were tested for significance by using a χ^2-test. Given the small sample size, we split the patients into three groups based on the most commonly reported drugs of concern: cannabis only, alcohol only and multiple psychoactive substances. In our sample, none of the patients declared using stimulants. On the same basis, we created three diagnostic groups to classify co-occurring psychiatric conditions according to the main psychiatric diagnosis identified in our sample: affective disorders, psychotic disorders and personality disorders.

Differences in the demographic and clinical variables between genders were examined by using a Fisher's exact test and a t-test for independent samples. The corresponding χ^2 values, odds ratios and 95% confidence intervals (CI_{95}) are reported. Furthermore, logistic regression was also employed to test binary variables. Initiation insomnia (binary variable, presence of insomnia as reference) was defined as the presence of difficulties falling asleep occurring more than 3 nights/week, when normal sleep conditions are present. Superficial (or fragmented) sleep was defined as the feeling of frequent awakenings or shallow sleep (presence of fragmented sleep as reference). Maintaining insomnia was defined as difficulties in maintaining sleep or early morning awakenings (presence of these symptoms as reference). Beginning of sleep disturbances was classified as before or after the initiation of substance abuse (before as reference).

The categorical variables were analyzed using categorical factor analysis. Principal component analysis for categorical data allowed us to analyze the probable association between categorical data. In the second step, to assess the main factor associated with sleep perception, we separately analyzed the data for men and women through a multivariate regression analysis.

3. Results

3.1. Demographics

Out of the 43 patients (mean age 42.6 ± 10.2 years old), 68% were male and all but one (African, cannabis user) were Caucasians. The demographic data are presented in Table 1.

Table 1. Demographic characteristics of the sample by gender and primary substance of concern. Results are presented as number and percentage (%). Significant χ^2-test results are marked in bold. OR- Odds ratio

	Cannabis Users N (%)			Alcohol Users N (%)			Multiple Substances Users N (%)		
	All	Men	Women	All	Men	Women	All	Men	Women
Marital status - married	3 (7.5%)	1 (3.4%)	2 (15.4%)	9 (22.5%)	7 (25.9%)	2 (15.4%)	6 (15.0%)	5 (18.5%)	1 (7.7%)
Marital status - divorced	2 (5.0%)	2 (6.9%)	0	7 (17.5%)	4 (11.1%)	3 (22.6%)	7 (17.5%)	5 (18.5%)	2 (15.4%)
Marital status - never married	2 (5.0%)	1 (3.4%)	1 (7.7%)	3 (7.5%)	2 (7.4%)	1 (7.7%)	4 (10.0%)	2 (7.4%)	2 (15.4%)
Employment status - employed	3 (6.9%)	2 (6.9%)	1 (7.1%)	11 (25.5%)	10 (34.4%)	1 (7.1%)	7 (16.2%)	6 (20.7%)	1 (7.1%)
Employment status -unemployed	4 (9.3%)	2 (6.9%)	2 (14.3%)	8 (18.6%)	3 (10.3%)	5 (35.7%)	10 (23.2%)	6 (20.6%)	4 (28.5%)
Academic achievement - low	0	0	0	1 (2.3%)	0	1 (7.1%)	6 (13.9%) *	5 (17.2%)	1 (7.1%)
Academic achievement - normal	6 (13.9%)	4 (13.7%)	2 (14.2%)	15 (34.8%)	11 (37.9%)	4 (28.5%)	11 (25.5%)	7 (24.1%)	4 (28.5%)
Academic achievement - high	1 (2.3%)	0	1 (7.1%)	3 (6.9%)	2 (6.9%)	1 (7.1%)	0	0	0

*chi squared 7.45; OR 13.64, *p* = 0.006

Most cannabis and alcohol users had a normal education level, while multiple substances users had a lower education degree. We found no association between alcohol use and the demographic data (see Table 1).

3.2. The Substance of Use and Co-Occurrent Psychiatric Disorders

All included patients used at least one substance of abuse or dependence according to the International Classification of Diseases, ICD-10 criteria. We found different use patterns as a function of co-occurrent psychiatric diagnoses (χ^2 24.495, *p* < 0.001). The preferred substance of use was cannabis for 15.9% of patients, 66.6% with a diagnostic of a psychotic disorder. Alcohol was the substance of use for 43.2% of patients, 63.2% with a co-occurrent affective disorder. Polysubstance users mainly had a personality disorder diagnosis (58.8%). Table 2 presents the distribution of substance of use as a function of co-occurrent psychiatric disorder.

Table 2. Substance abuse by co-occurrent psychiatric disorder. Unadjusted odds ratios and 95% confidence intervals are presented. Significant results are marked in bold.

Primary Drug of Concern	Diagnosis	Substance Use (%)	No Substance Use (%)	Odds Ratio	95% Confidence Interval
Cannabis	Psychotic disorder	57.1	5.5	**22.67**	**2.86–179.18**
	Affective disorder	28.5	58.3	0.29	0.04–1.67
	Personality disorder	14.3	36.1	0.29	0.03–2.72

Table 2. Cont.

Primary Drug of Concern	Diagnosis	Substance Use (%)	No Substance Use (%)	Odds Ratio	95% Confidence Interval
Alcohol	Psychotic disorder	0	25	0.07	0.01–1.38
	Affective disorder	84.2	29.1	12.95	2.84–58.92
	Personality disorder	15.8	45.8	0.22	0.05–0.96
Multiple substances	Psychotic disorder	11.8	15	0.73	0.11–4.52
	Affective disorder	29.4	69.2	0.19	0.04–0.70
	Personality disorder	58.8	15.4	7.86	1.86–33.09

No gender differences were found for the association between the primary substance of concern and psychiatric diagnosis (multivariate regression analysis, Supplementary Table S1)

3.3. Psychiatric Diagnosis and Medication

The mean reported duration since the first main psychiatric diagnosis was 12.4 +/− 3.2 years, with no significant differences between men and women. The mean reported duration of psychoactive substance use was 14 +/− 2.4 years (data from 23 patients only).

In our sample, more men than women had a personality disorder ($p = 0.10$). The anxiety symptoms evaluated by GAD-7 were more intense and more frequent among the men (χ^2-test, $p = 0.04$).

In total, 62.8% of patients had experienced psychotropic treatment before admission, and 37.2% took sleep-inducing medication, which continued during the withdrawal period. The mean duration of the actual admission was 20.4 days.

Half of the patients had had at least one relapse to their substance of use, and 25.6% were hospitalized for decompensation of their main psychiatric disorder in the past two years.

3.4. Sleep Characteristics

Half of the patients declared having sleep difficulties for more than 10 years, with problems implementing coping strategies. The main reported sleep problem was difficulty falling asleep, with cannabis and alcohol users declaring higher sleep onset latency compared with polysubstance users (53.4 ± 5.3 and 51.2 ± 3.2, respectively, versus 40.2 ± 5.3 minutes).

In total, 71.5% of cannabis users and 68.4% of alcohol users declared starting their substance use after the development of insomnia, while for most polysubstance users (64.7%), drug use was not related to the development of sleep disturbances (χ^2-test 5.46, $p = 0.046$).

Most of the patients (69%) declared fragmented or superficial sleep. Persistent insomnia symptoms were present in 63.3% of patients, with a trend toward a higher frequency among patients with depression as their main psychiatric diagnosis ($p = 0.1$).

Men had higher risk for developing initiation insomnia symptoms (Table 3) and this risk increased even more after adjusting for psychiatric disorder and substance of abuse, while women were more exposed to maintaining insomnia symptoms. After adjusting for demographic covariates (education, marital status or employment), these results are no longer significant.

Table 3. Gender effect on insomnia and the onset of sleep complaints.

	OR	95% Confidence Interval	
		Lower	Upper
Initiation insomnia			
Unadjusted model	5.16	1.134	23.494

Table 3. Cont.

	OR	95% Confidence Interval	
		Lower	Upper
Model 1	9.71	1.47	64.08
Model 2	0.00	0	.
Maintaining insomnia	0.23	0.003	0.988
Unadjusted model	0.04	0.001	1.005
Model 1	0.16	0.022	1.201
Model 2	0.00	0	
Superficial sleep or frequent awakenings			
Unadjusted model	0.29	0.059	1.454
Model 1	0.16	0.022	1.201
Model 2	0.00	0	
Onset of sleep disturbance after onset of SUD			
Unadjusted model	2.28	0.548	9.517
Model 1	2.57	0.464	14.268
Model 2	0.00	0	

Logistic regression analysis (female gender as reference). Model 1 is adjusted for substance of use, main psychiatric diagnostic and the presence of anxiety. Model 2 is adjusted for substance of abuse, main psychiatric diagnostic, the presence of anxiety and socio-demographic variables (marital status, employment status, education). OR—odds ratio; SUD—substance use disorder.

Overall, the mean subjective sleep duration was diminished (6.05 ± 0.22 hours) and reported sleep latency increased (48.3 ± 3.2 minutes). Consequently, sleep efficiency was slightly reduced (84.1 ± 9.3%.). The crude unadjusted analysis showed that women declared better sleep quality and a better daytime functioning than men did, with the latter association close to statistical significance (see Table 4 for details), although these differences disappeared after controlling for confounders (substance of use, main psychiatric diagnosis and age) (Supplementary Table S2).

In our sample, 71.5% of cannabis users and 68.4% of alcohol users declared starting the substance use after the development of insomnia, equally associating the use of these substances as to correct their initiation insomnia. After controlling for multiple confounding factors (age, gender and psychotropic medication), this association was no longer statistically significant.

For all patients but two, the Epworth sleepiness scale score was inferior to 10 points (8.4 ± 2.4).

3.5. PSQI Domains

In our sample, the total PSQI score was altered in both genders (mean 9.8 +/− 4.21) with no differences between men and women (t-test, independent samples, p = non significant (ns), with 74% of the patients having a PSQI score higher than 5.

The domain analysis showed no gender differences in any of the measures except for sleep quality and the presence of anxiety (Table 4). Although not statistically significant, we noted a trend for lower subjective sleep duration and more altered daytime functioning in men (Table 4).

Table 4. Gender impact on analyzed variables [1].

	All	Men (n = 29)	Women (n = 14)	p-Value
Age [1]		40.65 (9.78)	45.64 (10.8)	0.158
Epworth [1]		9.10 (4.1)	6.73 (3.2)	0.526

Table 4. *Cont.*

	All	Men (*n* = 29)	Women (*n* = 14)	*p*-Value
Sleep onset latency (min) [1]	48.3 (3.2)	43.77 (21.7)	50.46 (28.37)	0.158
Sleep duration (hours) [1]	6.06 (0.22)	6.01 (1.54)	6.26 (1.75)	0.663
Sleep efficiency (%) [1]	84.1 (9.30)	82.36 (14.01)	86.83 (12.95)	0.702
PSQI-total score [1]	9.84 (4.2)	10.54 (3.85)	8.3 (4.73)	0.209
PSQI domains [2]				
Sleep disturbances - 0	9.30%	2.33%	6.98%	
Sleep disturbances - 1	34.88%	23.26%	11.63%	
Sleep disturbances - 2	41.86%	30.23%	11.63%	
Sleep disturbances - 3	13.95%	11.63%	2.33%	0.244
Sleep onset latency - 0	19.51%	9.76%	9.76%	
Sleep onset latency - 1	31.71%	21.95%	9.76%	
Sleep onset latency - 2	41.46%	31.71%	9.76%	
Sleep onset latency - 3	7.32%	4.88%	2.44%	0.621
Daytime dysfunction - 0	20.93%	11.63%	9.30%	
Daytime dysfunction - 1	32.56%	20.93%	11.63%	
Daytime dysfunction - 2	34.88%	25.58%	9.30%	
Daytime dysfunction - 3	11.63%	9.30%	2.33%	0.067
Sleep efficiency - 0	47.22%	30.56%	16.67%	
Sleep efficiency - 1	16.67%	8.33%	8.33%	
Sleep efficiency - 2	22.22%	22.22%	0	
Sleep efficiency - 3	13.89%	11.11%	2.78%	0.159
Sleep medication - 0	20.93%	13.95%	6.98%	
Sleep medication - 1	18.61%	6.98%	11.63%	
Sleep medication - 2	30.23%	20.93%	9.30%	
Sleep medication - 3	30.23%	25.58%	4.65%	0.169
Sleep quality - 0	25.58%	6.98%	18.61%	
Sleep quality - 1	23.26%	9.30%	13.95%	
Sleep quality - 2	30.23%	18.61%	11.63%	
Sleep quality - 3	20.93%	16.28%	4.65%	0.04
Sleep duration - 0	35.90%	20.51%	15.39%	
Sleep duration - 1	10.26%	5.13%	5.13%	
Sleep duration - 2	35.90%	33.33%	2.56%	
Sleep duration - 3	17.95%	7.69%	10.26%	0.06
Insomnia – present [2]	63.46%	44.19%	18.28%	0.332
Anxiety symptoms – present [2]	88.23%	70.58%	17.64%	**0.019**

Continuous variables were analyzed using t-test for independent samples; [2] categorical variables were tested using chi-squared test. Significant results are marked in bold.

Patients reporting insomnia symptoms had a higher PSQI score, had lower sleep duration (Table 5) and more frequently used sleep medication (OR 3.2, CI_{95} 0.7 to 5.6).

Table 5. Impact of insomnia symptoms on subjective continuous sleep parameters.

Variable	Insomnia Symptoms	Mean Difference	95.00% Confidence Interval		t	df	p-Value
			Lower Limit	Upper Limit			
PSQI score	absent	−4.4	−7.08	−1.72	−3.354	30	**0.002**
	present						
PSQI sleep onset latency (min)	absent	−23.4	−37.5	−9.29	−3.359	38	**0.002**
	present						
PSQI sleep efficiency	absent	2.19	−7.02	11.42	0.485	32	0.631
	present						
PSQI sleep duration (h)	absent	0.91	−0.12	1.95	1.787	37	0.082

Results from a *t*-test for independent samples. Significant *p* values are marked in bold. PSQI: Pittsburgh Sleep Quality Index.

Cannabis users reported more frequently impaired sleep onset latency compared with multiple substance users (OR 1.58, CI$_{95}$ 0.14 to 2.80), while alcohol use was associated more frequently with initiation and maintaining sleep difficulties compared with the same group (OR 2.90, CI$_{95}$ 0.25 to 5.70), even if statistical significance disappeared after correcting for confounding factors.

Interestingly, subjective daytime functioning was, overall, not altered as a consequence of poor sleep (χ^2 4.30, $p = 0.23$).

The principal component analysis for categorical data run on sleep and main psychiatric diagnosis variables retained six dimensions explaining 79.16% of the variability (Supplementary Table S3). The first dimension loaded sleep medication use, presence of sleep disturbances, difficulties falling asleep and low sleep quality. Cannabis use associated with altered sleep quality and increased sleep onset latency. Alcohol and cannabis use loaded on the fourth dimension, together with superficial sleep, and diminished sleep duration and increased sleep latency. Intriguingly, multiple substance use was associated with better sleep efficiency. Initiation and maintaining insomnia loaded with alcohol use.

In a second step, we looked at demographic variables which may impact the results and this analysis retained two major dimensions with a significant eigenvalue (>1) suggesting that men had more severe insomnia symptoms, were more anxious and had a higher total PSQI score (Supplementary Table S3).

4. Discussion

This preliminary study subjectively assessed patient sleep patterns one month prior to on-demand admission for controlled withdrawal in the absence of decompensation of the main psychiatric diagnosis.

The distribution of the primary substance of use related to the psychiatric diagnoses in our sample was consistent with the data previously published in the literature.

The global prevalence of insomnia symptoms was significantly higher compared with the general population and also congruent with the data described previously [31,34]. While insomnia prevalence in the general population is higher among women, the higher prevalence of insomnia symptoms among the men in our sample could be associated with their higher incidence of anxiety. As expected, anxiety is highly associated with sleep initiation difficulties.

As already suggested previously [10], the association between the investigated sleep parameters and the specific substance of use was minor, indicating that disturbed sleep is highly prevalent among patients using a substance, regardless of the type of substance, although those consuming alcohol or cannabis declared increased sleep onset latency.

Interestingly, patients using multiple substances (almost 60% of them with a personality disorder diagnosis) did not associate the use of substances or relapse with sleep difficulties.

It is important to note that none of our patients used stimulants, which may impact sleep in a different manner. While before testing the effect of potential confounding variables, cannabis and alcohol users declared altered sleep, the polysubstance users did not. The lack of the association between sleep disturbances and multiple substance use may be due to the effect of the different substances used masking the presence of sleep initiation or maintaining difficulties.

Even though it is generally assumed that chronic altered sleep quality could potentiate the impact of substance use on cognitive function [35], the absence of daytime functioning alteration by poor sleep in our sample is a puzzling issue worth exploring further. Equally, although the data relating substances of use to an underlying psychiatric diagnosis are globally in line with those already published (likewise for the higher prevalence of sleep problems compared with the general population), the predominance of insomnia symptoms in men together with the higher presence of anxiety in this group warrant further study.

As addictive behavior was engaged in more than half of the patients prior to the onset of their sleep problems, we maintain the bidirectional link between sleep disturbances and the use of psychoactive substances. Due to the cross-sectional nature of this study, it is impossible to elaborate more on this relationship here. The complex factors moderating/mediating this bidirectional relationship deserve further investigation.

Several limiting factors affect the results of this study:

First, the sample size is small compared with the high variability of main psychiatric diagnosis and substance of use. Fourteen patients had a personality disorder diagnosis (four borderline, four antisocial, three avoidant and three dependent), and a small number of patients in each category did not permit a detailed analysis.

Moreover, patients did not fill in questionnaires about the severity of their addiction one month prior to admission, and this factor could have added significant information.

Finally, the retrospective design of the study, based mainly on patient reports, does not allow a more objective evaluation of certain data, especially the chronologic appearance of the disorders (as the diagnostic delay for some psychiatric troubles is well known). A recall bias in collecting subjective data due to the nature of the study and of the administered questionnaires could have impacted the results.

Due to the high variability of the clinical status of patients for a better analysis, future inclusion criteria should be more restrictive, and a bigger sample should be included.

5. Conclusions

Independently of the main psychiatric diagnosis and other parameters, dual disorder patients face significant sleep disturbances with low sleep quality. Implementing detailed sleep evaluations and proposing different strategies to diminish such sleep problems seem to be highly important in the evolution of these patients. Further studies and follow-up studies could offer an answer to the role of sleep in addiction and dual disorders and support the importance of a good quality of sleep, together with stabilizing the main psychiatric disorder, in diminishing the frequency or the severity of the use of psychoactive substances among these patients.

While still in its beginnings, research advances on sleep disturbances in the context of substance use and dual disorders may greatly improve the knowledge of substance use disorders etiology and, therefore, find new methods of prevention and treatment.

Supplementary Materials: The following are available online at http://www.mdpi.com/2077-0383/9/6/2015/s1, Table S1: Multivariate regression analysis, model adjusted for gender and gender interaction; Table S2: Multivariate regression: multivariate analysis estimating diagnostic impact on analyzed parameters—fully adjusted model; Table S3—CATPCA—principal components analysis for categorical data; Figure S1. Time line of data collection.

Author Contributions: Each author has made a substantial contribution to the work, has approved the submitted version and agrees to be personally accountable. All authors have read and agreed to the published version of the manuscript.

Funding: This research received no external funding

Acknowledgments: The authors thank Ornella Passoni et Karolina Jassiak for their contribution in data collection.

Conflicts of Interest: The authors declare no conflict of interest.

References

1. Gregory, A.M.; Sadeh, A. Sleep, emotional and behavioral difficulties in children and adolescents. *Sleep Med. Rev.* **2012**, *16*, 129–136. [CrossRef] [PubMed]
2. Gao, X.; Meng, L.-X.; Ma, K.-L.; Liang, J.; Wang, H.; Gao, Q.; Wang, T. The bidirectional causal relationships of insomnia with five major psychiatric disorders: A Mendelian randomization study. *Eur. Psychiatry* **2019**, *60*, 79–85. [CrossRef]
3. Charrier, A.; Olliac, B.; Roubertoux, P.; Tordjman, S. Clock Genes and Altered Sleep–Wake Rhythms: Their Role in the Development of Psychiatric Disorders. *Int. J. Mol. Sci.* **2017**, *18*, 938. [CrossRef] [PubMed]
4. Akers, K.G.; Cherasse, Y.; Fujita, Y.; Srinivasan, S.; Sakurai, T.; Sakaguchi, M. Concise Review: Regulatory Influence of Sleep and Epigenetics on Adult Hippocampal Neurogenesis and Cognitive and Emotional Function. *STEM CELLS* **2018**, *36*, 969–976. [CrossRef] [PubMed]
5. Ford, D.E. Epidemiologic study of sleep disturbances and psychiatric disorders. An opportunity for prevention? *JAMA* **1989**, *262*, 1479–1484. [CrossRef] [PubMed]
6. Breslau, N.; Roth, T.; Rosenthal, L.; Andreski, P. Sleep disturbance and psychiatric disorders: A longitudinal epidemiological study of young Adults. *Boil. Psychiatry* **1996**, *39*, 411–418. [CrossRef]
7. Acker, J.; Richter, K.; Piehl, A.; Herold, J.; Ficker, J.H.; Niklewski, G. Obstructive sleep apnea (OSA) and clinical depression—prevalence in a sleep center. *Sleep Breath.* **2016**, *21*, 311–318. [CrossRef]
8. Cañellas, F.; de Lecea, L. Relaciones entre el sueño y la adicción [Relationships between sleep and addiction]. *Adicciones* **2012**, *24*, 287–290. [CrossRef]
9. Arnedt, J.T.; Conroy, D.A.; Brower, K.J. Treatment options for sleep disturbances during alcohol recovery. *J. Addict. Dis.* **2007**, *26*, 41–54. [CrossRef]
10. Magnee, E.H.B.; Oene, G.H.D.W.-V.; Wijdeveld, T.A.G.M.; Coenen, A.M.L.; De Jong, C.A.J. Sleep disturbances are associated with reduced health-related quality of life in patients with substance use disorders. *Am. J. Addict.* **2015**, *24*, 515–522. [CrossRef]
11. Crum, R.M.; Chan, Y.-F.; Storr, C.L.; Ford, D.E. Sleep Disturbance and Risk for Alcohol-Related Problems. *Am. J. Psychiatry* **2004**, *161*, 1197–1203. [CrossRef]
12. Dolsen, M.R.; Harvey, A.G. Life-time history of insomnia and hypersomnia symptoms as correlates of alcohol, cocaine and heroin use and relapse among adults seeking substance use treatment in the United States from 1991 to 1994. *Addiction* **2017**, *112*, 1104–1111. [CrossRef]
13. Roehrs, T.; Roth, T. Sleep Disturbance in Substance Use Disorders. *Psychiatr. Clin. North Am.* **2015**, *38*, 793–803. [CrossRef] [PubMed]
14. Roberts, R.E.; Roberts, C.R.; Duong, H.T. Chronic Insomnia and Its Negative Consequences for Health and Functioning of Adolescents: A 12-Month Prospective Study. *J. Adolesc. Heal.* **2007**, *42*, 294–302. [CrossRef] [PubMed]
15. Brower, K.J. Assessment and treatment of insomnia in adult patients with alcohol use disorders. *Alcohol* **2015**, *49*, 417–427. [CrossRef] [PubMed]
16. Eban-Rothschild, A.; Rothschild, G.; Giardino, W.J.; Jones, J.R.; De Lecea, L. VTA dopaminergic neurons regulate ethologically relevant sleep–wake behaviors. *Nat. Neurosci.* **2016**, *19*, 1356–1366. [CrossRef] [PubMed]
17. Valentino, R.J.; Volkow, N. Drugs, sleep, and the addicted brain. *Neuropsychopharmacology* **2019**, *45*, 3–5. [CrossRef]
18. James, M.H.; Mahler, S.V.; Moorman, D.E.; Aston-Jones, G. *A Decade of Orexin/Hypocretin and Addiction: Where Are We Now?* Springer Science and Business Media LLC: Berlin, Germany, 2017; Volume 33, pp. 247–281.
19. Conroy, D.A.; Arnedt, J.T. Sleep and Substance Use Disorders: An Update. *Curr. Psychiatry Rep.* **2014**, *16*, 487. [CrossRef]
20. Roncero, C.; Grau-López, L.; Díaz-Morán, S.; Miquel, L.; Martinez-Luna, N.; Casas, M. Evaluación de las alteraciones del sueño en pacientes drogodependientes hospitalizados. *Medicina Clínica* **2012**, *138*, 332–335. [CrossRef]
21. Mellinger, G.D.; Balter, B.; Uhlenhuth, E.H. Insomnia and its treatment: Prevalence and correlates. *Arch. Gen. Psychiatry* **1985**, *42*, 225–232. [CrossRef]
22. Ohayon, M.; Lemoine, P. Sommeil et principaux indicateurs d'insomnie dans la population générale française. *L'Encéphale* **2004**, *30*, 135–140. [CrossRef]

23. Yang, J.; Guo, Y.; Du, X.; Jiang, Y.; Wang, W.; Xiao, D.; Wang, T.; Lu, C.; Guo, L. Association between Problematic Internet Use and Sleep Disturbance among Adolescents: The Role of the Child's Sex. *Int. J. Environ. Res. Public Heal.* **2018**, *15*, 2682. [CrossRef] [PubMed]
24. Ogeil, R.P.; Phillips, J.G.; Rajaratnam, S.M.; Broadbear, J. Risky drug use and effects on sleep quality and daytime sleepiness. *Hum. Psychopharmacol. Clin. Exp.* **2015**, *30*, 356–363. [CrossRef]
25. Miquel, L.; Roncero, C.; García-García, G.; Barral, C.; Daigre, C.; Grau-López, L.; Bachiller, D.; Casas, M. Gender Differences in Dually Diagnosed Outpatients. *Subst. Abus.* **2013**, *34*, 78–80. [CrossRef]
26. Drapalski, A.L.; Bennett, M.; Bellack, A. Gender differences in substance use, consequences, motivation to change, and treatment seeking in people with serious mental illness. *Subst. Use Misuse* **2010**, *46*, 808–818. [CrossRef]
27. World Health Organisation. International Classification of Diseases 10th edition, Chapter V: Mental and Behavioral Disorders. 2019 Online Version. Available online: https://www.who.int/classifications/icd/en/bluebook.pdf (accessed on 15 January 2020).
28. Buysse, D.J.; Reynolds, C.F.; Monk, T.H.; Berman, S.R.; Kupfer, D.J. The Pittsburgh sleep quality index: A new instrument for psychiatric practice and research. *Psychiatry Res. Neuroimaging* **1989**, *28*, 193–213. [CrossRef]
29. Bastien, C. Validation of the Insomnia Severity Index as an outcome measure for insomnia research. *Sleep Med.* **2001**, *2*, 297–307. [CrossRef]
30. Johns, M.W. A New Method for Measuring Daytime Sleepiness: The Epworth Sleepiness Scale. *Sleep* **1991**, *14*, 540–545. [CrossRef]
31. Sateia, M.J. International Classification of Sleep Disorders-Third Edition. *Chest* **2014**, *146*, 1387–1394. [CrossRef]
32. Riemann, D.; Baglioni, C.; Bassetti, C.L.; Bjorvatn, B.; Groselj, L.D.; Ellis, J.; Espie, C.A.; Garcia-Borreguero, D.; Gjerstad, M.; Gonçalves, M.; et al. European guideline for the diagnosis and treatment of insomnia. *J. Sleep Res.* **2017**, *26*, 675–700. [CrossRef]
33. Spitzer, R.L.; Kroenke, K.; Williams, J.B.W.; Löwe, B. A Brief Measure for Assessing Generalized Anxiety Disorder. *Arch. Intern. Med.* **2006**, *166*, 1092–1097. [CrossRef] [PubMed]
34. Angarita, G.A.; Emadi, N.; Hodges, S.; Morgan, P.T. Sleep abnormalities associated with alcohol, cannabis, cocaine, and opiate use: A comprehensive review. *Addict. Sci. Clin. Pr.* **2016**, *11*, 9. [CrossRef] [PubMed]
35. Kenney, S.; Labrie, J.W.; Hummer, J.F.; Pham, A.T. Global sleep quality as a moderator of alcohol consumption and consequences in college students. *Addict. Behav.* **2012**, *37*, 507–512. [CrossRef] [PubMed]

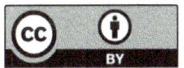

© 2020 by the authors. Licensee MDPI, Basel, Switzerland. This article is an open access article distributed under the terms and conditions of the Creative Commons Attribution (CC BY) license (http://creativecommons.org/licenses/by/4.0/).

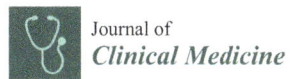 *Journal of* *Clinical Medicine*

Commentary

The Conceptual Framework of Dual Disorders and Its Flaws

Matteo Pacini [1], Angelo G. I. Maremmani [2,3,4] and Icro Maremmani [1,4,5,*]

1. G. De Lisio Institute of Behavioral Sciences, 56100 Pisa, Italy; paciland@virgilio.it
2. Department of Psychiatry, North-Western Tuscany Local Health Unit, Tuscany NHS, Versilia Zone, 55049 Viareggio, Italy; angelo.maremmani@uslnordovest.toscana.it
3. PISA-School of Experimental and Clinical Psychiatry, 56100 Pisa, Italy
4. Association for the Application of Neuroscientific Knowledge to Social Aims (AU-CNS), 55045 Pietrasanta, Lucca, Italy
5. Vincent P. Dole Dual Disorder Unit, 2nd Psychiatric Unit, Santa Chiara University Hospital, University of Pisa, 56100 Pisa, Italy
* Correspondence: icro.maremmani@med.unipi.it; Tel.: +39-050-993045

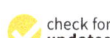

Received: 25 April 2020; Accepted: 1 July 2020; Published: 3 July 2020

Abstract: When psychiatric illness and substance use disorder coexist, the clinical approach to the patient is, unsurprisingly, awkward. This fact is due to a cultural context and, more directly, to the patient's psychiatric condition and addiction behaviors—a situation that does not favor a scientific approach. In dual disorder facilities, several types of professionals work together: counselors, social workers, psychologists, and psychiatrists. Treatment approaches vary from one service to another and even within the same service. It is crucial to provide dual disorder patients with multiple treatments, comprising hospitalization, rehabilitative and residential programs, case management, and counselling. Still, when treating dual disorder (DD) heroin use disorder (HUD) patients, it is advisable to follow a hierarchical algorithm. First, we must deal with addiction: by detoxification, whenever possible. This means starting most patients on anti-craving pharmacological maintenance, though aversion therapy may be appropriate for a few of them. Opiate antagonists may be used with heroin-addicted patients as long as those patients are only mildly ill. In contrast, agonist opioid medications, i.e., buprenorphine and methadone suit moderately and severely ill patients, respectively. Achieving control of mood instability or psychotic episodes is the next step, to be followed by a prevention strategy to counteract residual cravings and dominate mood disorders or psychotic episodes through long-term pharmacological maintenance that is focused on a double target.

Keywords: dual disorders; flaws; conceptual framework

Many different terms have been introduced to define the co-occurrence of a psychiatric disease and a substance use disorder. In the recent past, acronyms such as MICA (Mentally Ill Chemical Abusers or Mentally Ill Chemically Affected), MISA (Mentally Ill Substance Abusers), CAMI (Chemical Abuse and Mental Illness), and SAMI (Substance Abuse and Mental Illness) have been used [1]. Other innovations include 'Dual Diagnosis' and 'Concurrent Disorders' [2–6]. Currently, dual disorder (DD) is the term applied by the World Association on Dual Disorders to people who have an addictive disorder alongside a co-occurring mental one [7].

1. Dead Ends and Start Lines in Dual Disorder

Several studies or reviews have discussed the issue of the disease chronology of dual disorder. In other words, how can primary psychiatric disorders be distinguished from substance-induced transient or persistent disorders with similar symptoms? A DSM-based classification is of little help, since the exclusion of putative substance-induced disorders from a primary psychiatric category resulted in little attention being paid to these secondary disorders. Substance-induced disorders are, in fact, commonly regarded as difficult to handle, resistant to treatment, and are without any standard treatment algorithm. Similarly, it is not exactly clear what benefits can be gained by pressing the issue of whether a cluster of symptoms is substance induced or primary. Although it is true that the disorder may manifest itself later, the opposite hypothesis is true too. It is also important to carefully consider whether a cluster of substance-induced symptoms, like some psychotropic medications, can be contraindicated (as when antidepressants trigger bipolar episodes).

In any case, we continue to believe that this issue is a dead end for the following reasons. First, the assumption that substance-induced disorders are different from spontaneous ones is gratuitous. As far as we know, certain substance-induced psychiatric disorders may just be phenocopies of spontaneous versions of the same biological disorder. Moreover, the time overlap between onset periods may lead to overrating of the effect of a substance on the development of certain psychiatric disorders. These disorders would find a way to emerge, whether after a time interval or else gradually over time, in some cases showing a sharp profile of classic symptoms rather than a substance-filtered clinical picture. Lastly, the diagnosis of a "secondary" disorder does not automatically imply that detachment from the substance will lead to a stable extinction of symptoms. On the other hand, the persistence of symptoms long after detachment from substance use and the accomplishment of detoxification do not necessarily indicate a primary disorder. The emergence of psychiatric symptoms after the end of agonist opioid treatment may indicate a therapeutic effect of that kind of treatment on an independent psychiatric disorder, as in the case of methadone-withdrawal psychoses. These disorders are often hard to recognize during agonist treatment. They may be considered as transient withdrawal-related accidents rather than primary disorders that were initially masked within an illustration of severe chronic intoxication and then disappeared during anti-craving treatment.

Psychiatric disorders are heterogeneous, as they share no common source for all psychiatric symptoms. Instead of splitting a patient population into sharply defined clinical disorders (for instance, affective psychosis and methamphetamine use or panic disorder and alcoholism), most studies prefer to refer to obscure "all-in" categories, such as dual diagnosis, dual disorders, psychiatric comorbidity, and "psychiatric symptoms." Moreover, no distinction is drawn between different substance classes. The result is that we are forced to reason over treatment approaches to methamphetamine addicts with psychotic symptoms who are lumped together with opioid addicts, who have to cope with depression, or alcoholics, who have to contend with social phobia. We agree on the usefulness of a research "field" that resorts to grouping together all such conditions, as long as there is a common ground of clinical and biological knowledge. In general, research projects would achieve more if they were based on clearly defined targets and study populations.

Substance use disorders are heterogeneous, too, since not all clinical symptoms correspond to a chronic relapsing loss of control over use (i.e., addiction). Also, not all cases of poly-use have the same dynamics concerning primary addiction and any concurrent psychiatric disorder(s). In greater detail, we assessed patients with alcohol–heroin poly-use, cocaine–alcohol poly-use, and heroin–cocaine poly-use, comparing them with exclusive users of heroin, alcohol, and again heroin, respectively. In some cases, other minor substances, mostly cannabis and benzodiazepines, were involved too, even if their use had not been the original reason for treatment. Studies have agreed on indicating cocaine abuse as correlated with axis I bipolar disorder, whether it is combined with alcohol or heroin. On the other hand, the heroin–alcohol poly-use pattern is typical of highly cyclothymic subjects, whose data, however, remain below the threshold of clinical diagnosis [8–12]. Depressive disorders are unrelated to either combination. The heroin–alcohol combination often develops because of treatment omission, premature termination, or, simply, undermedication, so that it seems at first glance to be a surrogate or enhanced form of a common opioid-based drug disorder [13,14]. The cyclothymic profile is, in fact, the only profile that discriminates heroin- and alcohol-dependent patients from healthy controls [15,16].

Apart from addiction-centered studies, other authors have indicated stimulant use, possibly coupled with alcohol and cannabis, as peculiar to a bipolar diathesis. These authors proposed the concept of bipolar-stimulant spectrum disorders, going beyond the causal distinction between spontaneous, associated, and induced bipolar disorders [17].

2. Screening and Definition Criteria for Dual Disorder Heroin Addiction

In several studies, no psychiatric category is specified when reporting on the comorbidities of substance abusers; instead, authors refer to comorbid mental disturbance by drawing on syndrome names as labels or naming series of key symptoms. The foremost criterion for the screening of dual disorders should be the deviance of putative diagnosis from the stereotype of transient chronic intoxication, either during substance use or soon after detoxification. Such a stereotype varies according to which substance is accounted for, even if not defined during mixed poly-use phases. Nevertheless, the stereotype of heroin addiction has been reliably defined as the depressive–anxious–hypersensitive–somatic syndrome. This clinical picture runs parallel to acute opioid impairment (susceptibility to withdrawal) and the severity of the addiction. A variant of the same syndrome can be identified as the hypophoric syndrome ("reward deficit" syndrome) [18] following detachment from opiates or agonist treatment subtraction, otherwise known as the late withdrawal syndrome. This latter condition is well known to be an indicator of relapse, sensitive to opiate agonists, and worsened by antagonists. Italian authors have worked to ascertain the exact reasons why the above conditions should not be labeled as dual disorders or at least are not enough to authorize the recognition of an independent mood or anxiety disorder.

On the other hand, psychotic states, as well as substance-related excitement, are quite unlikely during opiate maintenance, even in patients who may be abusing cocaine during methadone maintenance [19].

European data on the prevalence of psychosis in AOT populations show a relatively low rate of schizophrenia or delusional disorder, regardless of the rate of global comorbidity. In the Netherlands, as many as 39% of opioid users in treatment do display psychotic symptoms, out of an 84% overall comorbidity rate, but current (acute) psychosis does not reach the 10% level. A small population Italian study on hospitalized substance abusers (heroin being featured as the primary substance) described the effects of methadone dose increase and the reduction of antipsychotics and mood stabilizers at discharge, under similar conditions for the length of stay in hospital and the kind of index diagnosis at admission [20]. On the whole, the current evidence favors the view that opioid agonist treatments have a therapeutic influence on psychotic states (an influence that is dependent on the doses being used), and that this link may mask the prevalence of psychotic disorders in populations maintained on over-standard doses.

3. Dual Disorder Patients and Treatment System

The medical approach to the dual disorder (DD) patient is inevitably awkward. This fact is due to a cultural context and involves both the patient's psychiatric condition and addiction behaviors. This predicament does not facilitate a scientific approach to psychiatric illness, in general, or, more forcefully, to addictive diseases. On the one hand, depression and worries about effectiveness are unlikely to restrain patients from resorting to medical services. On the other hand, environmental issues interfere with the correct treatment system. Patients are unlikely to know what kind of treatment is provided by which service. Some services, though effective, are only available in some areas, while others are only available if paid for; therefore, those addicts in some parts of a country have difficult issues to face.

When DD patients apply to an outpatient clinic to receive treatment for their addiction, it often happens that acute psychiatric disorders are misdiagnosed for substance-induced ones or, conversely, intoxication or withdrawal symptoms are misinterpreted as psychiatric illness. In the latter case, patients are usually transferred to psychiatric services. Paradoxically, the same happens with psychiatric patients who apply for treatment at psychiatric units, if they are also current substance use disorder (SUD) patients [21]. The frequency and intensity of psychiatric symptoms and substance-induced symptoms usually rise and fall. So, the need to buffer irregular acute variations on a basis comprising a dual disorder may catch the clinician's attention more than the need to control the independent aspects of the case, which will be addictive, psychiatric, and social. The result may be that the national health system becomes an impediment to patients seeking treatment, rather than a manner of offering them adequate health facilities. Currently, a correct approach to DD patients requires not only that attention be dedicated to the specific issues of each patient but also calls for a growing awareness of the continuing discrepancy between the health system, as it is, at present, implemented, and the needs of DD patients.

Several types of operators work together in psychiatric services: counselors, social workers, psychologists, psychiatrists, and others, on a case-by-case basis. Treatment strategies vary between services and within the same service. It is crucial to provide psychiatric patients with integrated treatments, comprising hospitalization, rehabilitative and residential programs, case management, and counseling, to satisfy the needs arising from both acute and chronic conditions. In some cases, psychotropic medications are used to treat psychiatric disorders and SUD at the same time. The frequency of use of nonmedical psychotropics in treating general psychiatric patients is low, whereas DD patients tend to abuse otherwise harmless agents, such as sedative tricyclic antidepressants [22,23] and antipsychotics [24–33]. Problems may, therefore, follow from the incautious prescription of psychotropic medication to addiction-prone patients. So, psychiatrists should extend their knowledge of substance-related medical issues, while physicians treating drug addicts should take the trouble to become knowledgeable about psychiatry, especially the use of psychotropic medications. As in general psychiatry, a variety of therapeutic solutions are available for the treatment of SUD patients. We can list agonist maintenance, therapeutic communities, short- and long-term detoxification programs, and self-help programs, which often utilize divergent basic principles and may be discordant with each other. Some programs require a patient's drug-free condition as indispensable to initiating treatment, whereas becoming drug-free is simply the long-term result of other programs. Methadone or buprenorphine maintenance therapy does not invariably aim at the complete elimination of heroin use. Controlled heroin use may be adequate, when no other programs are successful, as long as methadone maintenance ensures satisfactory personal and social recovery. The coverage of heroin-assisted treatment (HAT) in countries where it is available is modest when compared with other agonist maintenance treatments for heroin use disorder (HUD). Within the European Union, the role of HAT is negligible. A range of therapeutic, prevention, safety, and economic concerns about the possible negative effects of HAT, for patients and the treatment system, are debated in the light of pertinent research evidence [34–39]. None of these concerns are justified. Encouraging effects should predominate on the treatment system and public order. The HAT methodology has good outcomes for previously treatment-resistant HUD patients, besides deserving consideration as a safe, useful element in a comprehensive treatment system for HUD patients and, crucially, a cost-effective therapy [40].

Although the teams working in addiction medicine units comprise counselors, psychologists, psychiatrists, and physicians, other professionals may be involved too, offering a variety of ancillary skills. The integration, according to a biopsychosocial approach, of various professional skills, should be placed at the core of any service directed to combating addiction. Psychotropic medications are currently used to treat overdose and withdrawal symptoms in SUD patients, but some of these medications, especially disulfiram, naltrexone, and methadone, are effective on addiction too. Addiction controlling physicians are often knowledgeable about psychiatric medications, but a prejudice exists that any psychotropic medication is expected to induce dependence. Especially in countries with separate psychiatric and addiction units, many addiction physicians avoid prescribing psychotropic medications, whereas they should be skilled and knowledgeable in resorting to them and being able to choose the right type for specific psychopathological conditions. In this kind of service, unless DD patients are supported with effective treatment for their mental illness, the risk of relapse is destined to remain high.

Alcoholics Anonymous and Narcotics Anonymous—two types of self-help associations—may have much to offer to DD patients. Self-help interventions should not be considered as alternative treatment options but be integrated into a comprehensive treatment. On the other hand, speculative fears and misinformation may spread within self-help groups, if participants never go beyond reporting opinions based on personal experiences. In the United States, specific self-help programs for DD patients have been developed by focusing on the advancement of patients' compliance with psychopharmacological treatment.

DD patients commonly get in touch with their GPs, but they regularly get only minor attention. In Italy, e.g., GPs are likely to deal with DD patients by prescribing generic psychotropics, such as anxiolytics and antidepressants, but not abuse-targeting medications, such as disulfiram and naltrexone, whose use is limited to specialized programs. GPs are the category of physician that is most prone to prescribe benzodiazepines as anxiolytic drugs, although benzodiazepines carry the highest risk of nonmedical use. Generally speaking, GPs are most concerned about the complications of addiction, such as overdosing, withdrawal symptoms, or physical issues, rather than aiming for an intervention that targets the core of the addiction. There are only a few cases in which GPs are involved in the treatment of DD patients [41–44]

4. Case Management of Dual Disorder Patients

The public health system has constantly given patients the responsibility of presenting for treatment as a sign of being motivated to ask for treatment. More recently, the same issue has been introduced with reference to what is called "case management" (CM). Most DD patients are, in fact, reluctant to resort to local addiction units or are unable to benefit from available facilities. CM may be a crucial resource for SUD patients when the aim is to include patients in treatment programs and improve their retention in treatment. CM may also help attenuate the negative results of leaving treatment. Conversely, programs without a CM are more likely to be handicapped by hospitalization episodes and psychopathological crises, while the most complicated cases are unlikely to be successfully resolved. The main aim of CM is to encourage hesitant patients to request treatments and limit the negative impact of treatment breakdowns on the personal history of those patients. DD patients need to be followed up for both their conditions, addictive and psychiatric, by applying strategies formulated to fit the specific details of their condition. Patients as well as physicians should make a contribution to treatment. At present, physicians treat patients, who, in responding, tend to deny the presence or minimize the severity of their condition, often with excessive emphasis. DD patients require a very different method in accepting and complying with the treatment. It is prudent to avoid confrontation with particularly severe patients, such as psychotic ones, because they are unable to comply with the rules of the program until the severity of their condition has shown considerable improvement. Too often, addiction is regarded with a "here and now" attitude by physicians, who also tend to exaggerate the environmental aspects of co-present psychiatric disorders. SUD tends to be considered as symptomatic of previous psychic trauma, rather than having the status of an independent illness. Too often, treatment focuses on the psychotherapeutic resolution of some developmental age problem, in the mistaken supposition that addiction will remit once its background issues have been resolved. So far, the main outcome of this bias has been a perpetuation of the vicious circle of addiction.

Some treatment programs require patients to be drug free as a precondition for entering treatment. In most DD patients (such as people with schizophrenia), a drug-free state should only be considered as a possible long-term outcome of enhanced methadone maintenance. On the other hand, a drug-free condition may be useful for patients with depression or panic disorder, to allow an earlier, correct diagnosis and, later, more adequate treatment. For DD patients, imposing a preliminary drug-free condition to allow entry into treatment actually turns out to be an obstacle [45]. We, therefore, suggest that the concept of a "drug-free state" be redefined as a therapeutic goal to be approached step-by-step in parallel with an adequate treatment program. Homeless patients who dwell in highly drug-polluted environments cannot be expected to reach a drug-free condition after the imposition of a hard-and-fast deadline.

5. Towards a Hierarchical Approach to Dual Disorder Treatment

We consider three types of treatment models, i.e., sequential, parallel, and integrated, and we propose our hierarchical approach.

The sequential model has been the first one to be employed, and, up to the present time, has been the most frequently utilized. According to this model, the psychiatric and the addictive dimensions of the DD are approached in two different stages. Some clinicians reckon that the addiction should always be approached first and that it is possible to treat the comorbid psychiatric syndrome once any nonmedical use has ceased. Others claim that specific treatments for the psychiatric part of DD may be feasible even when there is the ongoing use of a substance before any specific intervention is taken to end addiction. Another view is that the decision on treatment priority should consider the severity of each condition, with precedence being given to the condition most urgently calling for treatment. For example, we could consider the case of a DD depressed HUD patient requesting treatment at a psychiatric clinic when still suffering from depression, while also participating in a specific program to cure his recurrent alcohol binges.

In the parallel model, the patient is enrolled in two programs simultaneously, the first treating the psychiatric part and the second focusing on addiction. A twelve-step program, may, for instance, be associated with psychiatric treatment under the supervision of mental health professionals. As with the sequential model, this model too consists of a combination of already ongoing programs. Psychiatrists deal with the psychiatric illness, while addiction physicians manage the addiction-related problems. The integrated model combines psychiatric and addiction treatments in a single program, which has been specifically tailored to meet the needs of DD patients. Theoretically, two distinct categories of physicians and skills should be involved, together with a twofold CM approach. This would allow patients to avoid being overwhelmed by the double danger of psychiatric and addictive relapses. Each of these treatment models has its pros and cons. Requirements for treatment adequacy vary with different states of comorbidity, symptom severity, and global functional impairment. The sequential and parallel models may best fit severely addicted patients who also suffer from a minor psychiatric disease. The main negative aspect of these approaches is that patients may receive contradictory information in the two different settings. By contrast, in our opinion, when a CM facility is available and is expressed through a single operator possessing the two sets of skills, which are appropriate to that specific setting, patients would get the full benefits of a binary, two-edged treatment approach [46].

The integrated model is an advanced one. Criteria have even been proposed to determine what constitutes an integrated treatment [47], with preliminary meta-analyses attesting to its efficacy beyond nonintegrated treatments [48].

In our opinion, when treating DD/HUD patients, it is advisable to follow a hierarchical algorithm [49]. According to our clinical experience, the addiction dimension should be dealt with first, by detoxifying patients, and, certainly, by starting most patients on anti-craving agonist maintenance. It should, in any event, be borne in mind that aversion therapy (e.g., disulfiram) may produce a good outcome for a few patients [50]. Opiate antagonists may be administered to HUD patients as long as those patients are only mildly ill, whereas agonist medications, i.e., buprenorphine and methadone suit moderately and severely ill patients, respectively [51,52]. Achieving control of mood instability or psychotic episodes is the next step. It should, eventually, be followed by a preventive strategy to counter residual cravings and breakthrough episodes of mood disorders or psychotic episodes by using long-term pharmacological maintenance with a double target [53,54]. Relapse prevention must never be understood as complete extinction, but as a trend towards a lower grade of severity, a reduction in frequency, while successfully delaying the possible occurrence of a relapse [55,56]. HUD patients should be considered as a population in which it is possible to register and study the effects of chronic opioid injury and its consequent opioid dysfunctions. The predated body of pharmacological knowledge about the psychiatric properties of methadone and buprenorphine seems to corroborate what emerged from the description of agonist opiate-treated DD/HUD patients by our research group [53,57–62]. The toxic properties of fast-acting opiates and the therapeutic properties of slow-acting ones prove to be crucial issues in HUD patients, whether they do or do not have DD. Methadone and buprenorphine should be recognized as psychoactive medications, with useful properties in the treatment of opiate addiction, having a wider therapeutic potential when heroin addiction is combined with a psychiatric disorder [20,49,57,59,61,63–73].

6. Conclusions

To sum up, dual disorders may be present in cases of intense affective discomfort, especially when patients are free from current intoxication or are emerging after a long period of well-being after discharge from opiate agonist treatment. In all other cases, an addiction-related profile should be considered first—a profile that is likely to be improved by opiate agonist initiation, dose increase, or reintroduction. Psychotic symptoms are more likely to indicate a dual disorder as being responsible for psychosis, except in situations of enforced acute withdrawal or acute psychotomimetic intoxication [74].

The intermingling between substance abuse and psychiatric risk disposition, or primary milder disorders, may lead to full-blown syndromes which would not have developed spontaneously, but do so because of exposure to at least one substance. In such cases, it is not always possible to ascertain the course of the associated disorder, especially when anti-craving therapies are used, which may have a dual effect. Otherwise, the course of the disorder in the absence of relapse will help to bring clarification. The latest clinical configuration should be accounted for the symptoms. For instance, a bipolar type 2 disorder ranking up to type 1 after substance abuse should be rated as bipolar 1. In any case, the course of the condition is expected to be more favorable in a substance-free condition [75].

Author Contributions: M.P., A.G.I.M. and I.M. contributed equally to the manuscript. All authors have read and agreed to the published version of the manuscript.

Funding: This paper received no external funding.

Conflicts of Interest: The authors declare no conflict of interest in writing this article.

References

1. Ries, R.K. *Assessment and Treatment of Patients with Coexisting Mental Illness and Alcohol and Other Drug Abuse. Treatment Improvement Protocol (TIP) Series 9*; Center for Substance Abuse Treatment: Rockville, MD, USA, 1994.
2. Buckley, P.F. Prevalence and consequences of the dual diagnosis of substance abuse and severe mental illness. *J. Clin. Psychiatry* **2006**, *67*, 5–9. [CrossRef]
3. Buckley, P.F.; Brown, E.S. Prevalence and consequences of dual diagnosis. *J. Clin. Psychiatry* **2006**, *67*, e01. [CrossRef]
4. Mueser, K.T.; Drake, R.E.; Wallach, M.A. Dual diagnosis: A review of etiological theories. *Addict. Behav.* **1998**, *23*, 717–734. [CrossRef]
5. Lehman, A.F.; Myers, P.; Corty, E.; Thompson, J.W. Prevalence and patterns of 'dual diagnosis' among psychiatric impatients. *Compr. Psychiatry* **1994**, *35*, 106–112. [CrossRef]
6. Baigent, M. Managing patients with dual diagnosis in psychiatric practice. *Curr. Opin. Psychiatry* **2012**, *25*, 201–205. [CrossRef] [PubMed]
7. Szerman, N.; Martinez-Raga, J.; Baler, R.; Roncero, C.; Vega, P.; Basurte, I.; Grau-Lopez, L.; Torrens, M.; Casas, M.; Franco, C.; et al. Joint Statement on Dual Disorders: Addictions and Other Mental Disorders. *Salud Ment.* **2017**, *40*, 245–247. [CrossRef]
8. Maremmani, I.; Pacini, M.; Perugi, G.; Deltito, J.; Akiskal, H. Cocaine abuse and the bipolar spectrum in 1090 heroin addicts: Clinical observations and a proposed pathophysiologic model. *J. Affect. Disord.* **2008**, *106*, 55–61. [CrossRef] [PubMed]
9. Pacini, M.; Maremmani, I.; Vitali, M.; Romeo, M.; Santini, P.; Vermeil, V.; Ceccanti, M. Cocaine Abuse in 448 Alcoholics: Evidence for a Bipolar Connection. *Addict. Disord. Treat.* **2010**, *9*, 164–171. [CrossRef]
10. Vitali, M.; Pacini, M.; Maremmani, I.; Romeo, M.; Ceccanti, M. Pattern of cocaine consumption in a sample of italian alcoholics. *Int. Clin. Psychopharmacol* **2011**, *26*, e98. [CrossRef]

11. Maremmani, A.G.I.; Pacini, M.; Bacciardi, S.; Ceccanti, M.; Maremmani, I. Current use of cannabis and past use of heroin as predictors of alcohol and concomitant cocaine use disorder. *Alcologia* **2015**, *22*, 36–40.
12. Maremmani, A.G.I.; Pacini, M.; Pani, P.P.; Ceccanti, M.; Bacciardi, S.; Akiskal, H.S.; Maremmani, I. Possible trajectories of addictions: The role of bipolar spectrum. *Heroin Addict. Relat. Clin. Probl.* **2016**, *18*, 23–32.
13. Maremmani, I.; Shinderman, M.S. Alcohol, benzodiazepines and other drugs use in heroin addicts treated with methadone. Polyabuse or undermedication? *Heroin Addict. Relat. Clin. Probl.* **1999**, *1*, 7–13.
14. Pacini, M.; Maremmani, A.G.I.; Ceccanti, M.; Maremmani, I. Former heroin-dependent alcohol use disorder patients. Prevalence, addiction history and clinical features. *Alcohol. Alcohol.* **2015**, *50*, 451–457. [CrossRef] [PubMed]
15. Pacini, M.; Maremmani, I.; Vitali, M.; Santini, P.; Romeo, M.; Ceccanti, M. Affective temperaments in alcoholic patients. *Alcohol* **2009**, *43*, 397–404. [CrossRef] [PubMed]
16. Maremmani, I.; Pacini, M.; Popovic, D.; Romano, A.; Maremmani, A.G.; Perugi, G.; Deltito, J.; Akiskal, K.; Akiskal, H. Affective temperaments in heroin addiction. *J. Affect. Disord.* **2009**, *117*, 186–192. [CrossRef]
17. Camacho, A.; Akiskal, H.S. Proposal for a bipolar-stimulant spectrum: Temperament, diagnostic validation and therapeutic outcomes with mood stabilizers. *J. Affect. Disord.* **2005**, *85*, 217–230. [CrossRef]
18. Martin, W.R.; Jasinski, D.R. Physiological parameters of morphine dependence in man, early abstinence, protracted abstinence. *J. Psychiatr. Res.* **1969**, *7*, 9–17. [CrossRef]
19. Maremmani, I.; Pani, P.P.; Mellini, A.; Pacini, M.; Marini, G.; Lovrecic, M.; Perugi, G.; Shinderman, M. Alcohol and cocaine use and abuse among opioid addicts engaged in a methadone maintenance treatment program. *J. Addict. Dis.* **2007**, *26*, 61–70. [CrossRef] [PubMed]
20. Pacini, M.; Maremmani, I. Methadone reduces the need for antipsychotic and antimanic agents in heroin addicts hospitalized for manic and/or acute psychotic episodes. *Heroin Addict. Relat. Clin. Probl.* **2005**, *7*, 43–48.
21. Lovrecic, M.; Lovrecic, B.; Dernovsek, M.Z.; Tavcar, R.; Maremmani, I. Unreported double frequency of heroin addicts visiting psychiatric services and addiction treatment services. *Heroin Addict. Relat. Clin. Probl.* **2004**, *6*, 27–32.
22. Haddad, P. Do antidepressants have any potential to cause addiction? *J. Psychopharmacol.* **1999**, *13*, 300–307. [CrossRef] [PubMed]
23. Haddad, P.; Anderson, I. Antidepressants aren't addictive: Clinicians have depended on them for years. *J. Psychopharmacol.* **1999**, *13*, 291–292. [CrossRef] [PubMed]
24. Hanley, M.J.; Kenna, G.A. Quetiapine: Treatment for substance abuse and drug of abuse. *Am. J. Health Syst. Pharm.* **2008**, *65*, 611–618. [CrossRef] [PubMed]
25. Morin, A.K. Possible intranasal quetiapine misuse. *Am. J. Health Syst. Pharm.* **2007**, *64*, 723–725. [CrossRef]
26. Hussain, M.Z.; Waheed, W.; Hussain, S. Intravenous quetiapine abuse. *Am. J. Psychiatry* **2005**, *162*, 1755–1756. [CrossRef]
27. Murphy, D.; Bailey, K.; Stone, M.; Wirshing, W.C. Addictive potential of quetiapine. *Am. J. Psychiatry* **2008**, *165*, 918. [CrossRef]
28. Pierre, J.M.; Shnayder, I.; Wirshing, D.A.; Wirshing, W.C. Intranasal quetiapine abuse. *Am. J. Psychiatry* **2004**, *161*, 1718. [CrossRef]
29. Pacini, M.; Santucci, B.; Maremmani, I. Requests for quetiapine from jailed substance abusers: Are they a form of abuse or self-medication in response to long-term opioid dysphoria? *Heroin Addict. Relat. Clin. Probl.* **2014**, *16*, 35–40.
30. Paparrigopoulos, T.; Karaiskos, D.; Liappas, J. Quetiapine: Another drug with potential for misuse? A case report. *J. Clin. Psychiatry* **2008**, *69*, 162–163. [CrossRef]
31. McLarnon, M.E.; Fulton, H.G.; MacIsaac, C.; Barrett, S.P. Characteristics of quetiapine misuse among clients of a community-based methadone maintenance program. *J. Clin. Psychopharmacol.* **2012**, *32*, 721–723. [CrossRef]
32. Galyuk, T.M.; de Backer, G.; de Jong, C.A.; Beers, E.; Loonen, A.J. [Abuse of quetiapine. Two addicted patients with borderline personality disorder]. *Ned. Tijdschr. Geneeskd.* **2009**, *153*, 674–676. [PubMed]
33. Reeves, R.R.; Brister, J.C. Additional evidence of the abuse potential of quetiapine. *South Med. J.* **2007**, *100*, 834–836. [CrossRef]
34. Bammer, G.; Dobler-Mikola, A.; Fleming, P.M.; Strang, J.; Uchtenhagen, A. The heroin prescribing debate: Integrating science and politics. *Science* **1999**, *284*, 1277–1278. [CrossRef] [PubMed]

35. Rehm, J.; Gschwend, P.; Steffen, T.; Gutzwiller, F.; Dobler-Mikola, A.; Uchtenhagen, A. Feasibility, safety, and efficacy of injectable heroin prescription for refractory opioid addicts: A follow-up study. *Lancet* **2001**, *358*, 1417–1423. [CrossRef]
36. Fischer, B.; Rehm, J.; Kirst, M.; Casas, M.; Hall, W.; Krausz, M.; Metrebian, N.; Reggers, J.; Uchtenhagen, A.; van den Brink, W.; et al. Heroin-assisted treatment as a response to the public health problem of opiate dependence. *Eur. J. Public Health* **2002**, *12*, 228–234. [CrossRef] [PubMed]
37. Guttinger, F.; Gschwend, P.; Schulte, B.; Rehm, J.; Uchtenhagen, A. Evaluating long-term effects of heroin-assisted treatment: The results of a 6-year follow-up. *Eur. Addict. Res.* **2003**, *9*, 73–79. [CrossRef] [PubMed]
38. Uchtenhagen, A.A. Heroin maintenance treatment: From idea to research to practice. *Drug Alcohol Rev.* **2011**, *30*, 130–137. [CrossRef]
39. Strang, J.; Groshkova, T.; Uchtenhagen, A.; van den Brink, W.; Haasen, C.; Schechter, M.T.; Lintzeris, N.; Bell, J.; Pirona, A.; Oviedo-Joekes, E.; et al. Heroin on trial: Systematic review and meta-analysis of randomised trials of diamorphine-prescribing as treatment for refractory heroin addictiondagger. *Br. J. Psychiatry* **2015**, *207*, 5–14. [CrossRef]
40. Uchtenhagen, A. The role and function of heroin-assisted treatment at the treatment system level. *Heroin Addict. Relat. Clin. Probl.* **2017**, *19*, 17–24.
41. Maremmani, I.; Barra, M.; Bignamini, E.; Consoli, A.; Dell'Aera, S.; Deruvo, G.; Fantini, F.; Fasoli, M.G.; Gatti, R.; Gessa, G.L.; et al. Clinical foundations for the use of methadone. Italian Consensus Panel on Methadone Treatment. *Heroin Addict. Relat. Clin. Probl.* **2002**, *4*, 19–31.
42. Michelazzi, A.; Vecchiet, F.; Cimolino, T. General Practitioners and Heroin Addiction. Chronicle of a Medical Practice. *Heroin Addict. Relat. Clin. Probl.* **1999**, *1*, 39–42.
43. Michelazzi, A.; Vecchiet, F.; Leprini, R.; Popovic, D.; Deltito, J.; Maremmani, I. GPs' office based Metadone Maintenance Treatment in Trieste, Italy.Therapeutic efficacy and predictors of clinical response. *Heroin Addict. Relat. Clin. Probl.* **2008**, *10*, 27–38.
44. Michelazzi, A.; Vecchiet, F.; Maremmani, I. Clinical Foundation for the Use of Methadone in General Practitioner's Office. Italy as Case Study. In *The Principles and Practice of Methadone Treatment*; Maremmani, I., Ed.; Pacini Editore Medicina: Pisa, Italy, 2009; pp. 217–226.
45. Pacini, M.; Maremmani, I. Malleus maleficarum. the superstition of psychosocially centred intervention in addictive diseases. Heroin Addiction as case study. *Heroin Addict. Relat. Clin. Probl.* **2013**, *15*, 9–18.
46. Hoelscher, J.K.; Sprick, W. Integrating home care into a community healthcare system: One agency's experience. *Home Healthc. Nurse Manag.* **1999**, *3*, 11–17. [PubMed]
47. Mueser, K.T.; Noordsy, D.L.; Drake, R.E.; Fox, L. *Integrated Treatment for Dual Disorders: A Guide to Effective Practice*; Guilford Press: New York, NY, USA, 2003.
48. Karapareddy, V. A Review of Integrated Care for Concurrent Disorders: Cost Effectiveness and Clinical Outcomes. *J. Dual Diagn.* **2019**, *15*, 56–66. [CrossRef] [PubMed]
49. Maremmani, I.; Perugi, G.; Pacini, M.; Akiskal, H.S. Toward a unitary perspective on the bipolar spectrum and substance abuse: Opiate addiction as a paradigm. *J. Affect. Disord.* **2006**, *93*, 1–12. [CrossRef] [PubMed]
50. Fuller, R.K.; Gordis, E. Does disulfiram have a role in alcoholism treatment today? *Addiction* **2004**, *99*, 21–24. [CrossRef]
51. Dematteis, M.; Auriacombe, M.; D'Agnone, O.; Somaini, L.; Szerman, N.; Littlewood, R.; Alam, F.; Alho, H.; Benyamina, A.; Bobes, J.; et al. Recommendations for buprenorphine and methadone therapy in opioid use disorder: A European consensus. *Expert Opin. Pharmacother.* **2017**, *18*, 1987–1999. [CrossRef]
52. Maremmani, I.; Gerra, G. Buprenorphine-based regimens and methadone for the medical management of opioid dependence: Selecting the appropriate drug for treatment. *Am. J. Addict.* **2010**, *19*, 557–568. [CrossRef]
53. Maremmani, A.G.I.; Rovai, L.; Bacciardi, S.; Rugani, F.; Pacini, M.; Pani, P.P.; Dell'Osso, L.; Akiskal, H.S.; Maremmani, I. The long-term outcomes of heroin dependent-treatment-resistant patients with bipolar 1 comorbidity after admission to enhanced methadone maintenance. *J. Affect. Disord.* **2013**, *151*, 582–589. [CrossRef]
54. Maremmani, A.G.I.; Pallucchini, A.; Rovai, L.; Bacciardi, S.; Spera, V.; Maiello, M.; Perugi, G.; Maremmani, I. The long-term outcome of patients with heroin use disorder/dual disorder (chronic psychosis) after admission to enhanced methadone maintenance. *Ann. Gen. Psychiatry* **2018**, *17*, 14. [CrossRef] [PubMed]

55. Bizzarri, I.V.; Casetti, V.; Sanna, L.; Maremmani, A.G.I.; Rovai, L.; Bacciardi, S.; Piacentino, D.; Conca, A.; Maremmani, I. Agonist Opioid Treatment as historical comprehensive treatment ('Dole & Nyswander' methodology) is associated with better toxicology outcome than Harm Reduction Treatment. *Ann. Gen. Psychiatry* **2016**, *1*, 5–34.
56. Maremmani, I.; Pacini, M.; Lubrano, S.; Giuntoli, G.; Lovrecic, M. Harm reduction and specific treatments for heroin addiction. Different approaches or levels of intervention?. An illness-centred perspective. *Heroin Addict. Relat. Clin. Probl.* **2002**, *4*, 5–11.
57. Maremmani, I.; Zolesi, O.; Agueci, T.; Castrogiovanni, P. Methadone doses and psychopathological symptoms during methadone maintenance. *J. Psychoact. Drugs* **1993**, *25*, 253–256. [CrossRef]
58. Maremmani, A.G.; Rovai, L.; Rugani, F.; Bacciardi, S.; Dell'Osso, L.; Maremmani, I. Substance abuse and psychosis. The strange case of opioids. *Eur. Rev. Med. Pharmacol. Sci.* **2014**, *18*, 287–302. [PubMed]
59. Bizzarri, J.V.; Conca, A.; Maremmani, I. Does a buprenorphine augmentation control manic symptoms in bipolar disorder with a past history of heroin addiction? A case report. *Heroin Addict. Relat. Clin. Probl.* **2014**, *16*, 49–54.
60. Maremmani, I.; Canoniero, S.; Pacini, M. Methadone dose and retention in treatment of heroin addicts with Bipolar I Disorder comorbidity. Preliminary Results. *Heroin Addict. Relat. Clin. Probl.* **2000**, *2*, 39–46.
61. Maremmani, I.; Zolesi, O.; Aglietti, M.; Marini, G.; Tagliamonte, A.; Shinderman, M.; Maxwell, S. Methadone dose and retention during treatment of heroin addicts with Axis I psychiatric comorbidity. *J. Addict. Dis.* **2000**, *19*, 29–41. [CrossRef] [PubMed]
62. Maremmani, I.; Pacini, M.; Lubrano, S.; Perugi, G.; Tagliamonte, A.; Pani, P.P.; Gerra, G.; Shinderman, M. Long-term outcomes of treatment-resistant heroin addicts with and without DSM-IV axis I psychiatric comorbidity (dual diagnosis). *Eur. Addict. Res.* **2008**, *14*, 134–142. [CrossRef] [PubMed]
63. Maremmani, I. When a New Drug Promotes the Integration of Treatment Modalities: Suboxone and Harm Reduction. *Heroin Addict. Relat. Clin. Probl.* **2008**, *10*, 5–12.
64. Maremmani, A.G.I. Is opioid agonist treatment the only way to treat the psychopathology of heroin addicts? [Letter]. *Heroin Addict. Relat. Clin. Probl.* **2013**, *15*, 57–60.
65. Maremmani, A.G.I.; Pani, P.P.; Rovai, L.; Bacciardi, S.; Rugani, F.; Dell'Osso, L.; Pacini, M.; Maremmani, I. The effects of agonist opioids on the psychopathology of opioid dependence. *Heroin Addict. Relat. Clin. Probl.* **2013**, *15*, 47–56.
66. Maremmani, I.; Pacini, M.; Lovrecic, M.; Lubrano, S.; Perugi, G. Maintenance Therapy with opioid agonist for heroin addicted patients. Usefulness in the treatment of comorbid psychiatric diseases. In *Maintenance Treatment of Heroin Addiction. Evidence at the Crossroads*; Waal, H., Haga, E., Eds.; Cappelen Akademisk Forlag: Oslo, Norway, 2003; pp. 221–233.
67. Pacini, M.; Maremmani, I. What have we learned from the Agonist Opioid Treatment of dual disorder heroin addicts? *Addict. Disord. Treat.* **2017**, *16*, 164–174. [CrossRef]
68. Maremmani, I.; Pacini, M.; Lubrano, S.; Canoniero, S.; Lovrecic, M.; Perugi, G. Clinical Foundation for the Use of Methadone in Dual Diagnosis Patients. In *The Principles and Practice of Methadone Treatment*; Maremmani, I., Ed.; Pacini Editore Medicina: Pisa, Italy, 2009; pp. 153–180.
69. Maremmani, I.; Zolesi, O.; Castrogiovanni, P. Psychosocial and psychopathological features as predictors of response to long term and high dosages methadone treatment. In *Drug Addiction & AIDS*; Loimer, N., Schmid, R., Springer, A., Eds.; Springer: Wien, Austria, 1991; pp. 230–237.
70. Pani, P.P.; Maremmani, I.; Pacini, M.; Lamanna, F.; Maremmani, A.G.; Dell'osso, L. Effect of psychiatric severity on the outcome of methadone maintenance treatment. *Eur. Addict. Res.* **2011**, *17*, 80–89. [CrossRef] [PubMed]
71. Maremmani, A.G.; Rovai, L.; Pani, P.P.; Pacini, M.; Lamanna, F.; Rugani, F.; Schiavi, E.; Dell'osso, L.; Maremmani, I. Do methadone and buprenorphine have the same impact on psychopathological symptoms of heroin addicts? *Ann. Gen. Psychiatry* **2011**, *10*, 17. [CrossRef] [PubMed]
72. Maremmani, I.; Pacini, M.; Pani, P.P. Effectiveness of buprenorphine in double diagnosed patients. Buprenorphine as psychotropic drug. *Heroin Addict. Relat. Clin. Probl.* **2006**, *8*, 31–48.
73. Maremmani, I.; Rolland, B.; Somaini, L.; Roncero, C.; Reimer, J.; Wright, N.; Littlewood, R.; Krajci, P.; Alho, H.; D'Agnone, O.; et al. Buprenorphine dosing choices in specific populations: Review of expert opinion. *Expert Opin. Pharm.* **2016**, *17*, 1727–1731. [CrossRef]

74. Maremmani, I.; Pacini, M.; Pani, P.P.; Perugi, G.; Deltito, J.; Akiskal, H. The mental status of 1090 heroin addicts at entry into treatment: Should depression be considered a 'dual diagnosis'? *Ann. Gen. Psychiatry* **2007**, *6*, 31. [CrossRef]
75. Akiskal, H.S.; Pinto, O. The evolving bipolar spectrum. Prototypes I, II, III, and IV. *Psychiatr. Clin. N. Am.* **1999**, *22*, 517–534. [CrossRef]

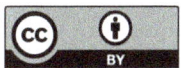

© 2020 by the authors. Licensee MDPI, Basel, Switzerland. This article is an open access article distributed under the terms and conditions of the Creative Commons Attribution (CC BY) license (http://creativecommons.org/licenses/by/4.0/).

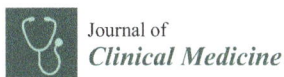

Review

Concurrent Disorder Management Guidelines. Systematic Review

Syune Hakobyan [1,*], Sara Vazirian [1], Stephen Lee-Cheong [2], Michael Krausz [1], William G. Honer [1] and Christian G. Schutz [1]

1. Department of Psychiatry, The University of British Columbia, Vancouver, BC V6T 1Z4, Canada; Sara.Vazirian@alumni.ubc.ca (S.V.); Michael.Krausz@ubc.ca (M.K.); William.Honer@ubc.ca (W.G.H.); Christian.Schutz@ubc.ca (C.G.S.)
2. Department of Public Health, King's College London, London WC2R 2LS, UK; stephenleecheong@gmail.com
* Correspondence: Syune.Hakobyan@alumni.ubc.ca; Tel.: +1-604-562-7991

Received: 29 May 2020; Accepted: 22 July 2020; Published: 28 July 2020

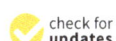

Abstract: Concurrent disorder refers to a diverse set of combinations of substance use disorders and mental disorders simultaneously in need of treatment. Concurrent disorders are underdiagnosed, undertreated, and more complex to manage, practicing the best recommendations can support better outcomes. The purpose of this work is to systematically assess the quality of the current concurrent disorders' clinical recommendation management guidelines. Literature searches were performed by two independent authors in electronic databases, web, and gray literature. The inclusion criteria were English language clinical management guidelines for adult concurrent disorders between 2000 and 2020. The initial search resulted in 8841 hits. A total of 24 guidelines were identified and assessed with the standardized guidelines assessment tool: AGREE II (Appraisal of Guidelines for Research and Evaluation). Most guidelines had acceptable standards, however, only the NICE guidelines had all detailed information on all AGREE II Domains. Guidelines generally supported combinations of treatments for individual disorders with a very small evidence base for concurrent disorders, and they provided little recommendation for further structuring of the field, such as level of complexity or staging, or evaluating different models of treatment integration.

Keywords: concurrent disorder; co-occurring disorder; dual diagnosis; dual pathology; addiction comorbidity; comorbid substance abuse; comorbid illicit use; comorbid addiction; comorbid mental illness; coexisting mental illness

---

1. Introduction

Concurrent disorder (also called dual diagnosis, co-occurring disorder, comorbidity) refers to a specific form of multimorbidity within the area of mental health, where at least one substance use disorder and at least one non-substance-bound mental disorder is simultaneously in need of treatment. The World Health Organization (WHO) defined dual diagnosis as the co-occurrence of a psychoactive substance use disorder and another psychiatric disorder in the same individual [1]. The European Monitoring Centre for Drugs and Drug Addiction (EMCDDA) defined comorbidity/dual diagnosis as the temporal coexistence of two or more psychiatric disorders as defined by the International Classification of Diseases, one of which is problematic substance use. To describe the co-occurring mental health and substance use disorders, other terms have been used as well. The Canadian accepted term is "concurrent disorder" [2]. The US-American accepted term is "co-occurring disorders" [3]. The term "comorbidity" is used in Australia; however, recently more descriptive terms have been used: "coexisting mental health and substance use disorders" or "coinciding mental illness and substance abuse". The term "coexisting problems" is used in New Zealand. "Chemically affected

Mental Illness" (CAMI), "Mental Illness Chemically Affected" (MICA), "Substance Affected Mentally Ill" (SAMI), "Mental Illness Substance Affected" (MISA), "Mental Illness Substance Use Disorder" (MISUD), and "Individuals with Co-Occurring Psychiatric and Substance Use Disorders" (ICOPSD) are other terms used to describe the same condition [4]. The term "dual diagnosis" is frequently used in the United Kingdom, Australia, Spain, and Spanish speaking countries. Adding to the confusion, the term "dual diagnosis" is applied for concurrent intellectual or developmental disorders with mental health disorders in Canada. For the purpose of this work the intellectual and developmental disabilities with mental health concerns that are considered as a "dual diagnosis" or "concurrent disorder", will not be considered or discussed.

In mental health, the focus of research and guidelines has been on individual disorders, despite concurrent disorders being common and seemingly increasing [5]. Substance use disorders and non-substance-related mental disorders are frequently chronic, requiring long-term care. Greater severity of a single psychiatric disorder increases the risk of developing concurrent disorders. This also means that in general the frequency of comorbidity increases from population-based studies, to outpatient studies, to inpatient studies. In population-based studies, approximately one-fourth of people with anxiety or major depressive disorders are expected to have an overlapping substance use disorder in their lifetime [6,7]. Similarly, half of the people with bipolar disorder or schizophrenia will experience a substance use disorder [8]. Studies generally exclude tobacco dependence, otherwise the numbers would be substantially higher.

People with concurrent disorders tend to be underdiagnosed and undertreated, whilst experiencing a high burden of morbidity and mortality. There are big gaps between the need for substance use disorders, mental disorders treatment, and delivered services. Unmet need for treatment is more for substance use disorders. Psychiatrists are often uninvolved with the management of substance use disorders, and general or addiction physicians treating substance use disorders do not necessarily diagnose psychiatric disorders. The treatment of psychiatric disorders and substance use disorders is separated in many countries, with different treatment traditions, separate organizations within the healthcare system, separate treatment providers, and separate funding. Individuals with concurrent disorders are not only more complex to diagnose and treat, but they are also at higher risk of additional multimorbidity, becoming socially marginalized, entangled with the legal system, and subject to stigma [9]. Both mortality and morbidity are increased in those with concurrent disorders. The main causes are premature drug-related death [10] and increased risk of suicide [11,12]. Increased utilization of healthcare services has been demonstrated, despite the demonstrated treatment gap. For example, in a Canadian cohort study, individuals with concurrent disorders had significantly higher odds of Emergency Department use (Adjusted odds ratio [AOR] D 1.71; 95% confidence interval [CI]), 1.4–2.11, hospitalization (AOR D 1.45; 95% CI, 1.16–1.81), and primary care visits (AOR D 1.34; 95% CI, 1.05–1.71) than those with either substance use disorder or non-substance-related mental disorders [13].

The mechanisms of development of concurrent disorders are complex, however, frequently both conditions share neurological pathways, overlapping underlying genetic risk factors, as well as common "environmental" risk factors. People with concurrent disorders are frequently part of a highly vulnerable population—with multiple biological, psychological, and social risk factors; as a consequence, the course of both types of conditions can be more severe and complicated due to multiple persistent risk factors [14–16]. Additionally, the impact of substance use disorders and non-substance-use mental disorders interact, affecting the course and prognosis of both [15,17]. As a result, the management of concurrent disorders is quite complex.

The traditional approach in healthcare systems has been, and still is to address each issue separately, with limited or no standards to simultaneously address both components of concurrent disorder within the same care team. Traditional treatment methods of sequential or uncoordinated parallel care are nowadays considered obsolete. Despite new coordinated and integrated treatment approaches constituting the current standard, the majority of healthcare systems have yet to adapt.

There are still many barriers to the management and delivery of services for concurrent disorder [18–22]. In Canada for example, models for service delivery evolved unevenly, coordination and integration of care were limited by challenges related to the implementation of collaborative care and the need for local networks to foster service coordination and policy accountability [23,24].

The last 20 years have seen some developments, with the creation of new journals (e.g., the Journal of Dual Diagnosis) and new societies (e.g., the World Association of Dual Diagnosis). While the need for improved care for concurrent disorders is clear, the process of adapting the healthcare system to efficiently care for these individuals seems to have been slow. Clinical management guidelines are an important tool, developed to help facilitate evidence-based treatment practice.

Our purpose was to systematically review the most current clinical management guidelines for concurrent disorders and explore their scope, approach, structure, knowledge limitations, and consistency, in order to make suggestions for the future.

It is important to understand the scope of the guidelines and what they address: issues and populations. The target primary and secondary audiences may include: patients living with concurrent disorders, pharmacists, and other healthcare professionals who manage these conditions. In addition, methodological issues and issues with potential bias such as funding, the role in the design or conduct of the study, collection, analysis, and interpretation of the data or preparation, review, or approval of the guideline will be addressed.

2. Materials and Methods

The protocol for this systematic review was prepared according to the PRISMA-P checklist [25,26]. The review was registered in the international register—PROSPERO (International Prospective Register of Ongoing Systematic Reviews, http://www.crd.york.ac.uk/prospero).

To identify relevant guidelines, literature searches were carried out by two independent reviewers: S.H. and S.V. (in case of disagreement S.L.C. was involved and, if any discrepancy, C.S. advised) in the following electronic databases and websites: MEDLINE (via Ovid), EMBASE (via Ovid), PsycINFO, CINAHL, Trip, JouleCMA, DynaMed, SIGN, UpToDate, NICE Guidelines, and CADTH. All reviewers had completed medical training and had experience in working with individuals with concurrent disorders. Additionally, a web search for other gray literature and relevant reference lists was done. Researchers and clinicians in the field were also contacted to provide any known information about the available guidelines. All the searches were set between 1 January 2000 and 18 March 2020. Samples of keywords/MESH terms are attached in Supplementary file. The inclusion criteria were to consider all published or unpublished English language formal clinical management guidelines of concurrent disorders for the appraisal of guidelines with the AGREE II (Appraisal of Guidelines for REsearch and Evaluation) tool. The AGREE (Appraisal of Guidelines for REsearch and Evaluation) instrument was developed to address the issue of variability in guideline quality, which assesses the methodological rigor and transparency of guideline development. The original AGREE tool has been refined to AGREE II [27]. In addition, guidelines addressed to all relevant professionals, patients, and their families were considered for review, but not appraised with the AGREE II. For the purpose of this work, intellectual/developmental disabilities occurring simultaneously with mental health concerns, described as "dual diagnosis" or "concurrent disorder", were not considered. Accordingly, the exclusion criteria were: reviews of concurrent disorder management, non-English guidelines, literature addressing persons with neurodevelopmental disorders, and literature published earlier than 1 January 2000.

The search conducted revealed a total of 8841 results, comprising an electronic database search and a gray literature search. There were 8041 results from the electronic database search, which were all imported to RefWorks. After duplicate deletion, 6420 results remained. The results of the gray literature and website search (in total 800 results) were not uploaded to the RefWorks. Whenever possible, the removal of duplicate results was done manually and assessed with the same approach. From both sources, the electronic database and gray literature searches, the study titles, abstracts, and full papers were examined by both authors (S.H. and S.V.) to identify eligible studies based on the inclusion criteria. Decisions of the two authors were recorded separately and in case of disagreement, were discussed. In the absence of consensus, a decision was made by the third reviewer (S.L.C.), and finally, by the supervisory author (C.G.S.). All titles were scanned (8841) and if relevant to concurrent disorders, abstracts were read (275), and were classified for inclusion to appraise into YES, MAYBE, and NO groups. Electronic database search results were manually sorted within RefWorks, while gray literature results were manually sorted outside of it. In the YES and MAYBE groups, 75 full papers (55 from an electronic database + 20 * from gray literature) were read. A full-text review was performed for the 75 selected studies and recorded into a study selection form, documenting the reason for the exclusion and inclusion of each study. After this process, 55 papers remained that fulfilled inclusion criteria and were considered for the qualitative analysis. After full assessment, 24 papers fully fulfilled the inclusion criteria and were included in the final analysis (Figure 1: PRISMA Flow Diagram 1, Table 1). The AGREE II instrument was used to report the guidelines.

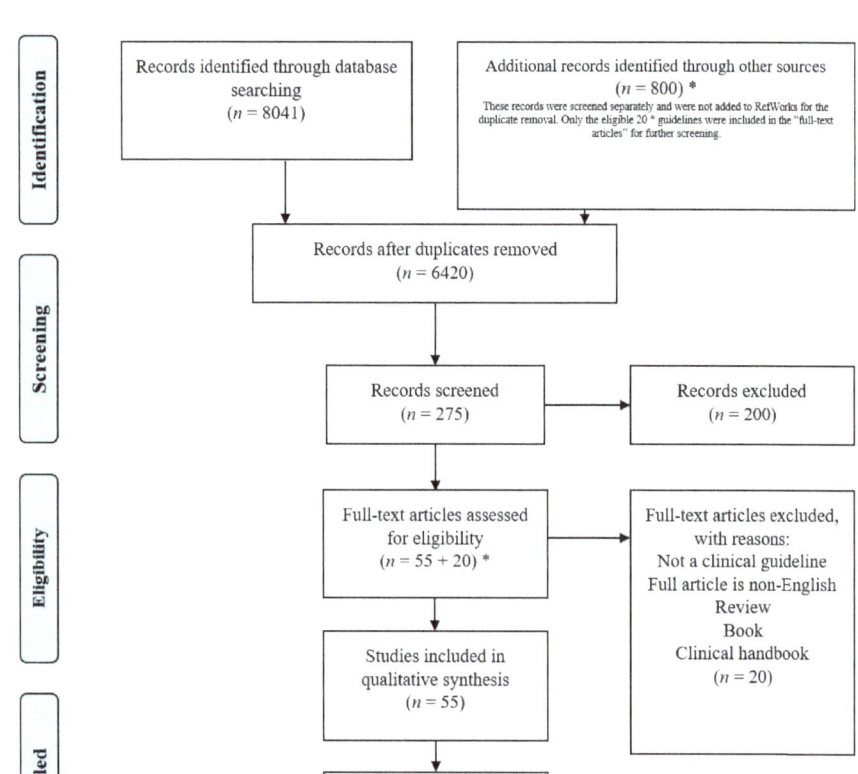

Figure 1. PRISMA 2009. Flow Diagram 1.

3. Results

In total, 24 clinical guidelines developed for concurrent disorders were included in the final analysis for appraisal by AGREE II (Table 1).

There were four Australian, one Brazilian, four Canadian, three UK, four EU, two New Zealand (one joint with Australia), five American, and one collaborative guidelines. The search yielded many different forms of information resources to manage concurrent disorders, but they were not included in this study to be appraised by AGREE II, as they were not formal clinical management guidelines. However, some of them were very comprehensive on concurrent disorder management information [1]. In addition, guidelines that were not addressed to physicians but for counselors [52] and those that were addressed to the patients and families [53–55], were not included. The Scottish National guideline on schizophrenia addressed concurrent disorders management only briefly, and therefore was not included in the appraisal list [56]. Similarly, toolkit [30], handbooks [57–62], reviews of current literature [19,63–66], reviews of recommendations [67,68], or adopted summaries of other guidelines [69] were not considered for inclusion within the appraisal. Lastly, some of the papers that provided concurrent disorders management related information were not included because they were only consensus recommendations for the standard of care development and suggestions for service delivery implementation [46,70–87].

Overall quality according to the AGREE II for the majority of guidelines was average (Tables 2 and 3). Only four of the guidelines were of low quality and rated low with the AGREE II appraisal. Almost all guidelines clearly described their scope and purpose in great detail. Stakeholder involvement from different groups representing the range of views and preferences of all target groups were not considered by approximately half of the guidelines. A concern was that almost half of the guidelines showed some weaknesses in the rigor needed to comply with the standards required for developing evidence-based guidelines. Guidelines should be revised regularly to provide up to date support, however information regarding guideline updates was regularly missing.

Guidelines need to be clear and make the most important information easily identifiable. While most guidelines were clear about the recommendations, emphasis on key recommendations was often absent.

Applicability constituted perhaps the weakest domain with the most deficiencies in most guidelines: issues such as resource implications were almost never discussed, neither were issues of monitoring and/or auditing.

Lastly, information on editorial independence was missing or not clearly defined in many of the guidelines. Half of the guidelines provided no information recording this important aspect of guideline development, with failure to address competing interests of the guideline development group members.

The four Australian guidelines were all developed by the Australian Government Health Departments. All of them comprehensively covered all the questions concerning scope, purpose, and stakeholder involvement. One of the guidelines was specifically developed for primary care workers. However, none of the guidelines were developed with the maximum possible rigor. In some circumstances, information was not presented as clearly as needed for clinical practice. The implication for the resources of applying the recommendations was limited. Lastly, none of the guidelines had sufficient information on editorial independence.

Guidelines from the Brazilian Association of Studies on Alcohol and Other Drugs (ABEAD) for diagnosis and treatment of psychiatric comorbidity with alcohol and other substance dependence described clearly the scope and purpose of the guideline. However, classic guideline components including grading the evidence level and key recommendations were not mentioned. Assessment of this guideline using the AGREE II standards showed that for all domains, the information could be presented in a clearer format.

Table 1. Concurrent disorder guidelines included for the appraisal with the AGREE II (Appraisal of Guidelines for Research and Evaluation) tool (last reviewed 18 March 2020).

	Title	Developed by	Country	Year	Population Targeted
1	Comorbidity of Mental Disorders and Substance Use: A Brief Guide for The Primary Care Clinician [28]	Australian Government. Drug and Alcohol Services South Australia	Australia	2008	People with mental disorders and substance use
2	NSW Clinical Guidelines for the Care of Persons with Comorbid Mental Illness and Substance Use Disorders in Acute Care Settings [29]	NSW Department of Health	Australia	2009	People with comorbid mental health and substance use disorders
3	Queensland Health Dual Diagnosis Clinical Guidelines. Co-Occurring Mental Health and Alcohol and Other Drug Problems [30]	Queensland Health	Australia	2010	People with comorbid mental health and substance use disorders
4	Guidelines on The Management of Co-Occurring Alcohol and Other Drug and Mental Health Conditions in Alcohol and Other Drug Treatment Settings [31]	NHMRC Centre of Research Excellence in Mental Health and Substance Use National Drug and Alcohol Research Centre University of New South Wales	Australia	2016	Patients with alcohol and other drugs dependence and mental health conditions
5	Guidelines of The Brazilian Association of Studies on Alcohol and Other Drugs (ABEAD) for Diagnosis and Treatment of Psychiatric Comorbidity with Alcohol and Other Substance and Dependence [32]	Brazilian Association of Studies on Alcohol and Other Drugs	Brazil	2017	Alcohol and drug-dependent patients suffering from comorbid psychiatric disorders
6	Best Practices Concurrent Mental Health and Substance Use Disorders [33]	CAMH	Canada	2002	People with mental health with a substance use disorder
7	The Canadian Network for Mood and Anxiety Treatments (CANMAT) Task Force Recommendations for the Management of Patients with Mood Disorders and Comorbid Substance Use Disorders [34]	CANMAT	Canada	2012	People with mood disorders and comorbid substance use disorders
8	Concurrent Disorders Guidelines. A Supplement to The Provincial Addictions Treatment Standards [35]	Regional Health Authorities of Newfoundland and Labrador	Canada	2015	People with concurrent disorders
9	Canadian Schizophrenia Guidelines: Schizophrenia and Other Psychotic Disorders with Coexisting Substance Use Disorders [36]	CPA	Canada	2017	People with schizophrenia and other psychotic disorders with coexisting substance use disorders
10	Coexisting Severe Mental Illness (Psychosis) and Substance Misuse: Assessment and Management in Healthcare Settings [37]	NICE	UK	2011	People with coexisting severe mental illness (psychosis) and substance misuse
11	BAP Updated Guidelines: Evidence-Based Guidelines for the Pharmacological Management of Substance Abuse, Harmful Use, Addiction, and Comorbidity: Recommendations from BAP [38]	BAP	UK	2012	People with substance abuse, harmful use, addiction, and comorbidity
12	Coexisting Severe Mental Illness and Substance Misuse: Community Health and Social Care Services [39]	NICE	UK	2016	People with coexisting severe mental illness and substance misuse
13	EPA Guidance on Tobacco Dependence and Strategies for Smoking Cessation in People with Mental Illness [40]	EPA	EU	2013	People with tobacco dependence and mental illness

Table 1. Cont.

	Title	Developed by	Country	Year	Population Targeted
14	Guideline for Screening, Diagnosis, and Treatment of ADHD in Adults with Substance Use Disorders [41]	Belgian Universities and Hospital Collaborators	Belgium	2017	People with attention deficit hyperactivity disorder with substance use disorders
15	Dual Diagnosis: An Integrated Approach to Treatment: Evidence-Based Clinical Practice Guidelines [42]	Andalusian Health System Hospital	Spain	2019	People with dual diagnosis
16	Psychiatric Comorbidity in Alcohol Use Disorders: Results from The German S3 Guidelines [43]	German Association for Psychiatry, Psychotherapy, and Psychosomatics (DGPPN) and the German Association for Addiction Research and Therapy (DG-Sucht)	Germany	2017	People with psychiatric comorbidity in alcohol use disorders
17	The Assessment and Management of People with Coexisting Mental Health and Substance Use Problems [44]	New Zealand Ministry of Health	New Zealand	2010	People with coexisting mental health and substance use problems
18	Royal Australian and New Zealand College of Psychiatrists Clinical Practice Guidelines for the Management of Schizophrenia and Related Disorders [45]	Royal Australian and New Zealand College of Psychiatrists	New Zealand and Australia	2016	People with schizophrenia and related disorders
19	Improving the Care of Individuals with Schizophrenia and Substance Use Disorders: Consensus Recommendations [46]	Consensus Meeting	USA	2005	Individuals with schizophrenia and substance use disorders
20	Substance Abuse Treatment for Persons with Co-Occurring Disorders [47]	U.S. Department of Health and Human Services Substance Abuse and Mental Health Services Administration Center for Substance Abuse Treatment	USA	2005	People with co-occurring disorders
21	Substance Abuse: Clinical Issues in Intensive Outpatient Treatment [48]	U.S. Department of Health and Human Services Substance Abuse and Mental Health Services Administration Center for Substance Abuse Treatment	USA	2005	People with co-occurring disorders
22	Co-Occurring Posttraumatic Stress Disorder and Substance Use Disorder: Recommendations for Management and Implementation in the Department of Veterans Affairs [49]	Department of Veterans Affairs	USA	2011	People with co-occurring posttraumatic stress disorder and substance use disorder
23	Treatment of PTSD and Comorbid Disorders [50]	International Society for Traumatic Stress Studies	USA	2009	People with posttraumatic stress disorder and comorbid disorders
24	World Federation of Societies of Biological Psychiatry (WFSBP) Guidelines for Biological Treatment of Schizophrenia Part 3: Update. 2015. Management of Special Circumstances: Depression, Suicidality, Substance Use Disorders and Pregnancy and Lactation [51]	World Federation of Societies of Biological Psychiatry (WFSBP)	Collaboration of different countries	2015	People with schizophrenia and substance use disorders

Table 2. Full version of the AGREE II instrument (Strongly Disagree—1, Strongly Agree—7).

GUIDELINES (Please See Table 1: Included Guidelines)	1	2	3	4	5	6	7	8	9	10	11	12	13	14	15	16	17	18	19	20	21	22	23	24
DOMAIN 1. SCOPE AND PURPOSE																								
1. The overall objective(s) of the guideline is (are) specifically described.	6	7	7	6	5	7	6	7	7	7	7	7	6	7	6	7	6	7	7	7	7	6	6	7
2. The health question(s) covered by the guideline is (are) specifically described.	6	7	7	6	5	7	6	7	7	7	7	7	6	7	4	6	2	7	5	7	5	6	5	7
3. The population (patients, public, etc.) to whom the guideline is meant to apply is specifically described.	6	7	6	7	5	7	6	7	6	7	7	7	5	7	5	7	6	7	7	6	6	7	6	7
DOMAIN 2. STAKEHOLDER INVOLVEMENT																								
4. The guideline development group includes individuals from all relevant professional groups.	6	6	6	6	3	7	5	6	6	6	7	7	5	3	1	7	4	7	3	7	7	2	3	6
5. The views and preferences of the target population (patients, public, etc.) have been sought.	3	6	4	7	2	7	5	5	5	7	7	5	7	3	3	1	6	3	6	1	2	7	1	2	3
6. The target users of the guideline are clearly defined.	6	7	5	7	3	7	5	6	5	7	7	7	6	7	5	6	4	7	7	6	6	7	7	7
DOMAIN 3. RIGOR OF DEVELOPMENT																								
7. Systematic methods were used to search for evidence.	4	6	4	5	3	5	6	6	6	7	7	7	7	3	7	3	7	3	6	2	5	3	7
8. The criteria for selecting the evidence are clearly described.	7	6	4	6	2	5	6	3	5	7	7	7	6	7	3	6	5	6	1	5	5	6	1	7
9. The strength and limitations of the body of evidence are clearly described.	6	5	4	5	1	4	6	2	6	7	7	7	6	6	2	5	4	5	2	5	6	7	6	7
10. The methods for formulating the recommendations are clearly described.	5	6	4	3	1	5	6	2	6	7	7	5	7	1	6	4	7	4	5	5	5	5	5	7
11. The health benefits, side effects, and risks have been considered in formulating the recommendations.	6	7	6	2	3	5	6	5	6	7	7	7	5	5	3	5	2	7	5	3	2	3	2	6
12. There is an explicit link between the recommendations and the supporting evidence.	5	4	4	2	1	4	6	3	4	7	5	7	5	6	1	7	1	7	2	2	2	7	7	7
13. The guideline has been externally reviewed by experts prior to its publication.	2	4	2	1	1	3	3	2	7	7	5	7	4	6	3	4	1	7	6	4	4	5	1	5
14. A procedure for updating the guideline is provided.	5	6	1	7	1	3	2	2	5	7	7	7	4	2	1	2	1	2	1	2	2	7	1	2
DOMAIN 4. CLARITY OF PRESENTATION																								
15. The recommendations are specific and unambiguous.	5	5	4	4	3	5	4	3	6	7	6	7	6	7	3	7	6	7	7	4	5	5	3	7
16. The different options for management of the condition or health issue are clearly presented.	6	5	6	7	5	5	5	3	6	7	6	7	6	6	2	6	4	7	5	2	5	2	5	6
17. Key recommendations are easily identifiable.	3	6	6	5	1	6	2	2	6	7	6	7	4	4	6	6	7	7	7	5	6	4	6	7
DOMAIN 5. APPLICABILITY																								
18. The guideline describes facilitators and barriers to its application.	6	5	4	7	2	4	4	3	5	7	7	7	4	5	2	3	5	3	7	5	5	6	2	2
19. The guideline provides advice and/or tools on how the recommendations can be put into practice.	7	6	6	3	2	4	4	5	6	7	6	7	4	5	2	3	5	4	7	5	6	6	2	2
20. The potential resource implications of applying the recommendations have been considered.	3	4	5	4	3	4	3	3	5	7	5	7	4	2	1	3	4	4	5	5	5	6	1	1
21. The guideline presents monitoring and/or auditing criteria.	2	3	2	2	1	3	2	2	3	7	3	7	3	1	1	2	2	2	2	1	2	5	1	1

Table 2. *Cont.*

GUIDELINES (Please See Table 1: Included Guidelines)	1	2	3	4	5	6	7	8	9	10	11	12	13	14	15	16	17	18	19	20	21	22	23	24
DOMAIN 6. EDITORIAL INDEPENDENCE																								
22. The views of the funding body have not influenced the content of the guideline.	4	4	2	4	4	4	4	3	6	7	3	7	4	4	3	6	2	5	3	6	6	3	2	6
23. Competing interests of guideline development group members have been recorded and addressed.	1	1	1	1	1	7	1	6	2	7	7	6	2	1	7	1	7	1	5	6	1	5	1	7
1. Rate the overall quality of this guideline. Lowest possible quality—1 Highest possible quality—7	5	5	5	5	5	3	5	4	6	7	6	7	5	5	3	6	6	5	3	6	4	5	3	6
OVERALL CALCULATED BY DOMAIN AVERAGE	5	5	5	5	5	4	5	5	4	6	7	6	7	5	5	3	6	3	4	3	4	4	3	4
2. I would recommend this guideline for use. Yes—1, Yes with Modifications—2, No—3	2	2	2	2	2	2	2	2	2	2	2	2	1	2	2	2	2	2	2	2	2	2	2	2

NOTES

Table 3. Short version of the Agree II instrument (Strongly Disagree—1, Strongly Agree—7).

GUIDELINES (Please See Table 1: Included Guidelines)	1	2	3	4	5	6	7	8	9	10	11	12	13	14	15	16	17	18	19	20	21	22	23	24
DOMAIN 1. SCOPE AND PURPOSE	6	7	7	6	5	7	6	7	7	7	7	7	6	7	5	7	5	7	6	7	6	7	6	7
DOMAIN 2. STAKEHOLDER INVOLVEMENT	5	6	6	5	7	3	7	5	6	6	6	7	4	4	2	6	4	7	4	5	7	3	4	5
DOMAIN 3. RIGOR OF DEVELOPMENT	5	6	4	4	2	4	5	3	6	7	7	7	5	6	2	5	3	5	3	4	4	6	3	6
DOMAIN 4. CLARITY OF PRESENTATION	5	5	5	5	3	5	4	3	6	7	6	7	5	6	4	6	6	7	6	4	5	4	5	7
DOMAIN 5. APPLICABILITY	5	5	4	4	2	4	3	3	5	7	5	7	4	3	2	3	4	3	5	4	5	6	2	2
DOMAIN 6. EDITORIAL INDEPENDENCE	3	3	2	3	6	3	5	3	7	7	5	7	5	3	2	7	2	6	2	6	6	2	2	7
1. Rate the overall quality of this guideline. Lowest possible quality—1 Highest possible quality—7	5	5	5	5	4	5	5	4	6	7	6	7	5	5	3	6	3	4	3	4	4	4	3	4
2. I would recommend this guideline for use. Yes—1, Yes with Modifications—2, No—3	2	2	2	2	2	2	2	2	2	1	2	1	2	2	2	2	2	2	2	2	2	2	2	2

NOTES

Canadian guidelines were developed by Health Canada, CANMAT, and included adapted guidelines based on UK parent guidelines. All clearly described their scope and purpose and involved stakeholders from the relevant fields in the process. However, all other domains showed room for improvement. Canadian Schizophrenia Guidelines: "Schizophrenia and Other Psychotic Disorders with Coexisting Substance Use Disorders" developed for people with schizophrenia and other psychotic disorders with coexisting substance use disorders was appraised, receiving nearly maximum scores in all domains. However, it was addressing only schizophrenia and other psychotic disorders.

UK guidelines were developed by NICE (National Institute for Health and Care for Excellence) and BAP (The British Association for Psychopharmacology). Both NICE guidelines comprehensively covered all the aspects of guideline development and scored the maximum. The guideline NG58 "Coexisting Severe Mental Illness and Substance Misuse: Community Health and Social Care Services", was addressed to and developed for community health and social care services, and was also included in an assessment with the AGREE II, as it was recommended to read in conjunction with NICE CG 120 Clinical Guideline "Coexisting Severe Mental Illness (Psychosis) and Substance Misuse: Assessment and Management in Healthcare Settings". The guideline NG 58 was not directly addressed to clinicians and was for the wider health and social care needs, such as employment and housing. However, both these guidelines covered different biopsychosocial aspects of concurrent disorders management with the same approach and therefore appraising them together was appropriate. Both NICE guidelines scored the highest possible with AGREE II. "BAP Updated Guidelines: Evidence-Based Guidelines for the Pharmacological Management of Substance Abuse, Harmful Use, Addiction and Comorbidity: Recommendations from BAP" were extremely clear on the scope and were developed with the utmost rigor and scored close to the possible maximum, with only minimal missing information.

The four European guidelines had very different scopes. They were developed rigorously in all domains according to the AGREE II tool assessment, however they could all be improved with clarification. "Psychiatric Comorbidity in Alcohol Use Disorders: Results from The German S3 Guidelines" developed by The German Association for Psychiatry, Psychotherapy, and Psychosomatics (DGPPN) and The German Association for Addiction Research and Therapy (DG-Sucht) for people with psychiatric comorbidity in alcohol use disorders, were the best-scored guidelines, with applicability being the main domain requiring significant improvement.

The two New Zealand guidelines had findings similar to the Australian guidelines with some domains requiring improvements. One of the guidelines was created in partnership with the Australian Government.

There were five guidelines developed in the USA. With a very different scope, they had similar overall rigor of development in all domains. However, not all clearly described information on editorial independence.

The collaborative guideline created by different stakeholders, provided a very clear scope. However, all other domains of information could be improved with minor additional information.

4. Discussion

This review collected all concurrent disorder English language guidelines developed over the last 20 years. Ten guidelines were developed between 2000 and 2010 and 14 between 2011 and 2020. Eight of the 14 were developed in the last five years, suggesting an increasing trend or recognition of importance. All guidelines struggled with a limited evidence base, as the pool of evidence showed limited expansion.

All guidelines were ICD/DSM based. They generally discussed specific combinations of disorders, often differentiating illicit substances and alcohol use disorders. This differentiation is consistent with established treatment providing agencies. The focus of most guidelines was on combining evidence-based interventions targeting substance use disorders with evidence-based interventions targeting non-substance-related mental disorders. Some guidelines included tobacco use disorders, while others did not. Gambling, which only recently has become part of the substance use and addiction section of the DSM and ICD, was generally not included.

Aside from the specific combination of disorders, there was little additional conceptualization of concurrent disorders. Attempts to develop psychopathological approaches that go beyond the count of symptoms are still in its infancy: e.g., the HiTOP model [88], played no role in the current conceptualization of concurrent disorders and played no role in the development of the guidelines.

There have been some attempts to develop specific models of concurrent or multimorbidity interventions, such as "patient-centered medical homes" or "Assertive Community Teams". These attempts were sometimes mentioned but have not been considered in the guidelines as of yet. Similarly, attempts to classify approaches and levels of integration of services such as the "Levels of Collaboration. Mental Health/Primary Care Integration Options" developed by ACCT (Addiction Technology Center Transfer Network), also seem to have not become standardized enough to be utilized in guidelines [89]. None of the approaches to develop and operationalize different levels of integration have become standard enough to be included.

The level of organization of integration of care seems to not have moved beyond very basic recommendations, such as sequential, parallel, and integrated models. The sequential model suggests treating one condition, then the other. The parallel model suggests receiving mental health treatment from mental health services plus separately receiving addiction treatment from addiction services. Integrated treatment models offer one team providing mental health and addiction services within the same setting. Current evidence seems to suggest that the sequential model is obsolete, while the integrated treatment models may provide the best outcomes for the management of concurrent disorders [90]. A recent systematic review revealed that integrated models of care are more effective than conventional, nonintegrated models. Integrated models demonstrated superiority to standard care models through reductions in substance use disorders and improvement of mental health in patients with concurrent disorders. The review revealed similar findings to other studies, which indicated that the integrated model is more cost-effective than standard care [91]. Addressing both issues in an integrated manner may help to achieve better outcomes. All guidelines promoted the benefits of integrated, however, with different levels of details.

Similar in terms of simplicity and intuitiveness to the characterization of the sequential/parallel and integrated approaches is the four-quadrant framework for concurrent disorders. The four-quadrant framework has been developed to address the variability of concurrent disorders. Being a spectrum of disorders ranging from high prevalence with low impact, to low prevalence with high impact, results in considerable variation. As a result, this framework provides a model of substantial diversity in the individual treatment needs of the various people who experience concurrent disorders [92,93]. The four-quadrant model was mentioned in two guidelines developed by the U.S. Department of Health and Human Services, but played no role in specific guideline recommendations.

In order to address the level of care needs, such as indicated in a simple fashion in the four-quadrant model, an evidence-based approach to assessing severity, complexity, and need of care would be necessary. This can be in the form of staging, which has been recommended for individual disorders, but not for concurrent disorders. For example, staging has been recommended for the development of more targeted specific treatments in primary, secondary, and tertiary care settings. As concurrent disorders are closely related to severity and complexity, staging may be an issue of specific interest to concurrent disorders. However, none of the guidelines discussed or introduced staging or any similar form of determining specific levels of care.

5. Conclusions

Overall, specific evidence for the management of concurrent disorders continues to be rare, making it necessary for guidelines to often rely on combining evidence for individual disorders. Some studies in concurrent disorder patients indicate that certain approaches working in individual disorders are less or not effective in concurrent disorders, such as SSRIs in alcohol-dependent individuals with major depressive disorder. There is also some evidence that some medication may work better, such as clozapine for individuals suffering from schizophrenia and substance use disorder.

As current evidence suggests that better outcomes of concurrent disorder management can be achieved with integrated management approaches, broader application appears warranted. However, integrated approaches in current medical systems are rare. Furthermore, it seems that higher functionality in patients appears to allow for less integration of treatment for different disorders. Guidelines rarely allow for graded approaches and generally lack any recommendations regarding grading or staging.

Based on available evidence of this review of current guidelines quality, some of the subsections in practically all guidelines can be improved. Furthermore, certain important aspects that are essential for treatment planning are not addressed by any guideline, including the specifics of a concurrent disorder framework, the "matching" of treatment needs, and the evaluation or "staging" of the severity.

Supplementary Materials: The following are available online at http://www.mdpi.com/2077-0383/9/8/2406/s1, EMBASE/Ovid Search Terms Used and Results; MEDLINE/Ovid Search Terms Used and Results; PsychINFO Search Terms Used and Results and CINAHL Search Terms Used and Results.

Author Contributions: Conceptualization: C.G.S. and S.H. Methodology: S.H. and C.G.S. Writing—original draft preparation: S.H. and C.G.S. Writing—review and editing: All authors. Literature search, selection, and appraisal of guidelines: S.H and S.V. Supervision: C.G.S. All authors have read and agreed to the published version of the manuscript.

Funding: This research received no funding other than S.H. as a Ph.D. student received a Four-Year Fellowship from The University of British Columbia Graduate and Postdoctoral Studies.

Conflicts of Interest: All authors declare no conflicts of interest.

References

1. Torrens, M.; Mestre-Pintó, J.-I.; Domingo-Salvany, A. *Comorbidity of Substance Use and Mental Disorders in Europe*; The European Centre for Drugs and Drug Addiction: Lisabon, Portugal, 2015.
2. Skinner, W.W.J.; O'Grady, P.O.C.; Bartha, C.; Parker, C. *Concurrent Substance Use and Mental Health Disorders. An Information Guide*; Centre for Addiction and Mental Health: Toronto, ON, Canada, 2010; ISBN 978-1-77052-604-4.
3. Co-Center for Excellence (COCE). *Definitions and Terms Relating to Co-Occurring Disorders*; Overview Paper 1; Co-Occurring Center for Excellence (COCE): Rockville, MD, USA; Substance Abuse and Mental Health Services Administration (SAMHSA): Rockville, MD, USA, 2007.
4. Dual Diagnoses Overview Series. 2017. Available online: http://www.dualdiagnosis.org.au/home/images/documents/1._Terminology.pdf (accessed on 20 March 2020).
5. Kessler, R.C. The Epidemiology of Dual Diagnosis. *Biol. Psychiatry* **2004**, *56*, 730–737. [CrossRef] [PubMed]
6. Conway, K.P.; Compton, W.; Stinson, F.S.; Grant, B.F. Lifetime comorbidity of DSM-IV mood and anxiety disorders and specific drug use disorders: Results from the National Epidemiologic Survey on Alcohol and Related Conditions. *J. Clin. Psychiatry* **2006**, *67*, 247–257. [CrossRef] [PubMed]
7. Regier, D.A. Comorbidity of mental disorders with alcohol and other drug abuse. Results from the Epidemiologic Catchment Area (ECA) Study. *JAMA* **1990**, *264*, 2511–2518. [CrossRef] [PubMed]
8. Khan, S. Concurrent Mental and Substance Use Disorders in Canada. Statistics Canada, Catalogue no. 82-003-X. *Health Rep.* **2017**, *28*, 3–8. [PubMed]
9. Todd, J.; Green, G.; Harrison, M.; Ikuesan, B.A.; Self, C.; Baldacchino, A.; Sherwood, S. Defining dual diagnosis of mental illness and substance misuse: Some methodological issues. *J. Psychiatr. Ment. Health Nurs.* **2004**, *11*, 48–54. [CrossRef] [PubMed]
10. Fridell, M.; Bäckström, M.; Hesse, M.; Krantz, P.; Perrin, S.; Nyhlén, A. Prediction of psychiatric comorbidity on premature death in a cohort of patients with substance use disorders: A 42-year follow-up. *BMC Psychiatry* **2019**, *19*, 150. [CrossRef]
11. Aharonovich, E.; Liu, X.; Nunes, E.; Hasin, D.S. Suicide Attempts in Substance Abusers: Effects of Major Depression in Relation to Substance Use Disorders. *Am. J. Psychiatry* **2002**, *159*, 1600–1602. [CrossRef]
12. Appleby, L. Drug misuse and suicide: A tale of two services. *Addiction* **2000**, *95*, 175–177. [CrossRef]

13. Zhang, L.; Norena, M.; Gadermann, A.; Hubley, A.; Russell, L.; Aubry, T.; To, M.J.; Farrell, S.; Hwang, S.; Palepu, A. Concurrent Disorders and Health Care Utilization Among Homeless and Vulnerably Housed Persons in Canada. *J. Dual Diagn.* **2018**, *14*, 21–31. [CrossRef]
14. Mueser, K.T.; Drake, R.E.; Wallach, M.A. Dual diagnosis: A review of etiological theories. *Addict. Behav.* **1998**, *23*, 717–734. [CrossRef]
15. Ross, S.; Peselow, E. Co-Occurring Psychotic and Addictive Disorders. *Clin. Neuropharmacol.* **2012**, *35*, 235–243. [CrossRef] [PubMed]
16. National Institute on Drug Abuse (NIDA). *Common Comorbidities with Substance Use Disorders*; National Institute on Drug Abuse (NIDA): Baltimore, MD, USA, 2018.
17. Santucci, K. Psychiatric disease and drug abuse. *Curr. Opin. Pediatr.* **2012**, *24*, 233–237. [CrossRef] [PubMed]
18. Canaway, R.; Merkes, M. Barriers to comorbidity service delivery: The complexities of dual diagnosis and the need to agree on terminology and conceptual frameworks. *Aust. Health Rev.* **2010**, *34*, 262. [CrossRef]
19. Drake, R.E.; Essock, S.M.; Shaner, A.; Carey, K.B.; Minkoff, K.; Kola, L.; Lynde, D.; Osher, F.C.; Clark, R.E.; Rickards, L. Implementing Dual Diagnosis Services for Clients With Severe Mental Illness. *Psychiatr. Serv.* **2001**, *52*, 469–476. [CrossRef] [PubMed]
20. Drake, R.E.; Wallach, M.A.; McGovern, M.P. Special Section on Relapse Prevention: Future Directions in Preventing Relapse to Substance Abuse Among Clients With Severe Mental Illnesses. *Psychiatr. Serv.* **2005**, *56*, 1297–1302. [CrossRef] [PubMed]
21. Ridgely, M.S.; Goldman, H.H.; Willenbring, M. Barriers to the Care of Persons With Dual Diagnoses: Organizational and Financing Issues. *Schizophr. Bull.* **1990**, *16*, 123–132. [CrossRef]
22. Flynn, P.M.; Brown, B.S. Co-occurring disorders in substance abuse treatment: Issues and prospects. *J. Subst. Abus. Treat.* **2008**, *34*, 36–47. [CrossRef]
23. Wiktorowicz, M.; Abdulle, A.; Di Pierdomenico, K.; Boamah, S.A. Models of Concurrent Disorder Service: Policy, Coordination, and Access to Care. *Front. Psychol.* **2019**, *10*. [CrossRef]
24. *A Systems Approach to Substance Use Services in Canada*; Canadian Centre on Substance Abuse: Ottawa, ON, Canada, 2013; ISBN 978-1-927467-20-6.
25. Moher, D.; Shamseer, L.; Clarke, M.; Ghersi, D.; Liberati, A.; Petticrew, M.; Shekelle, P.G.; Stewart, L.A. Preferred reporting items for systematic review and meta-analysis protocols (PRISMA-P) 2015 statement. *Syst. Rev.* **2015**, *4*, 1. [CrossRef]
26. Shamseer, L.; Moher, D.; Clarke, M.; Ghersi, D.; Liberati, A.; Petticrew, M.; Shekelle, P.; Stewart, L.A. The PRISMA-P Group Preferred reporting items for systematic review and meta-analysis protocols (PRISMA-P) 2015: Elaboration and explanation. *BMJ* **2015**, *349*, g7647. [CrossRef]
27. Brouwers, M.C.; Kerkvliet, K.; Spithoff, K. The AGREE Reporting Checklist: A tool to improve reporting of clinical practice guidelines. *BMJ* **2016**, *352*. [CrossRef] [PubMed]
28. Gordon, A. *Comorbidity of Mental Disorders and Substance Use: A Brief Guide for the Primary Care Clinician*; Drug and Alcohol Services South Australia: Adelaide, Australia, 2008.
29. Mental Health Branch. *NSW Clinical Guidelines for the Care of Persons with Comorbid Mental Illness and Substance Use Disorders in Acute Care Settings*; NSW Department of Health: New South Wales, Australia, 2009.
30. Queensland Health. *Dual Diagnosis Clinical Guidelines Co-Occurring Mental Health and Alcohol and Other Drug Problems*; Queensland Health: Brisbane, Australia, 2010.
31. Marel, C.; Mills, L.K.; Kongston, R.; Gournay, L.; Deady, M.; Lambkin-Kay, F.; Baker, A.; Teesson, M. *Guidelines on The Management of Co-Occurring Alcohol and Other Drug and Mental Health Conditions in Alcohol and Other Drug Treatment Settings*, 2nd ed.; NHMRC Centre of Research Excellence in Mental Health and Substance Use: Sydney, Australia; National Drug and Alcohol Research Centre: Randwick, Australia; University of New South: Sydney, Australia, 2016.
32. Zaleski, M.; Laranjeira, R.R.; Marques, A.C.P.R.; Ratto, L.; Romano, M.; Alves, H.N.P.; Soares, M.B.D.M.; Abelardino, V.; Kessler, F.H.P.; Brasiliano, S.; et al. Guidelines of the Brazilian Association of Studies on Alcohol and Other Drugs (ABEAD) for diagnosis and treatment of psychiatric comorbidity with alcohol and other substance and dependence. *Int. Rev. Psychiatry* **2017**, *29*, 254–262. [CrossRef] [PubMed]
33. Centre for Addiction and Mental Health. *Best Practices Concurrent Mental Health and Substance Use Disorders*; Health Canada: Ottawa, ON, Canada, 2002.

34. Beaulieu, S.; Saury, S.; Sareen, J.; Tremblay, J.; Schütz, C.G.; McIntyre, R.S.; Schaffer, A. The Canadian Network for Mood and Anxiety Treatments (CANMAT) task force recommendations for the management of patients with mood disorders and comorbid substance use disorders. *Ann. Clin. Psychiatry* **2012**, *24*, 38–55. [PubMed]
35. Rush, B. *Concurrent Disorders Guidelines. A Supplement to the Provincial Addictions Treatment Standards*; Regional Health Authorities of Newfoundland and Labrador: Happy Valley-Goose Bay, NL, Canada, 2015.
36. Crockford, D.; Addington, N. Canadian Schizophrenia Guidelines: Schizophrenia and Other Psychotic Disorders with Coexisting Substance Use Disorders. *Can. J. Psychiatry* **2017**, *62*, 624–634. [CrossRef] [PubMed]
37. Coexisting Severe Mental Illness (Psychosis) And Substance Misuse: Assessment and Management in Healthcare Settings. Clinical Guideline. 2011. Available online: www.nice.org.uk/guidance/cg120 (accessed on 20 March 2020).
38. Lingford-Hughes, A.R.; Welch, S.; Peters, L.; Nutt, D.J. BAP updated guidelines: Evidence-based guidelines for the pharmacological management of substance abuse, harmful use, addiction and comorbidity: Recommendations from BAP. *J. Psychopharmacol.* **2012**, *26*, 899–952. [CrossRef]
39. Coexisting Severe Mental Illness and Substance Misuse: Community Health and Social Care Services and NICE Guideline. 2016. Available online: www.nice.org.uk/guidance/ng58 (accessed on 20 March 2020).
40. Rüther, T.; Bobes, J.; De Hert, M.; Svensson, T.H.; Mann, K.; Batra, A.U.; Gorwood, P.; Möller, H.J. EPA guidance on tobacco dependence and strategies for smoking cessation in people with mental illness. *Eur. Psychiatry* **2014**, *29*, 65–82. [CrossRef]
41. Matthys, F.; Stes, S.; Brink, W.V.D.; Joostens, P.; Möbius, D.; Tremmery, S.; Sabbe, B. Guideline for Screening, Diagnosis and Treatment of ADHD in Adults with Substance Use Disorders. *Int. J. Ment. Health Addiction* **2014**, *12*, 629–647. [CrossRef]
42. Torres, G.N. Dual Diagnosis: A Theoretical Approximation from Review of Literature. *J. Drug Abus.* **2019**, *5*, 4. [CrossRef]
43. Preuss, U.W.; Gouzoulis-Mayfrank, E.; Havemann-Reinecke, U.; Schäfer, I.; Beutel, M.; Hoch, E.; Mann, K.F. Psychiatric comorbidity in alcohol use disorders: Results from the German S3 guidelines. *Eur. Arch. Psychiatry Clin. Neurosci.* **2017**, *268*, 219–229. [CrossRef]
44. Todd, C.; Te Ariari, O.T.O. *The Assessment and Management of People with Co-Existing Mental Health and Substance Use Problems*; Ministry of Health: Wellington, New Zealand, 2010; ISBN 978-0-478-35912-1.
45. Galletly, C.; Castle, D.; Dark, F.; Humberstone, V.; Jablensky, A.; Killackey, E.; Kulkarni, J.; McGorry, P.; Nielssen, O.; Tran, N. Royal Australian and New Zealand College of Psychiatrists clinical practice guidelines for the management of schizophrenia and related disorders. *Aust. New Zealand J. Psychiatry* **2016**, *50*, 410–472. [CrossRef]
46. Ziedonis, D.M.; Smelson, D.; Rosenthal, R.N.; Batki, S.L.; Green, A.I.; Henry, R.J.; Montoya, I.; Parks, J.; Weiss, R.D. Improving the Care of Individuals with Schizophrenia and Substance Use Disorders: Consensus Recommendations. *J. Psychiatr. Prac.* **2005**, *11*, 315–339. [CrossRef] [PubMed]
47. Center for Substance Abuse Treatment. *Substance Abuse Treatment for Persons With Co-Occurring Disorders*; Treatment Improvement Protocol (TIP) Series 42 DHHS Publication No. (SMA) 05-3922; Substance Abuse and Mental Health Services Administration: Rockville, MD, USA, 2005.
48. Center for Substance Abuse Treatment. *Substance Abuse: Clinical Issues in Intensive Outpatient Treatment*; Treatment Improvement Protocol (TIP) Series 47. DHHS Publication No. (SMA) 06-4182; Substance Abuse and Mental Health Services Administration: Rockville, MD, USA, 2006.
49. Bernardy, N.C.; Hamblen, J.L.; Friedman, M.J.; Kivlahan, D.R. Co-occurring Posttraumatic Stress Disorder and Substance Use Disorder: Recommendations for Management and Implementation in the Department of Veterans Affairs. *J. Dual Diagn.* **2011**, *7*, 242–261. [CrossRef]
50. Foa, B.E. Treatment of PTSD and Comorbid Disorders. In *Effective Treatments for PTSD*, 2nd ed.; Foa, B.E., Keane, M.T., Friedman, J.M., Cohen, A.J., Eds.; The Guilford Press: New York, NY, USA, 2009.
51. Hasan, A.; Falkai, P.; Wobrock, T.; Lieberman, J.; Glenthøj, B.; Gattaz, W.F.; Thibaut, F.; Möller, H.-J.; WFSBP Task Force on Treatment Guidelines for Schizophrenia. World Federation of Societies of Biological Psychiatry (WFSBP) Guidelines for Biological Treatment of Schizophrenia Part 3: Update 2015 Management of special circumstances: Depression, Suicidality, substance use disorders and pregnancy and lactation. *World J. Biol. Psychiatry* **2015**, *16*, 142–170. [CrossRef]

52. Skinner, W.J.W. *Treating Concurrent Disorders: A Guide for Counsellors*; Centre for Addiction & Mental Health: Toronto, ON, Canada, 2004; ISBN 9780888684998.
53. Skinner, W.J.W.; O'Grady, P. A Family Guide to Concurrent Disorders. Centre for Addiction and Mental Health: Toronto, ON, Canada, 2007. Available online: www.camh.net/About_Addiction_Mental_Health/Concurrent_Disorders/CD_priority_projects.html (accessed on 29 May 2020).
54. Dennis, C.D.; Douathy, A. *Addiction and Mood Disorders-A Guide for Clients and Families*; Oxford University Press: Oxford, UK, 2006.
55. O'Grady, P.C.; Skinner, W.J.W. *Partnering with Families Affected by Concurrent Disorders: Facilitators' Guide*; Centre for Addiction and Mental Health: Toronto, ON, Canada, 2007; Available online: www.camh.net/About_Addiction_Mental_Health/Concurrent_Disorders/cd_facilitator_guide0607.pdf (accessed on 20 March 2020).
56. Scottish Intercollegiate Guidelines Network (SIGN). *Management of Schizophrenia*; SIGN: Edinburgh, Scotland, 2013; (SIGN publication no. 131).
57. Geert, D.; Franz, M. *Co-occurring Addictive and Psychiatric Disorders. A Practice-Based Handbook from a European Perspective*; Springer: New York, NY, USA, 2015; ISBN1 978-3-642-45374-8. ISBN2 978-3-642-45375-5 (eBook). [CrossRef]
58. Bellack, S.A.; Bennett, E.; Gearon, S.J. *Behavioral Treatment for Substance Abuse in People with Serious and Persistent Mental Illness: A Handbook for Mental Health Professionals*; Routledge: Abingdon, UK, 2007; ISBN 0-415-95283-2.
59. Baker, A.; Velleman, R. *Clinical Handbook of Co-Existing Mental Health and Drug and Alcohol Problems*; Routledge: Abingdon, UK, 2007; ISBN 13 978-1-58391-775-6.
60. Back, E.S.; Foa, B.E.; Killen, K.T.; Mills, L.K.; Teesson, M.; Cotton, D.B.; Carroll, M.K.; Brady, T.K. *Concurrent Treatment of PTSD and Substance Use Disorders Using Prolonged Exposure (COPE): Patient Workbook; Therapist Guide*; Oxford University Press: New York, NY, USA, 2014; ISBN 978-0-19-933451-3.
61. Gray, K.M.; Upadhyaya, H.P. Tobacco smoking in individuals with attention-deficit hyperactivity disorder. *CNS Drugs* **2009**, *23*, 661–668. [PubMed]
62. Nunes, V.E.; Selzer, J.; Levounis, P.; Davies, A.C. *Substance Dependence and Co-Occurring Psychiatric Disorders-Best Practices for Diagnosis and Clinical Treatment*; Civic Research Institute Inc.: Princeton, NJ, USA, 2010; p. 1414.
63. Torrens, M.; Martínez-Sanvisens, D.; Martínez-Riera, R.; Bulbena, A.; Szerman, N.; Ruiz, P. Dual diagnosis: Focusing on depression and recommendations for treatment. *Addiction Disord. Treat.* **2011**, *10*, 50–59. [CrossRef]
64. Ekleberry, C.S. Integrated Treatment for Co-Occurring Disorders. In *Personality Disorders and Addiction*; Routledge: Abingdin, UK, 2009; ISBN 978-0-7890-3692-6.
65. Baandrup, L.; Rasmussen, J.Ø.; Klokker, L.; Austin, S.; Bjørnshave, T.; Bliksted, V.; Fink-Jensen, A.; Fohlmann, A.H.; Hansen, J.P.; Nielsen, M.K.; et al. Treatment of adult patients with schizophrenia and complex mental health needs–A national clinical guideline. *Nord. J. Psychiatry* **2015**, *70*, 231–240. [CrossRef]
66. Ronis, R.J. Best Practices for Co-Occurring Disorders. *J. Dual Diagn.* **2005**, *1*, 83. [CrossRef]
67. Watkins, K.E.; Hunter, S.B.; Burnam, M.A.; Pincus, H.A.; Nicholson, G. Review of Treatment Recommendations for Persons With a Co-occurring Affective or Anxiety and Substance Use Disorder. *Psychiatr. Serv.* **2005**, *56*, 913–926. [CrossRef]
68. Pennay, A.; Cameron, J.; Reichert, T.; Strickland, H.; Lee, N.K.; Hall, K.; Lubman, D.I. A systematic review of interventions for co-occurring substance use disorder and borderline personality disorder. *J. Subst. Abus. Treat.* **2011**, *41*, 363–373. [CrossRef]
69. Ghani, S. *Introduction to Magellan's Adopted Clinical Practice Guidelines for the Assessment and Treatment of Patients with Substance Use Disorders*; Magellan Health Inc.: Phoenix, AZ, USA, 2006–2018.
70. Ministry of Health. *Service Delivery for People with Co-Existing Mental Health and Addiction Problems. Integrated Solutions*; Ministry of Health: Wellington, New Zealand, 2010; ISBN 978-0-478-35919-0.
71. Minkoff, K. Best Practices: Developing Standards of Care for Individuals With Co-occurring Psychiatric and Substance Use Disorders. *Psychiatr. Serv.* **2001**, *52*, 597–599. [CrossRef]
72. Minkoff, K.; Cline, C.A. Developing Welcoming Systems for Individuals with Co-Occurring Disorders. *J. Dual Diagn.* **2005**, *1*, 65–89. [CrossRef]
73. Minkoff, K.; Cline, C.A. Dual Diagnosis Capability: Moving from Concept to Implementation. *J. Dual Diagn.* **2006**, *2*, 121–134. [CrossRef]

74. Minkoff, K. An Integrated Model for the Management of Co-Occurring Psychiatric and Substance Disorders in Managed-Care Systems. *Dis. Manag. Health Outcomes* **2000**, *8*, 251–257. [CrossRef]
75. Alberta Health Services. Enhancing concurrent capability: A Toolkit for Managers and Staff. In *Integrated Treatment Planning*; Alberta Health Services: Edmonton, AB, Canada, 2016.
76. Kelly, T.M.; Daley, D.C. Integrated treatment of substance use and psychiatric disorders. *Soc. Work. Public Health* **2013**, *28*, 388–406. [CrossRef] [PubMed]
77. Noordsy, D.L.; Fox, L.; Drake, E.R.; Mueser, T.K.; Smith, F.L. *Integrated Treatment for Dual Diagnosis Disorders: A Guide to Effective Practice*; The Guilford Press: New York, NY, USA, 2003; ISBN 1-57230-850-8.
78. Barreira, P.; Espey, B.; Fishbein, R.; Moran, D.; Flannery, R.B. Linking substance abuse and serious mental illness service delivery systems: Initiating a statewide collaborative. *J. Behav. Health Serv. Res.* **2000**, *27*, 107–113. [CrossRef]
79. Brousselle, A.; Lamothe, L.; Mercier, C.; Perreault, M. Beyond the limitations of best practices: How logic analysis helped reinterpret dual diagnosis guidelines. *Eval. Program Plan.* **2007**, *30*, 94–104. [CrossRef]
80. Dua, T.; Barbui, C.; Clark, N.; Fleischmann, A.; Poznyak, V.; Van Ommeren, M.; Yasamy, M.T.; Ayuso-Mateos, J.L.; Birbeck, G.L.; Drummond, C.; et al. Evidence-Based Guidelines for Mental, Neurological, and Substance Use Disorders in Low-and Middle-Income Countries: Summary of WHO Recommendations. *PLoS Med.* **2011**, *8*, e1001122. [CrossRef]
81. Westermeyer, J.J.; Weiss, D.R.; Ziedonis, M.D. *Integrated Treatment for Mood and Substance Use Disorders*; Johns Hopkins University Press: Baltimore, MD, USA, 2003.
82. Keyser, D.J.; Watkins, K.E.; Vilamovska, A.M.; Pincus, H.A. Focus on alcohol & drug abuse: Improving service delivery for individuals with co-occurring disorders: New perspectives on the quadrant model. *Psychiatr. Serv.* **2008**, *59*, 1251–1253.
83. American Society of Addiction Medicine. Public policy statement on co-occurring addictive and psychiatric disorders. *J. Addiction Dis.* **2001**, *20*, 121–123. [CrossRef]
84. Drake, R.E.; Mueser, K.T.; Brunette, M.F. Management of persons with co-occurring severe mental illness and substance use disorder: Program implications. *World Psychiatry* **2007**, *6*, 131–136.
85. Perron, B.; Bunger, A.C.; Bender, K.; Vaughn, M.G.; Howard, M.O. Treatment guidelines for substance use disorders and serious mental illnesses: Do they address co-occurring disorders? *Subst. Use Misuse* **2010**, *45*, 1262–1278. [CrossRef] [PubMed]
86. Lowe, A.L.; Abou-Saleh, M.T. The British experience of dual diagnosis in the national health service. *Acta Neuropsychiatr.* **2004**, *16*, 41–46. [CrossRef]
87. United Kingdom Department of Health. *Mental Health Policy Implementation Guide. Dual Diagnosis Good Practice Guide*; Department of Health Publications: London, UK, 2002.
88. Ruggero, C.J.; Kotov, R.; Hopwood, C.J.; First, M.; Clark, L.A.; Skodol, A.E.; Mullins-Sweatt, S.N.; Patrick, C.J.; Bach, B.; Cicero, D.C.; et al. Integrating the Hierarchical Taxonomy of Psychopathology (HiTOP) into clinical practice. *J. Consult. Clin. Psychol.* **2019**, *87*, 1069–1084. [CrossRef] [PubMed]
89. Stanley, S.; Gotham, J.H.; Johnson, K.; Padwa, H.; Murphy, D.; Krom, L. *ATTC White Paper: Integrating Substance Use Disorder and Health Care Services in An Era of Health Reform*; Addiction Technology Center Transfer Network: Kansas City, MS, USA, March 2015.
90. Burnam, M.A.; Watkins, K.E. Substance Abuse With Mental Disorders: Specialized Public Systems And Integrated Care. *Health Aff.* **2006**, *25*, 648–658. [CrossRef] [PubMed]
91. Karapareddy, V. A Review of Integrated Care for Concurrent Disorders: Cost Effectiveness and Clinical Outcomes. *J. Dual Diagn.* **2019**, *15*, 56–66. [CrossRef] [PubMed]
92. Ries, R. Clinical Treatment Matching Models for Dually Diagnosed Patients. *Psychiatr. Clin. N. Am.* **1993**, *16*, 167–175. [CrossRef]
93. McDonell, M.; Kerbrat, A.H.; Comtois, K.A.; Russo, J.; Lowe, J.M.; Ries, R.K. Validation of the Co-occurring Disorder Quadrant Model. *J. Psychoact. Drugs* **2012**, *44*, 266–273. [CrossRef]

© 2020 by the authors. Licensee MDPI, Basel, Switzerland. This article is an open access article distributed under the terms and conditions of the Creative Commons Attribution (CC BY) license (http://creativecommons.org/licenses/by/4.0/).

MDPI
St. Alban-Anlage 66
4052 Basel
Switzerland
Tel. +41 61 683 77 34
Fax +41 61 302 89 18
www.mdpi.com

Journal of Clinical Medicine Editorial Office
E-mail: jcm@mdpi.com
www.mdpi.com/journal/jcm

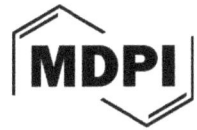

Ingram Content Group UK Ltd.
Milton Keynes UK
UKHW050213140423
420118UK00004B/134